The Kid.

The kidney
Physiology & pathophysiology
Seldin & Giebisch
Raven Press

Prostaglandins

MODERN PHARMACOLOGY-TOXICOLOGY

A Series of Monographs and Textbooks

1 A Guide to Molecular Pharmacology-Toxicology, Parts I and II *Edited by R. M. Featherstone*
2 Psychopharmacological Treatment: Theory and Practice *Edited by Herman C. B. Denber*
3 Pre- and Postsynaptic Receptors *Edited by Earl Usdin and William E. Bunney, Jr.*
4 Synaptic Receptors: Isolation and Molecular Biology *Eduardo De Robertis*
5 Methods in Narcotics Research *Edited by Seymour Ehrenpreis and Amos Neidle*
6 Horizons in Clinical Pharmacology *Edited by Roger F. Palmer*
7 Synthetic Antidiarrheal Drugs: Synthesis–Preclinical and Clinical Pharmacology *Edited by Willem Van Bever and Harbans Lal*
8 Receptors and Mechanism of Action of Steroid Hormones, Parts I and II *Edited by Jorge R. Pasqualini*
9 Hormone-Receptor Interaction: Molecular Aspects *Edited by Gerald S. Levey*
10 Structure and Function of Monoamine Enzymes *Edited by Earl Usdin, Norman Weiner, and Moussa B. H. Youdin*
11 Receptors in Pharmacology *Edited by John R. Smythies and Ronald J. Bradley*
12 Noncatecholic Phenylethylamines (in two parts) *Edited by Aron D. Mosnaim and Marion E. Wolf*

13 Biochemistry of Mental Disorders: New Vistas *Edited by Earl Usdin and Arnold J. Mandell*

14 Developments in Opiate Research *Edited by Albert Herz*

15 Cadmium Toxicity *Edited by John H. Mennear*

16 Body Temperature: Regulation, Drug Effects, and Therapeutic Implications *Edited by Peter Lomax and Edward Schönbaum*

17 Interferon and Interferon Inducers: Clinical Applications *Edited by Dale A. Stringfellow*

18 The Spinal Cord and Its Reaction to Traumatic Injury: Anatomy–Physiology–Pharmacology–Therapeutics *Edited by William F. Windle*

19 Hypertension Research: Methods and Models *Edited by Frederick M. Radzialowski*

20 Endorphins: Chemistry, Physiology, Pharmacology, and Clinical Relevance *Edited by Jeffrey B. Malick and Robert M. S. Bell*

21 Prostaglandins: Organ- and Tissue-Specific Actions *Edited by Stan Greenberg, Philip J. Kadowitz, and Thomas F. Burks*

Prostaglandins

ORGAN- AND TISSUE-SPECIFIC ACTIONS

Editors

Stan Greenberg
University of South Alabama
Mobile, Alabama

Philip J. Kadowitz
Tulane University
New Orleans, Louisiana

Thomas F. Burks
University of Arizona
Tucson, Arizona

MARCEL DEKKER, INC. New York and Basel

Library of Congress Cataloging in Publication Data
Main entry under title:

Prostaglandins, organ- and tissue-specific actions.

(Modern pharmacology-toxicology ; 21)
Includes indexes.
1. Prostaglandins--Physiological effect. I. Greenberg, Stanley, [date]. II. Kadowitz, Philip J., [date]. III. Burks, Thomas F. IV. Series.
[DNLM: 1. Cardiovascular systems--Physiology. 2. Prostaglandins--Physiology. W1 MO167T v.21 / QU 90 P9695]
QP801.P68P729 612'.405 82-5165
ISBN 0-8247-1682-5 AACR2

MARCEL DEKKER, INC.
270 Madison Avenue, New York, New York 10016

Current printing (last digit):
10 9 8 7 6 5 4 3 2 1

PRINTED IN THE UNITED STATES OF AMERICA

Dedication

This volume is dedicated to William R. Wilson, M.D., teacher, clinician, researcher, mentor, and friend, whose untimely death on May 1, 1975 was felt by the scientific community and his friends. It is our sincerest wish that his son Jeff and his wife Charlotte, who suffered the greatest loss and sadness, realize that the ideals and teachings of Bill will continue to be carried on within the scientific community by each of the students who had the pleasure of working with and knowing him. Bill commanded respect and loyalty out of admiration, not fear. Though in many positions of power, he utilized his influence for constructive rather than destructive purposes. In the years that we knew him he spoke well of many persons and spoke ill of none. He never achieved the national prominence of many scientists, but helped many others to achieve this goal. He devoted himself to his family, his students, and his university, and was a success with all three. Few men can tread in his path.

Foreword

Nearly 50 years have passed since the dual reports of von Euler and Goldblatt outlined the smooth-muscle stimulating activity of extracts from seminal fluid. Von Euler first referred to this new class of pharmacological agents as prostaglandins. These pioneering results also demonstrated activity involving vascular smooth muscle. Once again we have seen the long lapse of time (perhaps 30 years) between the original observations and full appreciation by the scientific community of the implications for research. Why this delay? A solution would greatly facilitate the inquiries of science.

Though the synthesis of prostaglandin derivatives is not presented in this volume, let us not forget the contributions by synthetic organic chemists. Structural identification of prostaglandins was followed by the need to develop new synthetic procedures and technical skills. This effort received additional stimulation when it was recognized that wide variances in biological properties resulted from minor alterations in chemical structure.

This varying biological activity found for the prostaglandins as a class of agents is found to a lesser extent for a single chemical entity. Thus, as the authors indicate, there are conflicting reports in the literature concerning many aspects of prostaglandin research. One would expect wide variations in species' responsiveness when bioassaying prostaglandin compounds. Minor variations in experimental conditions may alter considerably the measured response of a living system. Thus, these compounds are challenging for both the chemist and biologist. Change either the structure or experimental procedure and the results will probably vary.

Prostaglandins represents the joint efforts of several leading researchers Emphasis is placed on the effects of these highly active agents on smooth muscle with special attention given to the cardiovascular system. Also included are excellent discussions of the role of prostaglandins in factors which modify the function of the cardiovascular system, such as neuronal, platelets, and ionic mechanisms. The authors have indicated clearly areas for future research with clear implications for better definition of disease and possible advances in therapeutics.

In prostaglandin research there can be little doubt concerning the rapid advances during the past 15 years. This volume includes (in relation to the cardiovascular system) numerous topics together with critical discussion. The authors have attempted to numerate carefully the responses in relation to dose (with various prostaglandins there are numerous examples of vasoconstriction or vasodilation depending on dosage). They have discussed the experimental results in relation to a defined tissue. Prostaglandins may increase or decrease the amount of norepinephrine released from adrenergic nerve terminals and thus modify the function of a vascular bed. Adrenergic neuronal activation promotes the synthesis of prostaglandins. Many mechanisms involved in neuronal transmission are unknown. Is a physiological role in neuronal transmission being exhibited by selective prostaglandins?

The authors have attempted to define the action of prostaglandins in terms of the molecular level. Whether these mechanisms involve Ca^{2+} channels and thus modify membrane conductance and/or contractile processes in muscle, or other possible mechanisms, is still to be determined.

All readers of this volume will expand their knowledge of this exciting and rapidly changing area of research. With each of the chapters, the reader will find many ideas and challenges for future research. It is through this process that scientists will gain new insights into basic biological function in health and disease. With this knowledge, improved therapy for many cardiovascular disorders should be forthcoming.

We are indeed fortunate that so many authors devoted their time to writing and editing this book. May their efforts be dedicated to the advancement of knowledge.

The University of Iowa John P. Long

Preface

Scientific study of the prostaglandins has previously occurred in more-or-less distinct and identifiable stages. For two decades following their initial discovery, interest was rightfully focused upon prostaglandin assay techniques, chemical structures, and synthesis. Subsequently, during the 1950s and 1960s, research efforts became increasingly concerned with the physiological and biochemical aspects of prostaglandin actions. It became evident that prostaglandins affected intracellular concentrations of cyclic nucleotides, contractile activity of smooth muscle, and gastric and intestinal secretory activities. Prostaglandins were studied intensively for possible therapeutic use in the treatment of reproductive disorders, respiratory diseases, cardiovascular diseases, and gastrointestinal diseases.

The pace of prostaglandin research increased rapidly in the third epoch, which resulted from the discovery that the nonsteroidal anti-inflammatory agents inhibit the synthesis of prostaglandins. Possible roles of prostaglandins in the pathophysiology of joint pain, inflammation, headache, hypertension, congenital heart disease, development of fever, and as gastrointestinal cytoprotective agents and modulators of motility became subjects of almost frantic investigation. Even more recently, intensive exploration of the powerful physiological action of the thromboxanes, prostacyclin, and endoperoxide prostaglandin intermediates may represent another quantum advance in the prostaglandin story and certainly has contributed to the rapid proliferation of data and ideas about prostaglandin actions. The rate of evolution of prostaglandin research is now moving too quickly to capture its image faithfully in a book; details of the picture are blurred.

It has become clearly evident, however, that the initiator and modulator roles of the prostaglandins cannot be properly appreciated without some basic understanding of the systems within which they exert their effects. Prostaglandins usually do not act alone, but interact, often in complex ways, with other modulator and control systems to bring about altered function of the cells that come under their influence. Most chapters of this book have been prepared to provide some conceptual basis for understanding the physiological and biochemical events upon which the actions of the prostaglandins are exerted, with emphasis on the cardiovascular system. The effects of the prostaglandins are thus considered in the framework of multiple regulatory influences upon target cells. The editors hope that the information and concepts presented will therefore endure in interest as considerable new knowledge about prostaglandin actions comes to light.

Acknowledgments

During the preparation of this volume the editors devoted a large amount of time to their task while decreasing the time usually spent with family, friends, and job. We gratefully acknowledge the support provided us by the faculty and staff of the Department of Pharmacology of the University of South Alabama, University of Texas Health Science Center in Houston, and Tulane Medical School. A special acknowledgment must go to Dr. Thomas M. Glenn, who provided the proper environment and continued encouragement for the completion of this volume. The editors also thank all contributors for their patience during the preparation of this volume. Finally, the editors express their deepest appreciation and respect for Dr. John P. Long, Professor and Chairman of Pharmacology at the University of Iowa, and the late William R. Wilson, whose influence, teachings, and approach to science are reflected in each of our chapters.

Stan Greenberg
Philip J. Kadowitz
Thomas F. Burks

Contributors

John A. Bevan, M.B. Professor, Department of Pharmacology, University of California at Los Angeles, Los Angeles, California

Michael J. Brody, Ph.D. Professor, Department of Pharmacology, The University of Iowa College of Medicine, Iowa City, Iowa

Thomas F. Burks, Ph.D. Professor and Head, Department of Pharmacology, University of Arizona, Health Sciences Center, College of Medicine, Tucson, Arizona

Kenneth E. Clark,* Ph.D. Department of Pharmacology, The University of Iowa College of Medicine, Iowa City, Iowa

Frederick A. Curro, D.M.D., Ph.D. Associate Professor and Chairman, Department of Pharmacology, Fairleigh Dickinson University, School of Dentistry, Hackensack, New Jersey, and Clinical Associate Professor, Department of Oral and Maxillofacial Surgery, New York University, College of Dentistry, New York, New York

Robert E. Druilhet,† Ph.D. Assistant Professor of Medicine, Department of Internal Medicine, The University of Texas Medical School at Houston, Houston, Texas

Peter P. Dukes, Ph.D. Division of Hematology-Oncology, Children's Hospital of Los Angeles, Los Angeles, California, and Associate Professor, Department of Pediatrics and Biochemistry, University of Southern California, School of Medicine, Los Angeles, California

Earl W. Dunham, Ph.D. Associate Professor, Department of Pharmacology, University of Minnesota Medical School, Minneapolis, Minnesota

---

*Current affiliation: Assistant Professor and Director of Research, Department of Obstetrics and Gynecology, University of Cincinnati, Cincinnati, Ohio

†Current affiliation: OBI Hughes

Thomas F. Ferris, M.D. Nesbitt Professor and Chairman, Department of Medicine, University of Minnesota, Minneapolis, Minnesota

Robert W. Gardier,* Ph.D. Director, Biomedical Sciences Doctoral Program, Wright State University, Dayton, Ohio

Stan Greenberg, Ph.D. Associate Professor, Department of Pharmacology, College of Medicine, University of South Alabama, Mobile, Alabama

Carl A. Gruetter,† Ph.D. Instructor, Department of Pharmacology, Tulane University School of Medicine, New Orleans, Louisiana

Francis J. Haddy, M.D., Ph.D. Professor and Chairman, Department of Physiology, Uniformed Services University of the Health Sciences, Bethesda, Maryland

Philip B. Hollander, Ph.D. Professor and Deputy Chairman, Department of Pharmacology, College of Medicine, The Ohio State University, Columbus, Ohio

Albert L. Hyman, M.D. Research Professor of Surgery and Adjunct Professor of Pharmacology, Department of Surgery, Tulane University, School of Medicine, New Orleans, Louisiana

Philip J. Kadowitz, Ph.D. Department of Pharmacology, Tulane University, School of Medicine, New Orleans, Louisiana

Walter M. Kirkendall, M.D. Director of Hypertension Unit, Department of Medicine, University of Texas at Houston, Houston, Texas

Gesina L. Longenecker, Ph.D. Associate Professor, Department of Pharmacology, College of Medicine, University of South Alabama, Mobile, Alabama

Margaret G. Northway,‡ Ph.D. Assistant Professor, Department of Pharmacology, Uniformed Services University of the Health Sciences, Bethesda, Maryland

*Current affiliation: Professor, Department of Pharmacology and Toxicology, Wright State University School of Medicine, Dayton, Ohio

†Current affiliation: Assistant Professor, Department of Pharmacology, Marshall University School of Medicine, Huntington, West Virginia

‡Current affiliation: Research Scientist, Department of Surgery, King's Hospital Medical School, London, England

Merrill L. Overturf, Ph.D. Associate Professor of Medicine, Department of Internal Medicine, The University of Texas Medical School at Houston, Houston, Texas

John H. Sanner, Ph.D. Research Fellow, Department of Biological Research, G. D. Searle and Company, Chicago, Illinois

Ernst Wm. Spannhake, Ph.D. Assistant Professor, Department of Pharmacology, Tulane University, School of Medicine, New Orleans, Louisiana

Kazunobu Sugawara,* Ph.D. Associate Professor, 2nd Department of Pharmacology, Nagasaki University School of Medicine, Nagasaki, Japan

Rocco C. Venuto, M.D. Assistant Professor, Department of Medicine, State University of New York at Buffalo, School of Medicine, Buffalo, New York

Richard P. White, Ph.D. Professor, Department of Pharmacology, University of Tennessee Center for the Health Sciences, Memphis, Tennessee

Ben G. Zimmerman, Ph.D. Professor, Department of Pharmacology, University of Minnesota Medical School, Minneapolis, Minnesota

*Current affiliation: Chief, Department of Pharmacy, Yamagata University Hospital, Yamagata, Japan

Contents

Prostaglandins

Part I
INTRODUCTION

1 Adrenergic Neurotransmission in Blood Vessels

JOHN A. BEVAN / University of California Center for Health Sciences, Los Angeles, California

THE ADRENERGIC NEUROEFFECTOR MECHANISM

The adrenergic control of the tone of vascular smooth muscle is regulated through the sympathetic nervous system, which includes the adrenal medulla. Postganglionic sympathetic fibers ramify in the adventitia of a blood vessel and usually form a plexus at the adventitiomedial junction. The density of this innervation is not uniform but varies from one regional bed to another, between vessels of different size in the same vascular bed, and even along the length of one particular vessel. In a few blood vessels the adrenergic nerves enter the medial muscle layer for varying depths. Probably because of the paucity of observations, the location of vessels showing such medial distribution of adrenergic nerves does not appear to conform to any pattern of functional significance.

Since most of the norepinephrine (NE) in the postganglionic sympathetic neurons is found in the nerve terminals, the NE content of a blood vessel reflects the amount of transmitter stored in the terminal varicosities of the adrenergic ground plexus. Acetylcholinesterase is frequently found at the adrenergic synapse: its function is unknown, although at some sites it may indicate the presence of cholinergic nerves. The adrenergic transmitter is synthesized within the varicosity. The rate-limiting step in synthesis is that from tyrosine to dopa, regulated by tyrosine hydroxylase. Thus the activity of this enzyme provides a measurement of the tissue's capacity to synthesize the transmitter. The NE synthesis rate can also be measured more directly using isotopic methods.

The relationship between the adrenergic varicosity and the closest smooth muscle cells is not the same in all blood vessels, but varies from 40 nm to approximately 2 μm. In general, the smaller the diameter of the vessel, the closer the nerve ending approximates to the first layer of smooth muscle cells. This parameter has profound influence on the concentration of transmitter at the α-adrenergic receptors within the cleft, the amount of transmitter that emerges from the cleft, and a number of other transmission parameters (see below). Transmitter release is regulated by a variety of feedback mechanisms, including a negative feedback system mediated by the transmitter itself through α_2-receptors in the presynaptic membrane. After release the majority of the transmitter is taken up again into the adrenergic nerves by a special transport mechanism. When the synaptic cleft is small, the biological effect of the transmitter is terminated by neuronal reuptake; however, when the cleft is wide, the action of the transmitter is terminated by processes operating in the tunica media: diffusion, extraneuronal uptake and binding, and extraneuronal metabolism by monoamine oxidase and catechol catechol-O-methyltransferase. Only the transmitter released from the adrenergic plexus that moves toward the tunica media is responsible for smooth muscle contraction. The proportion that passes centrifugally into the adventitia exerts no biological effect. The proportion of released transmitter that enters the smooth muscle layer is different in different vessels. In the steady state, the concentration of NE in the blood vessel wall is highest near the adrenergic nerve plexus and diminishes toward the intima.

Whereas the vascular smooth muscle cell population of a blood vessel from an adult animal is very stable, during growth the number of smooth muscle cells and thus the effector system upon which the transmitter acts increases. There is evidence that the adrenergic innervation not only influences vascular smooth muscle tone but exerts a trophic effect on the vascular smooth muscle cell, influencing the growth of the blood vessel. Conversely, vascular smooth muscle cells seem to influence their innervation. Other factors that influence vascular smooth muscle proliferation include intravascular pressure and hormones. Vascular smooth muscle cells also synthesize most the of collagen and elastin in the blood vessel wall. This process also appears to be modulated by sympathetic activity.

The consensus is that the adrenergic transmitter is released by exocytosis. The contents of one vesicle are probably not released from each varicosity with each nerve impulse that passes along the axon. After release the adrenergic transmitter diffuses across the synaptic cleft and reacts with α- and β-adrenergic receptors in the postsynaptic membrane. These receptors are not identical in all blood vessels; they differ in their sensitivity to the transmitter and other characteristics of their responsiveness to drugs. α-Adrenergic receptors mediate vasoconstriction; β-adrenergic receptors vasodilation. The ratio of α to β effects is not constant, and although α effects usually dominate the response, this is not always the case. Although most α-adrenergic receptors are markedly influenced by neurogenic transmitter, β-adrenergic receptors are significantly exposed to neurogenic transmitter only in a number of restricted sites.

The adrenergic transmitter effects on vascular smooth muscle vary from one blood vessel to another not only because of differences in transmitter kinetics and distribution and in the receptor population, but because of intrinsic properties of the vascular smooth muscle cells themselves. Some cells exhibit spontaneous rhythmic activity, others maintained intrinsic tone. In addition, the medial tissue of some vessels will conduct transmitter effects for varying distances along the length of the blood vessel. Furthermore, the coupling mechanism between the receptors and the contractile machinery is not uniform: sometimes several mechanisms operate simultaneously in the same vessel. Thus the precise effect of the transmitter depends on varying properties of the blood vessel upon which it acts.

The endothelial cells of the blood vessel, particularly the smaller ones, are often connected to the vascular smooth muscle cells by myoendothelial cell gap junctions, suggesting cellular interactions between the two types of cells. This implies the possibility of some functional continuity between these two tunicae.

FUNCTIONAL CONSEQUENCES OF VARIATION IN THE VASCULAR NEUROEFFECTOR MECHANISM

Although the vascular neuroeffector mechanism has been studied in detail in comparatively few vessels, there is ample evidence that a number of its components vary widely in vessels from different parts of the vasculature. The following is a brief synopsis of this variation; where possible the functional consequences of this variation are indicated or suggested.

Innervation Density. Density of adrenergic innervation of blood vessels, whether measured by fluorescence microscopy, norepinephrine content, or [^{3}H]norepinephrine uptake varies remarkably—from complete absence to an innervation, as in the cephalic and saphenous veins and some of the smaller pial arteries, which on a weight basis is as high as any other organ in the body. This variation is found in both arteries and veins and even in vessels from the same regional bed. There is preliminary evidence that the innervation density is a major determinant of the magnitude of the contractile response. Thus a densely innervated vessel is usually a vessel highly reactive to sympathetic activity—there are exceptions to this: for example, the cerebral vessels.

Innervation Distribution. Although most blood vessels receive an innervation restricted to the adventitiomedial junction, in a number of instances the adrenergic nerves penetrate into the media to varying depths, as in the rabbit saphenous artery and cephalic vein. Studies suggest that medially innervated tissues contract more to nerve activity than do junctionally innervated vessels and that their frequency-response curves have a lower threshold and rise more steeply. Thus the extent of change of vessel tone with change in sympathetic discharge rate, particularly at the lower physiological frequency range, is greater with medial than junctional innervation. The action of the transmitter in junctionally innervated vessels, unless the synaptic cleft is small, is limited by extraneuronal factors. In medially innervated vessels the transmitter action is terminated by neuronal uptake. The latter mechanism would be expected to provide a finer, faster adjustment to transmitter action.

Transmitter Concentration. The mean effective concentration of the transmitter at the α-adrenergic receptors on the closest vascular smooth muscle cells varies in different blood vessels from approximately 10^{-8} M to $> 10^{-5}$ M for neural activity at 10 Hz. This can be related at least in part to variation in cleft width. In blood vessels where the cleft width is narrow, there is some evidence that extrasynaptic transmitter concentrations are subthreshold, suggesting that transmitter effects are limited to within the synapse.

Feedback Regulation of Release. Based in part on studies from nonvascular tissue, there is evidence that the effectiveness of the negative feedback control of transmitter release in the adrenergic synapse mediated through presynaptic α-adrenergic receptors increases as cleft size decreases. Such a relationship might be predicted, as the released transmitter would tend to remain at a high concentration in the region of the presynaptic α-adrenergic receptors for a longer period of time when the cleft is narrow due to hindrances to diffusion. This mechanism would tend to offset the increase in transmitter concentration expected when the pre- and postsynaptic membranes are close to each other.

Neuronal Uptake of Transmitter. Data from various vascular and nonvascular sources can be interpreted to suggest that when the synaptic cleft is wide, neuronal reuptake removes transmitter molecules before they reach the postsynaptic membrane. Those which escape reuptake diffuse away from the varicosity to act on the α-adrenergic receptors, which are located essentially out of range of the reuptake process. This transmitter is disposed of by extraneuronal mechanisms. On the other hand, when the cleft is narrow, there is indirect evidence that the transmitter acts on smooth muscle cells prior to reuptake. This is another contributing factor to the differences in transmitter concentrations in blood vessels with differing size of cleft. Thus the dominant mechanism of transmitter disposition may change along the length of the vascular tree. Termination of biological effect by reuptake would confer upon the smaller blood vessels a much finer mechanism of neurogenic control than that enjoyed by the larger vessels where transmitter effects are terminated by slower processes.

Extraneuronal Distribution of Transmitter. The transmitter that escapes reuptake after release from a junctional plexus is free to diffuse toward the lumen and outward through the adventitia. The distribution between adventitia and media for the pulmonary artery of the rabbit is approximately 6:1. Clearly, this ratio depends both on the relative thickness and density of the two tunicae and the presence of possible diffusion barriers. It would be influenced by such processes as medial hyperplasia, as occurs in hypertension. Thickening of the media in the absence of other changes would tend to reduce the absolute amount of released norepinephrine entering the smooth muscles, resulting in a smaller sympathetic response.

Modulation of Transmission. Both the release of the adrenergic transmitter and its action on the postsynaptic α-adrenergic receptor can be dramatically modulated by the number of naturally occurring molecules, including angiotensin, histamine, serotonin, and prostaglandins. In the rabbit, sympathetic effects on the cerebral circulation, for example, are increased dramatically by histamine in concentrations that by themselves have little effect on vascular tone. Such effects are more important in some vascular beds than in others. There is some evidence that some modulating substances, such as acetylcholine, prostaglandins, and angiotensin, might be locally produced in the blood vessel wall. If such effects were region or blood vessel specific, they might confer on circulating substances differential circulatory action via the sympathetic mechanism.

Trophic Nerve-Muscle Interaction. Recent experiments suggest that the sympathetic nervous system can influence the development and thickness of the vascular wall, at least during growth. After denervation, the arterial wall becomes thinner, the rate of vascular smooth muscle cell proliferation diminishes, and the physical characteristics of its wall change. For this reason, such an artery has a lowered capacity to develop tone to norepinephrine than to its innervated companion.

α- and β-Adrenergic Receptor Characteristics and Ratio. In the rabbit cerebral circulation an unusual α-receptor is present. It is comparatively insensitive to norepinephrine, and on the basis of amine potency ratios and other studies it is not identical to that found elsewhere. It is also possible that different α effects can be obtained from the vascular smooth muscle on the inside and on the outside of the vessel wall. Such features suggest the possibility that circulating norepinephrine may act on a different population of α-receptors than are acted on by neurogenic norepinephrine, and that differential regional effects of circulating norepinephrine, epinephrine, and drugs may result, in part at any rate, from differing action on α-adrenergic receptors.

In most blood vessels studied to date, β-adrenergic receptor responses to either endogenous or exogenous norepinephrine seems comparatively small. However, in specific blood vessels, as for example, the coronary arteries and the facial vein of the rabbit, β effects may dominate the neurogenic contractile response.

Monoamine Oxidase (MAO and Catechol-O-Methyltransferase (COMT). Studies of a series of fetal and adult blood vessels suggest that the bulk of MAO and COMT activity is related to the mass of the blood vessel wall. Of the two enzymes, COMT seems more important in the degradation of norepinephrine that has entered the blood vessel wall. Although only a small proportion of the total vessel MAO is located in the neuron, this is of major functional signifiçance.

Myogenic Conduction, Spontaneous Rhythmic Activity, and Intrinsic Vascular Tone. The extent and spread of induced activity in the long axis of the smooth muscle system varies in different blood vessels by more than 1500%. Propagation tends to make a more important contribution to the NE response and the number of nexi and extent of spontaneous rhythmic activity to increase in smaller compared with larger blood vessels. In contrast to most, a number of vessels, including the facial vein of the rabbit and the basilar artery of the cat, increase their tone spontaneously in vitro. Such preparations relax to vasodilator drugs in vitro while others under the same circumstances do not, except after prior exposure to a vasoconstrictor agent.

Variation in the various factors included in this chapter account in part for differences in the threshold, extent, nature, and rate of response and recovery of vessels to changes in neural frequency and levels of circulating catecholamine.

ACKNOWLEDGMENT

The new research presented in this chapter was carried out under U.S. Public Health Service Grants HL-08359, HL-15805, and HL-20581.

BIBLIOGRAPHY

1. Bevan, J. A., Bevan, R. D., and Duckles, S. P. Adrenergic regulation of vascular smooth muscle. In Handbook of Physiology, Sec. 2: The Cardiovascular System, Vol. II: Vascular Smooth Muscle, D. F. Bohn, A. P. Somlyo, and H. V. Sparks (Eds.). American Physiological Society, Baltimore, pp. 515-566, 1980.
2. Bevan, J. A. Some bases of differences in vascular response to sympathetic activity—variations on a theme. Circ. Res. 45:161-171, 1979.
3. Burnstock, G., and Costa, M. Their organization, function and development in the peripheral nervous system. In Adrenergic Neurons. Wiley, New York, pp. 1-225, 1975.
4. Cliff, W. J. Blood Vessels. Cambridge University Press, New York, 1976.

5. de la Lande, I. S. Adrenergic mechanisms in the rabbit ear artery. Blood Vessels 12: 137-160, 1975.
6. Duckles, S. P., and Bevan, J. A. Pathophysiology of vasospasm. In Vascular Neuroeffector Mechanisms, J. A. Bevan, G. Burnstock, B. Johansson, R. A. Maxwell, and O. A. Nedergaard (Eds.). Karger, Basel, pp. 162-169, 1976.
7. Fleisch, J. H. Further studies on the effect of aging on β-adrenoceptor activity of rat aorta. Br. J. Pharmacol. 42:311-313, 1971.
8. Folkow, D., and Neil, E. Circulation. Oxford University Press, New York, 1971.
9. Furchgott, R. F. Postsynaptic adrenergiv receptor mechanisms in vascular smooth muscle. In Vascular Neuroeffector Mechanisms, J. A. Beva, G. Burnstock, B. Johansson, R. A. Maxwell, and O. A. Nedergaard (Eds.). Karger, Basel, pp. 131-142, 1976.
10. Gillespie, J. S. Uptake of noradrenaline by smooth muscle. Br. Med. Bull. 29:136-141, 1973.
11. Iversen, L. L. Catecholamine uptake processes. Br. Med. Bull. 29: 130-135, 1973.
12. Ljung, B. Physiological patterns of neuroeffector control mechanisms. In Vascular Neuroeffector Mechanisms (2nd Int. Symp., Odense, 1975). Karger, Basel, pp. 143-155, 1976.
13. Moran, N. C. Adrenergic receptors. In Handbook of Physiology, Sec. 7, Vol. VI, R. O. Greep and E. B. Astwood (Eds.). American Physiological Society, Washington, D.C., pp. 447-472, 1975.
14. Paton, D. M. Characteristics of uptake of noradrenaline by adrenergic neurons. In The Mechanism of Neuronal and Extraneuronal Transport of Catecholamines, D. M. Paton (Ed.), Raven Press, New York, pp. 49-66, 1976.
15. Smith, A. D., and Winkler, H. Fundamental mechanisms in the release of catecholamines. In Catecholamines, Vol. 33 of Handbook of Experimental Pharmacology, H. Blaschko and E. Muscholl (Eds.). Springer-Verlag, Berlin, pp. 538-617, 1972.
16. Somlyo, A. P., and Somlyo, A. V. Vascular smooth muscle: II. Pharmacology of normal and hypertensive vessels. Pharmacol. Rev. 22: 249-353, 1970.
17. Spector, S., Tarver, J., and Berkowitz, B. Effects of drugs and physiological factors in the disposition of catecholamines in blood vessels. Pharmacol. Rev. 24:191-202, 1972.
18. Starke, K., Endo, T., and Taube, H. D. Relative pre- and post-synaptic potencies of α-adrenoceptor agonists in the rabbit pulmonary artery. Naunyn-Schmiedebergs Arch. Pharmakol. 291:55-78, 1975.
19. Stjärne, L. Basic mechanisms and local feedback control of secretion of adrenergic and cholinergic neurotransmitters. In Handbook of Psychopharmacology, Vol. 6, L. L. Iverson, S. D. Iverson, and S. H. Snyder (Eds.). Plenum, New York, 1976.
20. Weiner, N. Regulation of norepinephrine biosynthesis. Annu. Rev. Pharmacol. 10:273, 1970.

2 Capillary Filtration

FRANCIS J. HADDY / Uniformed Services University of the Health Sciences, Bethesda, Maryland

Fluid transfer across the capillary membrane determines the distribution of extracellular water between the vascular and interstitial spaces. It is therefore a major determinant of the absolute blood volume and the interstitial fluid volume. The absolute blood volume influences venous return and therefore cardiac output. Interstitial fluid volume has little effect on function in many organs but can greatly alter the function of others, lung and brain for example. In this chapter the determinants of fluid transfer across the capillary membrane are reviewed, and then the effects of the prostaglandins upon these determinants and hence upon fluid transfer are briefly described. These effects are compared to those of histamine and bradykinin, agents well known for their ability to influence fluid transfer.

A detailed list of references to fluid transfer across the capillary membrane has recently been presented in another review (1). The list of references at the end of this chapter therefore includes only certain papers appearing since 1975.

PHYSICAL DETERMINANTS OF FLUID TRANSFER ACROSS THE CAPILLARY MEMBRANE

In 1896, Starling described fluid transfer across the capillary membrane using purely physical forces. Data generated since then have only served to quantitate these forces partially; they have not indicated the need to add new forces, physical or otherwise. The relevant physical forces are (1) capillary hydrostatic pressure, (2) interstitial fluid hydrostatic pressure, (3) plasma colloid osmotic pressure, and (4) interstitial fluid colloid osmotic pressure. These forces determine the rate of fluid flow across the capillary membrane and allow its calculation when capillary surface area and permeability to filtered fluid are known. The driving force for filtration is the hydrostatic pressure gradient, i.e., capillary hydrostatic pressure minus interstitial fluid hydrostatic pressure. The absorbing force is the colloid osmotic pressure gradient, i.e., plasma colloid osmotic pressure minus interstitial fluid colloid osmotic pressure. Filtration occurs at sites in the capillary where the hydrostatic pressure gradient exceeds the colloid osmotic pressure gradient and reabsorption occurs at sites where the reverse obtains. The hydrostatic pressure gradient decreases along the length of the capillary as capillary hydrostatic pressure dissipates; consequently, filtration is more likely at the arterial end of the capillary than at the venous end. However, filtration will occur along the entire length in capillaries with a high hydrostatic pressure gradient and reabsorption along the entire length in capillaries with a low capillary pressure gradient. Filtration will also occur along the entire length if the colloid osmotic pressure gradient is very low and reabsorption will occur along the entire length if it is very high. The determinants of these gradients are considered next.

Hydrostatic Pressure Gradient

The absolute magnitude of this gradient will be in doubt as long as there are two polarized groups of investigators, one believing that interstitial fluid pressure is subatmospheric in some tissues and the other believing that it is positive in all tissues. Regardless of the absolute magnitude of the gradient, large changes in it can occur rapidly as a result of alterations in capillary hydrostatic pressure.

Capillary Hydrostatic Pressure. Mean capillary hydrostatic pressure is immediately determined by the distensibility of the capillary and the volume of blood contained within it. Since the capillary is relatively nondistensible (to a large extent because of support provided by the basement membrane and ground substance), small changes in volume result in large changes in pressure. Volume is, in turn, determined by the relation between capillary inflow and outflow. Inflow is set by the aortic blood pressure and the resistance to blood flow through arteries; outflow is determined by the resistance to flow through veins and the right atrial pressure. A decrease in aortic pressure, venous resistance, or right atrial pressure will lower capillary hydrostatic pressure, whereas a decrease in arterial resistance will raise capillary pressure. Conversely, an increase in aortic pressure, venous resistance, or right atrial pressure will raise capillary hydrostatic pressure, whereas an increase in arterial resistance will lower the pressure. A variable rarely operates by itself, however; one or more of the others frequently move in a direction to maintain capillary hydrostatic pressure constant.

Aortic Pressure. Changes in aortic pressure have surprisingly little effect on capillary hydrostatic pressure in many vascular beds. This is because the resistance to flow through the arteriole is high and because this resistance automatically changes in a direction to antagonize the effect of the change in aortic pressure. Consequently, changes in aortic pressure have little effect on capillary inflow. This autoregulation or self-regulation is particularly prominent in the renal vascular bed, where changes in aortic pressure over the middle range have essentially no effect on capillary pressures and consequently on the rate of glomerular filtration or lymph flow from a hilar lymphatic vessel. Increases in arterial pressure are accompanied by active arteriolar constriction and decreases by active arteriolar dilation. Similar effects are seen in the mesenteric vascular bed, where only 15% of a reduction in arterial pressure is transmitted to microvessels, and in skeletal muscle, where net transcapillary fluid movement is essentially zero over a wide range of arterial pressure. Passive changes in venous caliber also contribute to the constancy of capillary pressure. For example, a reduction in aortic pressure, in addition to causing active arteriolar dilation, also causes passive venous constriction subsequent to a fall in venous transmural pressure. This raises venous resistance, which helps to prevent a fall in capillary pressure.

When aortic pressure rises or falls to levels where autoregulation is less prominent or absent, the effect on capillary pressure is greater. Even here, however, factors other than aortic pressure determine capillary hydrostatic pressure. For example, a large rise in aortic pressure will passively dilate both arteries and veins, the former tending to increase and the latter tending to decrease capillary pressure.

Arterial Resistance. This resistance is highly adjustable through active changes in the caliber of arterioles and precapillary sphinctors. Thus arterial resistance can have a large effect on capillary pressure. Indeed, closure of the precapillary sphinctor completely stops inflow into the capillary and drops capillary pressure to that prevailing in anastomotic vessels. However, secondary changes also tend to blunt the effects of alterations in arterial resistance on capillary hydrostatic pressure. For example, the fall in capillary hydrostatic pressure subsequent to arteriolar constriction is somewhat blunted by a rise in venous resistance. The latter occurs because the decreased venous inflow lowers venous pressure, which causes passive venous constriction. On the other hand, the rise in capillary hydrostatic pressure subsequent to arteriolar dilation is to a certain extent antagonized by a fall in venous resistance. This occurs because the increased venous inflow raises venous transmural pressure, which in turn passively distends the veins.

Venous Resistance. Changes in venous resistance can also cause large changes in capillary pressure. Closure of veins, with a tourniquet for example, can completely stop capillary outflow and raise capillary pressure almost to the level of aortic pressure. In this vascular section, passive changes are prominent because of the great compliance of veins over the low-pressure range. Active changes in caliber are also prominent, even in the larger veins.

In some vascular beds, particularly intestine, the effects of venous resistance on capillary pressure are tempered by changes in arterial resistance of the same sign. For example, in the dog forelimb, the effect of venous constriction with a tourniquet on capillary pressure is partially blunted by automatic arteriolar constriction as arteriolar transmural pressure rises. This reaction is called the venous-arteriolar response. It reduces capillary inflow, thereby tempering the effect of the reduced capillary outflow on capillary hydrostatic pressure. This should limit filtration. Lymph flow has been measured in the dog forelimb and hindlimb before and after constricting the veins with a tourniquet and the increase in lymph flow is surprisingly small.

Atrial Pressure. In these same vascular beds, the effect of atrial pressure on capillary pressure is tempered by changes in both arterial and venous resistance. An increase in outflow pressure both passively distends the veins and actively contricts arterioles (venous-arteriolar response). Both of these secondary changes tend to reduce capillary pressure and the net effect is a smaller increase than would be seen in their absence. In the feline mesenteric vascular bed, only 60% of an increase in venous pressure is reflected in microvessels. Consequently, the increase in filtration is less than would be seen in the absence of the secondary changes.

Other vascular beds, that in lung for example, do not exhibit a venous-arteriolar response. Consequently, only passive venous dilation limits the rise in capillary pressure on elevation of atrial pressure.

These secondary responses should signal caution in assigning a fixed relation between venous pressure and capillary pressure, as is done in the calculation of the capillary filtration coefficient in whole organs. The magnitude of the secondary responses varies between organs and even within the same organ with a change in conditions (administration of a vasoactive agent, for example).

Interstitial Fluid Hydrostatic Pressure. The absolute value of interstitial fluid hydrostatic pressure is controversial because of practical problems in its measurement. Histological study of connective tissue shows that the interstitial space between blood vessels consists of a meshwork of collagen fibers filled with ground substance. Two separate phases may be distinguished within the ground substance: a gel phase and a free-fluid phase. Unfortunately, under normal conditions of hydration, the dimensions of the latter in most tissues are much smaller than those of the smallest pipettes. Consequently, its pressure cannot be measured directly. Indirect methods of measurement, utilizing the implanted capsule and wick techniques for example, record negative pressures with respect to atmosphere in subcutaneous tissues (2,3). The value with the capsule technique is approximately minus 6 mmHg under conditions of normal hydration. It falls to much lower values with a small reduction in volume during dehydration (an average of -27 mmHg has been recorded during the dehydration caused by a high capillary colloid osmotic pressure) and rises to positive values with large increases in volume during overhydration (edema). Consequently, the tissue has been said to have a very low compliance over the normal and dehydrated range and a very high compliance over the hydrated range (2,3). It is hypothesized that the tissue solids (collagen fibers, hyaluronic acid fibrillae of the mucopolysaccharide gel) have form rigidity like a sponge and that under normal conditions of hydration the tissue spaces are mainly collapsed with the solid elements of the tissues compacted on each other. Their elastic nature causes a tendency for them to recoil back to their original volume, thus creating suction (negative pressure) in the fluid of the tissue spaces. On the other hand, over the hydrated range they are easily pushed apart. To quote from a recent publication (2): "Normally the interstitial fluid is continually pumped back into circulation by way of the lymphatics, and additional fluid is absorbed by osmosis into the capillaries due to the oncotic pressure of the capillaries. These two effects cause a continuous dehydrating state of the tissue spaces, which compacts the tissue elements. The cells are compacted against each other and the reticular filaments of the hyaluronic acid and collagen gel are also compacted. Because of this compacted state, the walls of the normal tissue spaces exhibit very little change in elastic distortion as the interstitial fluid pressure changes. On the other hand, when interstitial fluid pressure rises into the positive range, there is now excess fluid in the interstitial spaces. This enlarges the spaces and eliminates the compaction of the tissue elements. Now the only limiting restraints to change the interstitial fluid volume are the tensile elements of the tissues. In loose areolar tissue such as the subcutaneous spaces, the tensile elements are very weak in comparison with the elasic strength of the compaction elements (cells, collagen fibers, hyaluronic acid gel). Therefore in the positive pressure range the compliance becomes at least 25 times as great as it is in the negative pressure range. To state this another way, the elastic volume distortion of the tensile elements is at least 25 times as great for a given pressure change as is the elastic volume compression of the compaction elements. In other tissues of the body this great difference between the negative and positive pressure ranges is not apparent. For instance, in the kidneys, which have a very strong elastic tensile capsule, there is not this sudden change in compliance between the negative and positive pressure ranges. Likewise, in muscles, which lie in strong sheaths, the difference also is not so great."

On the other hand, pressures measured by the needle and balloon methods record positive pressures (3). In addition in the rabbit ear, pockets of free fluid large enough to accommodate a micropipette with a 0.5 μm tip diameter have been found and here the pressure is slightly positive. Furthermore, excised samples of rabbit skin placed on membrane osmometers, covered with large pore membranes (0.2 μm pore diameter) freely permeable to protein, give pressures approaching atmospheric and the pressure in large pore (4500 Å) osmometers chronically implanted in rabbit subcutaneous tissue averages only -1.2 mmHg (4). These observations and others which suggest the possibility that a pressure difference develops between the cavity of perforated capsules and the surrounding tissue spaces because of osmotic factors have led some investigators to question the validity of the perforated capsule technique for measuring the hydrostatic pressure in the free-fluid phase of the ground substance. Those that use the capsule technique counter by suggesting that the needle and balloon techniques measure total tissue pressure (interstitial fluid pressure + solid tissue pressure) rather than interstitial fluid pressure, and it is the latter which influences the rate of fluid movement across the capillary membrane (3). They also believe that the micropipette values represent measurements of pressure in naturally edematous spaces that have not yet been found in other tissues (3) and that the membranes which develop on the outer and inner surfaces of the capsule do not offer a substantial barrier to albumin and globulin (5). Thus the controversy over the pressure level in normally hydrated sucutaneous tissue continues.

In certain tissues, renal for example, interstitial fluid hydrostatic pressure is clearly positive because all methods of measurement, including the perforated capsule technique, record pressures in excess of atmospheric (6).

Colloid Osmotic Pressure Gradient

The magnitude of this gradient depends to a major extent on the difference in protein concentration between the plasma and interstitial fluid. This difference is determined by the permeability of the capillary membrane to plasma proteins. As will become apparent, other colloids also contribute to the colloid osmotic pressure of interstitial fluid and thus to the magnitude of the gradient.

Plasma Colloid Osmotic Pressure. This pressure is approximately 27 mmHg in humans and somewhat less in cat, dog, rabbit, and rat. The contribution of albumin is much greater than that of globulin because the albumin molecule is smaller than the globulin molecule and in most species is present in higher concentrations. For these reasons and others, in humans approximately 65% of plasma colloid osmotic pressure is attributable to albumin and only approximately 15% to globulin. In other species, dog for example, the concentration of globulin is more nearly equal to that of albumin and consequently its contribution to total osmotic pressure is somewhat greater than 15%.

The escape rate of protein from microvessels is determined by the permeability of their membranes to the protein molecules. Electron microscopic studies reveal two basic types of microvessels: those with continuous endothelium, as in muscle, and those with fenestrated endothelium, as in certain viscera (others have features of both basic types). They also reveal slitlike junctions between the endothelial cells and a large population of vesicles within the endothelial cells. About 60% of the vesicles open to the surface and they occasionally connect to form a patent transendothelial channel. Most of the fenestrae have diaphragms of unknown nature and porosity. A basement membrane is also visualized.

Studies with visible "probe" molecules suggest that the vesicles transport molecules across the endothelial cell. It is thought that albumin and globulin escape from the microvessels both via vesicles and fenestrae. Whether albumin also escapes via the slitlike intercellular junctions is still undecided. The vesicles and fenestrae are especially prominent in the venous portion of the microvessel, thereby accounting for the higher permeability of this segment to proteins (the venous portion of the capillary also has more surface area than does the arterial portion). The basement membrane seems to serve as an extra coarse filter behind the endothelium (it apparently contributes to the rigidity of the true capillary).

It is thought that vesicular transport is independent of microvascular pressure, but studies suggest that pore size increases as a function of this pressure. Perhaps this is related to the fact that the venous capillary and venule distend with pressure (the true capillary is relatively indistensible). Other evidence suggests that intercellular slit size is increased by certain substances, such as histamine and bradykinin, through rounding or contraction of the endothelial cells. It has been suggested that these same agents increase vesicular transport.

Interstitial Fluid Colloid Osmotic Pressure. As with interstitial fluid hydrostatic pressure, practical problems leave the absolute magnitude of this pressure in doubt. It is difficult to obtain pure samples of free interstitial fluid for analysis. It does appear, however, that its magnitude is considerably greater than has been realized.

As pointed out above, the interstitial space must be considered compartmented into a two-phase system, a gellike phase and a free-fluid phase. The gellike phase is composed mainly of mucopolysaccharides, immense molecules that form an entangled network sufficiently dense to impede markedly the transport of molecules even as small as those of water (7). Protein molecules are excluded from this phase and are found only in the free-fluid phase. Since the mucopolysaccharides exert an osmotic pressure of their own, as do the proteins in the free fluid, the partition of fluid between the two phases must be in equilibrium and must depend on the relative concentrations of mucopolysaccharides and protein. In an in vitro mixture of 0.6% mucopolysaccharides (hyaluronate) and 2% protein (albumin), concentrations thought to be similar to those in interstitium of skin and muscle, the partition of fluid between the gellike mucopolysaccharide compartment and the free fluid containing the protein is approximately 1:1 (7). This mixture exerts an osmotic pressure on the order of 10 mmHg, a value similar to that obtained in rabbit subcutaneous tissue with chronically implanted small pore (~15 Å) membrane osmometers and also similar to the "swelling" pressure of excised samples of rabbit skin placed on a small pore membrane osmometer (4).

Other evidence also suggests that the colloid osmotic pressure of the interstitium is not negligible in skin and skeletal muscle. Fluid sampled from subcutaneous tissue and skeletal muscle of the mature rat by the nylon wick method has colloid osmotic pressures and total protein concentrations approximately 50% of those in plasma (8). Fluid aspirated from capsules implanted in the subcutaneous tissue of dog and rabbit contains 1.9 and 2.5 g% protein, respectively. Fluid obtained from subcutaneous tissue of the rabbit by the liquid paraffin cavity technique contains roughly 1.9 g% protein (the samples also contain mucopolysaccharides). Fluid taken from large-pore (4500 Å) membrane osmometers implanted in subcutaneous tissue of the rabbit contains 3.7 g% protein (4). Lymph collected from the larger lymphatics draining skin and skeletal muscle also contains considerable quantities of protein. That derived from the skin and paw of the dog forelimb, for example, contains 2-3 g% protein. Both albumin and globulin are present, slightly more of the former. Even greater concentrations are found in lymph draining other tissues and organs (liver, intestine, lung, etc.). There is only one study of peripheral lymph. Fluid obtained from collecting lymph channels 80-300 μm in diameter, draining directly from the cat intestine, has a total protein concentration of 2.6 g% and a corresponding colloid osmotic pressure of 8.8 cm H_2O (9).

All of these findings suggest that the colloid osmotic pressure of the interstitium is considerably higher than has been realized. It therefore could serve as an osmotic buffer, constituting the first line of defense against edema formation. Elevation of venous pressure, for example, would dilute the osmotically active substances in the interstitium, thereby increasing the colloid osmotic pressure gradient across the capillary membrane (the force opposing filtration) and hence limiting the filtration.

If the interstitial fluid colloid osmotic pressure is in fact on the order of 10-12 mmHg in rabbit, rat, and dog subcutaneous tissue, the colloid osmotic pressure gradient is about 10 mmHg (in these species, plasma colloid osmotic pressure is about 20 mmHg). If it were now assumed that we are dealing with a capillary section where net fluid movement is zero (net filtration pressure is zero), an interstitial fluid hydrostatic pressure of -6 mmHg (as recorded by the capsule technique) implies a capillary hydrostatic pressure of only 4 mmHg. Micropuncture reveals much higher values in a variety of tissues (9-13), including skin and skeletal muscle (10, 11). If the latter measurements were in balanced capillaries (zero net filtration pressure), interstitial fluid pressure could not have been negative. If they were made in capillaries operating in the filtering mode (positive net filtration pressure), as seems likely from measurements of lymph flow in a number of laboratories, one of the two mechanisms that could create a negative interstitial fluid pressure was absent, namely net fluid reabsorption by the capillary. For interstitial fluid pressure to have been negative, it must be assumed that the lymphatic vessels pumped fluid out of the interstitial space faster than it entered the space from the capillaries. The existence of such an efficient pumping mechanism will be considered after a description of the lymphatic system.

The terminal lymphatics begin as blind-end endothelial tubes or saccules or as a network of delicate endothelial tubes. The endothelial wall is extraordinarily thin but lacks obvious discontinuities. The adjacent cells are extensively overlapped and lack adhesive devices in many areas (14). Within the cells are found plasmalemmal vesicles and cytoplasmic filaments. The vessels lack a continuous basal lamina and maintain a close relationship with the adjoining interstitium by way of anchoring filaments (14). The terminal lymphatic vessel is highly permeable to large molecules. When electron dense tracers are injected intravenously (ferritin, horseradish peroxidase), subsequent microscopic examination of the tissues reveals the presence of tracer particles within the interstitium and the lymphatic capillary lumen (14). These particles appear to gain access into the lymphatic capillaries both via the intercellular clefts of patent junctions and the plasmalemmal vesicles (14). In mesentery, dye-tagged albumin injected into the terminal lymphatic diffuses immediately into the interstitium (15). Contractile activity is inconsistent. The pressure in terminal lymphatic vessels of exteriorized mesentery is uniformly ambient (0 cm H_2O). Like the true blood capillary, the terminal lymphatic is not easily distended.

Collecting or effluent channels are formed by the confluence of terminal vessels. In the collecting vessels, the endothelial cells have close to tight junctions and a more continuous basement membrane. In contrast to the terminal mesenteric vessel, an injected bolus of dye-tagged albumin shows no evidence of diffusion into the tissue proper (15), indicating that the collecting channel is quite impermeable to protein [there is some evidence (9) that protein concentration increases due to water loss as the lymph flows centrally]. Other clear features are one-way flap valves, compliant thick walls, smooth muscle cells, anchoring filaments, and contractile activity. The latter undoubtedly is to a large extent attributable to the smooth muscle cells, but a contribution from the endothelial cells has not been ruled out since, as in the terminal vessels, the endothelial cell contains cytoplasmic filaments. Movement of lymph down the length of the collecting vessel apparently results both from active contraction and from passive contraction due to external compression. The valves assure unidirectional flow. In mesentery, pressures in the large collecting lymphatics have a broad range (0-14 cm H_2O) (9).

It has been suggested that the inner portion of the overlapping endothelial cell junction in the terminal vessel can open as a one-way-flap-valve system when the interstitial fluid pressure is higher than that of the lymphatic intraluminal pressure (14). Conversely, when the intraluminal pressure is equal to or higher than interstitial pressure, the one-way flap valve is closed (14). It has also been suggested that, following contraction of the terminal lymphatic (due to shortening of the cytoplasmic myofilaments), the anchoring filaments pull the capillaries open, again creating a suction cycle and thereby a negative interstitial fluid pressure (3). However, firm evidence for flap-valve action and contractile activity of the endothelium in the terminal lympathic is lacking. In fact, in mesentery and omentum of mammals, the lymphatic terminals are not spontaneously contractile. Thus it is not yet established that the terminal lymphatics can pump fluid from the interstitial spaces.

Crystalloid Osmotic Pressure

Transcapillary fluid flux can also be influenced by changes in the concentrations of small molecules to which the capillary membrane is very permeable. Fluid transiently moves into the capillary on sudden addition of sodium chloride or dextrose to blood, whereas it transiently moves out of the capillary on sudden addition to interstitial fluid. The fluid movement is to a large extent the direct result of the establishment of a crystalloid osmotic pressure gradient across the capillary membrane. The movement is transient because the gradient soon disappears. The amount of fluid moved depends on the number of molecules added per unit volume and the permeability of the membrane to the molecules added.

Under special conditions, the fluid movement can be sustained. A sustained effect requires that the addition be continuous to one side of the membrane and that there be an infinite sink on the other side of the membrane into which the substance can disappear. Continuous addition to interstitial fluid in a local area meets these requirements. Here fluid continues to move from blood to interstitial fluid because the crystalloid osmotic pressure gradient across the capillary is sustained. The gradient is sustained because the blood into which the substance diffuses is continually replaced.

Changes in crystalloid osmotic pressure can produce fluid movement indirectly via changes in Starling's forces. For example, intraarterial infusion of a hypertonic solution of sodium chloride in the dog forelimb (perfused with blood at a constant rate) produces a small gradual fall in forelimb weight. The limb continues to lose weight even after the osmolality of interstitial fluid should equal that in blood. The continued loss of weight indicates that fluid continues to move into the blood phase. This probably results from secondary changes of tissue fluid colloid osmotic and hydrostatic pressures. The increase in interstitial fluid osmolality withdraws fluid from cells. This in turn dilutes the colloid in the interstitial spaces and raises interstitial fluid hydrostatic pressure. Both of these changes then move fluid from the interstitial space into the capillary.

Surface Area

Changes in surface area will not influence the amount of fluid in the tissues unless Starling's forces are out of balance; i.e., addition or deletion of capillaries which are in balance with respect to fluid movement will not change the amount of fluid in the tissue spaces. It will, however, have a great effect if they are out of balance. For example, the addition of capillaries that are filtering due to a high capillary hydrostatic pressure will increase the amount of fluid in the tissue spaces.

Surface area can be changed by altering the number of open capillaries of the size of those that are already open. The former mechanism is more efficient. Precapillary sphinctors can add or subtract whole capillaries. On the other hand, the true capillary is not easily distended; only the venular end changes measurably in size when transmural pressure is increased.

EFFECTS OF PROSTAGLANDIN ON TRANSCAPILLARY FLUID FLUX

Relative to histamine and bradykinin, local administration of prostaglandin E_1 has little effect on the interstitial store of fluid in dog limbs. Intrabrachial infusion of histamine or bradykinin can increase forelimb weight as much as 20% in 30 min; inspection and palpation reveal gross edema (16-18). The pressures in small veins increase, as do lymph flow and lymph protein concentration (16-18). Thus the edema results both from an increase in capillary hydrostatic pressure (due to arteriolar dilation) and an increase in interstitial fluid colloid osmotic pressure (due to an increase in the permeability of the microvascular membrane to plasma proteins). By contrast, intraarterial infusion of prostaglandin E_1 in the same preparation has essentially no effect on limb weight, even with extremely high rates of infusion (19, 20). Small vein and, by inference, capillary hydrostatic pressures do not rise despite potent arteriolar dilation (the veins seem to dilate proportionately). Effects are similar in the canine hindlimb; intraarterial infusion of prostaglandin E_1 decreases resistance but has no effect on the store of fluid as judged by limb volume (21). Furthermore, subcutaneous injection of prostaglandins (E_1, E_2, $F_{2\alpha}$, A_2) in the canine hindpaw, while increasing lymph flow slightly, decreases the lymph-to-plasma concentration ratios for total protein, and dextran 110 and has no effect on sieving ratios (22). Subcutaneous administration of histamine in this preparation produces large increases in lymph flow, lymph-to-plasma concentration ratios, and sieving ratios (22).

On the other hand, in the cat ileum, intraarterial infusion of 5 μg/min PGE_1 increases lymph flow without decreasing the lymph-to-plasma ratio for protein (23) and, in the dog forelimb perfused at constant flow, intraarterial infusion of 2 to 32 μg/min PGE_1 not only increases lymph flow but also increases lymph total protein concentration (24). Furthermore, in the hamster cheek pouch, topical application of PGE_1, PGE_2, and $PGF_{2\alpha}$ visually increases the leakage of fluoroscein-labeled dextran (MW = 150,000) from the postcapillary venule (8.6-14.0 μm), much like histamine and bradykinin (25).

Thus, while there is evidence that certain of the prostaglandins can increase the permeability of the postcapillary venule to plasma proteins and increase water efflux from the microvasculature, there is also evidence that they fail to substantially increase the interstitial store of water. Apparently, the capacity of the lymphatics to remove the filtered fluid is not overwhelmed, as in the case of histamine and bradykinin. Perhaps this is related to lesser effects on capillary hydrostatic pressure and microvascular permeability to plasma proteins.

REFERENCES

1. Haddy, F. J., Scott, J. B., and Grega, G. J. Peripheral circulation: fluid transfer across the microvascular membrane. In International Review of Physiology. Cardiovascular Physiology II, Vol. 9, A. C. Guyton and A. W. Cowley (Eds.). University Park Press, Baltimore, pp. 63-109, 1976.
2. Guyton, A. C., Cowley, A. W., Jr., Young, D. B., Coleman, T. G., Hall, J. E., and DeClue, J. W. Integration and control of circulatory function. In International Review of Physiology. Cardiovascular Physiology II, Vol. 9, A. C. Guyton and A. W. Cowley (Eds.), University Park Press, Baltimore, pp. 341-385, 1976.
3. Guyton, A. C., Taylor, A. E., and Brace, R. A. A synthesis of interstitial fluid regulation and lymph formation. Fed Proc. 35:1881-1885, 1976.
4. Stromberg, D. D., and Wiederhielm, C. A. Interstitial fluid oncotic pressures in rabbit subcutaneous tissue. Am. J. Physiol. 231:888-891, 1976.
5. Granger, H. J., and Taylor, A. E. Permeability of connective tissue linings isolated from implanted capsules. Circ. Res. 36:222-228, 1975.
6. Ott, C. E., and Knox, F. G. Tissue pressure and fluid dynamics in the kidney. Fed. Proc. 35:1872-1875, 1976.
7. Wiederhielm, C. A., Fox, J. R., and Lee, D. R. Ground substance mucopolysaccharides and plasma proteins: their role in capillary water balance. Am. J. Physiol. 230:1121-1125, 1976.
8. Reed, R. K., and Aukland, K. Transcapillary hydrostatic and colloid osmotic pressures in immature rats. Acta Physiol. Scand. 96:37A-38A, 1976.
9. Hargens, A. R., and Zweifach, B. W. Transport between blood and peripheral lymph in intestine. Microvasc. Res. 11:89-101, 1976.
10. Landis, E. M. Micro-injection studies of capillary blood pressure in human skin. Heart 15:209-228, 1930.
11. Fronek, K., and Zweifach, B. W. Microvascular pressure distribution in skeletal muscle and the effect of vasodilation. Am. J. Physiol. 228: 791-796, 1975.

12. Richardson, D. R., and Coates, F. Effects of norepinephrine infusion (IV) on microvascular pressures and capillary blood flow in the mesentery. Microvasc. Res. 9:166-181, 1975.
13. Gore, R. W., and Bohlen, H. G. Pressure regulation in the microcirculation. Fed. Proc. 34:2031-2037, 1975.
14. Leak, L. V. The structure of lymphatic capillaries in lymph formation. Fed. Proc. 35:1863-1871, 1976.
15. Zweifach, B. W., and Prather, J. W. Micromanipulation of pressure in terminal lymphatics in the mesentery. Am. J. Physiol. 228:1326-1335, 1975.
16. Haddy, F. J., Scott, J. B., and Grega, G. J. Effects of histamine on lymph protein concentration and flow in the dog forelimb. Am. J. Physiol. 223:1172-1177, 1972.
17. Grega, G. J., Kline, R. L., Dobbins, D. E., and Haddy, F. J. Mechanism of edema formation by histamine administered locally into canine forelimbs. Am. J. Physiol. 223:1165-1171, 1972.
18. Kline, R. L., Scott, J. B., Haddy, F. J., and Grega, G. J. Mechanism of edema formation in canine forelimbs by locally administered bradykinin. Am. J. Physiol. 225:1051-1056, 1973.
19. Daugherty, R. M., Jr., Schwinghamer, J. M., Swindall, S., and Haddy, F. J. The effects of local and systemic infusion of prostaglandin E_1 on the skin and muscle vasculature of the dog forelimb. J. Lab. Clin. Med. 72:869, 1968.
20. Daugherty, R. M., Jr. Effects of iv and ia prostaglandin E_1 on dog forelimb skin and muscle blood flow. Am. J. Physiol. 220:392-396, 1971.
21. Greenberg, R. A., and Sparks, H. V. Prostaglandins and consecutive vascular segments of the canine hindlimb. Am. J. Physiol. 216:567-571, 1969.
22. Joyner, W. L. Effects of prostaglandins on macromolecular transport from blood to lymph in the dog. Am. J. Physiol. 232:H690-H696, 1977.
23. Granger, D. N., Shackleford, J. S., and Taylor, A. E. PGE_1-induced intestinal secretion: mechanism of enhanced transmucosal protein efflux. Am. J. Physiol. 236:E788-E796, 1979.
24. Maciejko, J. J., Gorman, A. N., and Grega, G. J. The effect of PGE_1 on lymph protein concentration in the canine forelimb of dogs anesthetized with pentobarbital. Microvasc. Res. 17:S146, 1979.
25. Svensjö, E. Characterization of leakage of macromolecules in postcapillary venules. Doctoral thesis, Uppsala University, 1978.

3 Prostaglandins and Vascular Smooth Muscle in Hypertension

STAN GREENBERG / University of South Alabama College of Medicine, Mobile, Alabama

With the discovery of the prostaglandin system (1) came the beginning of an exciting new series of ubiquitous, endogenous metabolites of fatty acid metabolism, the study of which has resulted in an insight into the mechanisms that may modulate such diverse processes as platelet aggregation, renal electrolyte excretion, anaphylaxis, neurotransmitter release, pain, atherosclerotic lesion formation, and inflammation, to name just a few. With the myriad of diverse effects produced by the individual components of the prostaglandin cascade on arterial pressure, vascular resistance, and renal function (see Chaps. 4-6), it was a foregone conclusion that the prostanoid system would soon be implicated in the pathogenesis or modulation of hypertensive vascular disease. Many theories have been formulated to explain a role for prostaglandins as a modulator or mediator of the increased arterial pressure and resistance accompanying this disease process. Among these are theories which invoke (1) decreased levels of vasodilator prostanoid metabolites, (2) deficiencies in renal salt-losing prostaglandins, (3) excesses of salt-retaining prostanoids, (4) aberrant prostaglandin production by the kidney, (5) aberrant prostaglandin production by the vascular smooth muscle (VSM), and (6) aberrant sensitivities of the kidney and vasculature to circulating or locally produced prostaglandins, to explain the ability of prostanoids to act as a mediator of the increased arterial pressure of hypertension.

Until the discovery of the rapid clearance of prostaglandins by the lung, the role of circulating prostaglandins in the pathogenesis of hypertension was an interesting aspect for study. This concept has given way to the idea that local production or degradation of prostanoids may be an important site of derangement of the prostanoid system in hypertension, because both the vascular smooth muscle and kidney, two essential organs in the pathogenesis of hypertension, synthesize and degrade their own prostaglandins. With the exciting discovery of the prostacyclin and thromboxane components of the prostaglandin-leucotriene tetrad, the possibility existed that deficiencies in the production of prostacyclin (PGI_2) by the vasculature may play an important part in the pathogenesis of hypertension. With the findings that prostacyclin production is increased in the established phase of hypertension and that the small vessels may produce PGE_2 whereas the larger vessels may synthesize primarily PGI_2, the possibility that PGI_2 may play a major role in the pathogenesis of hypertension appears unlikely. This chapter reviews the current thoughts on the role of renal and vascular prostaglandins as potential modulators and mediators of human and experimental hypertension. Current hypotheses will be examined and new suggestions put forward on the potential mechanisms by which these compounds may play a role in the pathogenesis and maintenance of hypertensive vascular disease.

PROSTAGLANDIN SYNTHESIS, METABOLISM, AND STORAGE

The prostaglandins are carbon 20-22 hydroxylated fatty acids derived from their precursor fatty acids, archidonic dihomo-γ-linoleic, and linolenic acids. Of these precursors, the bisenoic fatty prostaglandins appear to be the major components of phospholipids in the cell membrane, and as such, serve as the predominant source of fatty acids from which the prostanoids are derived (2-6). The trienoic acid pathway, discovered by Needleman et al. (7), utilizes eicosapentanoic acid as a substrate for the prostaglandin synthetase, whereas the monoenoic acid pathway utilizes primarily dihomo-γ-linoleic acid (Fig. 1). There is little evidence to support a major role for prostaglandins of the monoenoic class in the kidney or vasculature of humans, although PGE_1 is considered to be a major metabolite of prostaglandin metabolism in animals and humans. The trienoic acid pathway in experimental animals and humans is relatively new. Eskimos appear to synthesize mainly thromboxane A_3 and PGI_3, the former compound losing its potency to stimulate aggregation of platelets, while PGI_3 retains its vasodilator activity (8). The significance of the trienoic acid pathway in experimental animals and humans remains to be elucidated. The major prostanoid pathway in humans therefore appears to be the bisenoic acid pathway system and thus this chapter concentrates on this system in the heart, vasculature, and kidney. The monoenoic and trienoic systems have been reviewed briefly by Lefer (8) and the interested reader is referred to this article for further details.

SYNTHESIS AND RELEASE

The bisenoic prostaglandins are derived from the arachidonic acid bound in the cell membrane with phospholipids, as a result of the activation of phospholipase A_2, with a small amount of prostanoids derived from triglycerides, as a result of the action of lipases on these fatty acid esters. The arachidonic acid cleaved from the phospholipid or triglyceride is then acted on by the enzyme designated as prostaglandin cyclooxygenase, an oxygen-dependent enzyme system located presumably within the microsomal fraction of the homogenized cell, suggesting that it is linked to the cell membrane. The resultant product formed, prostaglandin endoperoxide PGG_2, appears to undergo further lipid peroxidation to the pivotal, endoperoxide intermediary compound PGH_2, from which the three major classes of prostanoids (prostaglandins, thromboxanes, and prostacyclin) are derived. Thus PGH_2 appears to be the most important compound in the overall biologic regulation of the prostanoid system. PGH_2 can act as a substrate for prostacyclin synthetase, the enzyme that results in the formation of PGI_2, with the resultant formation of this potent vasodilator and antiaggregatory agent. Prostacyclin is produced primarily within the blood vessel, both within the vascular endothelium and the smooth muscle cells. Prostacyclin then undergoes both spontaneous and enzymatic degradation to 6-keto-$PGF_{1\alpha}$ and 9, 15-dihydroprostaglandin E_2, inactivate metabolites of PGI_2, respectively. There is some evidence that 6-keto-$PGF_{1\alpha}$, which is biologically inactive, may be transformed by the liver into a potent, long-acting vasodilator compound, 6-keto-PGE_2. The significance of this finding remains to be elucidated (9-12).

PGH_2 can also be utilized by the enzyme thromboxane synthetase to form the potent vasoconstrictor and aggregatory agent thromboxane A_2 (TxA_2). TxA_2 is produced primarily by the platelets, with some recent evidence supporting a role for local production of TxA_2 by the cerebral, pulmonary, and systemic VSM of pigs, dogs, rabbits, and rats. Thromboxane A_2 is degraded to the inactive metabolite TxB_2, which, however, still retains bronchiolar and vascular smooth muscle stimulating activity in vivo and in vitro. While tranylcypromine and analogs of prostacyclin can inactivate prostacyclin synthetase, imidazole, OKY-1555, N-2-hydroxybenzyl-clonidine, and some Upjohn Co. analogs of thromboxane and archidonic acid appear to be able to inhibit the synthesis of thromboxanes. Recent evidence suggests that high concentrations of the antihypertensive vasodilator hydralazine may act to produce vasodilation by inhibiting the formation of thromboxane within the platelets (13-21). The primary bisenoic prostaglandins (PGA_2, PGB_2, PGC_2, PGD_2, PGE_2, and $PGF_{2\alpha}$) are also formed from PGH_2 by the enzyme prostaglandin synthetase, which is ubiquitously distributed throughout most organs and tissues of the body (22). These prostaglandins are subsequently metabolized within the organs of their production or within the lung, by a wide variety of enzyme systems, and the subsequently more polar, inactive prostanoids are excreted by the kidney (23). In addition, evidence exists to support the concept of an isomerase, present in kidney, blood vessel, and brain (24), which may allow for the conversions of prostaglandin E_2 to prostaglandin D_1. The interested reader is referred to some current reviews on prostaglandin metabolism for further information (22-27). The schema for the synthesis and degradation of prostaglandins are summarized in Figs. 1-3.

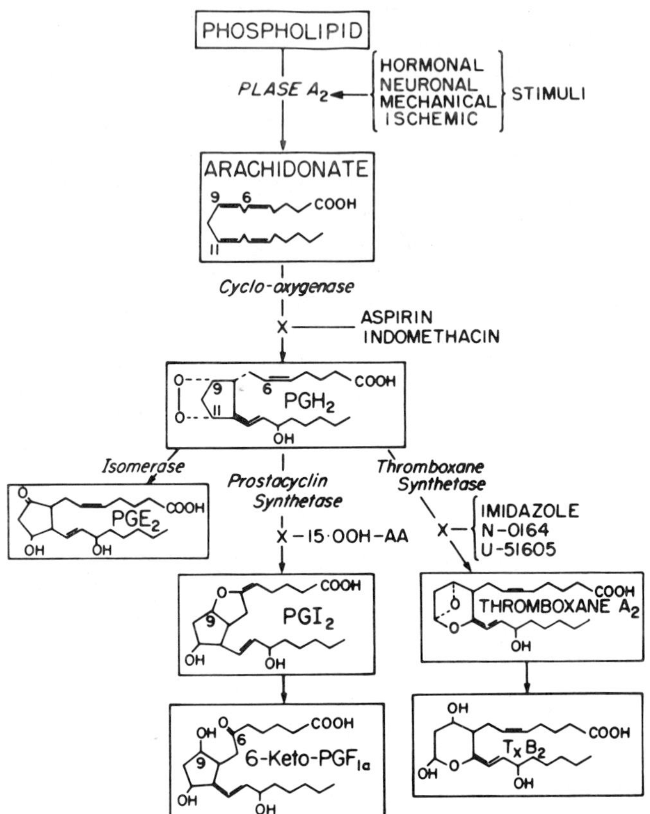

FIG. 1. Schema for prostaglandin biosynthesis. [Adapted from P. Needleman and W. R. Douglas, Biochemistry and Pharmacology of the Renal Prostaglandins. In Contemporary Issues in Nephrology, Vol. 4, B. M. Brenner and J. M. Stein (Eds.). Churchill Livingstone, New York, 1979.]

Inhibition of Prostaglandin Synthesis

The prostaglandin-synthesizing enzymes are believed to be microsomal or membrane-bound enzymes within the endoplasmic reticulum of the cell (22), whereas the enzymes involved in prostaglandin degradation are believed to be located in the cytosol (22). Once the prostanoid compound is formed, current evidence suggests that it is released to a limited extent, whereas most of the prostanoid is metabolized within the cell where it was synthesized. The lung appears to metabolize most of the circulating prostanoids (24). Since the prostaglandins do not seem to be stored within the organ of synthesis,

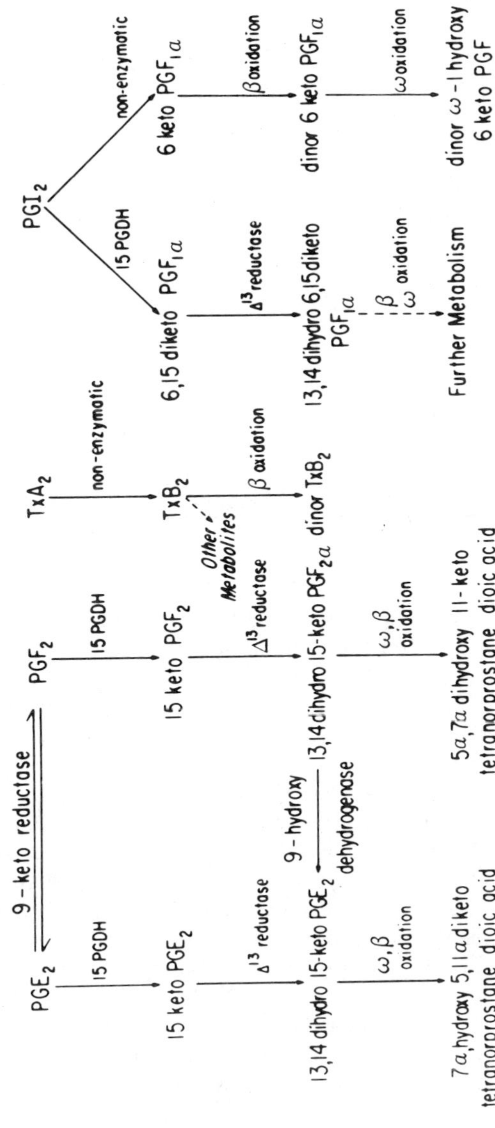

FIG. 2. Schema for prostaglandin degradation. [Adapted from P. Needleman and W. R. Douglas, Biochemistry and Pharmacology of the Renal Prostaglandins. In Contemporary Issues in Nephrology, Vol. 4, B. M. Brenner and J. M. Stein (Eds.). Churchill Livingstone, New York, 1979.]

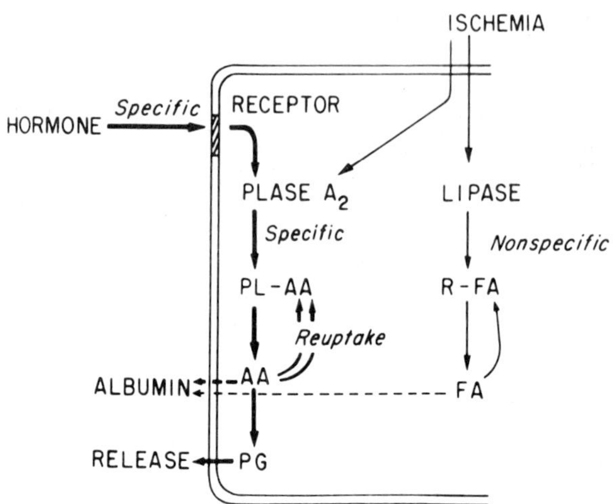

FIG. 3. Schema for prostaglandin activation. [Adapted from P. Needleman and W. R. Douglas, Biochemistry and Pharmacology of the Renal Prostaglandins. In Contemporary Issues in Nephrology, Vol. 4, B. M. Brenner and J. M. Stein (Eds.). Churchill Livingstone, New York, 1979.]

local changes in the synthesis and release of prostanoids will play more of a role in pathophysiologic effects of prostanoids than will defects in storage. More likely is the prospect that prostaglandins will play a local modulatory role at their site of synthesis and release than as circulating hormones. The one exception to this would be the thromboxanes. Since they are synthesized primarily in platelets, which enjoy the full extent of the cardiovascular system, aberrant mechanisms in platelet thromboxane synthesis can affect the entire cardiovascular system and the organs which the vasculature supplies. Since the prostaglandins are not stored within the cell (24-27), inhibition of the synthesis of the individual members of the prostanoid-leucotriene tetrad allows for the study of the role of individual members of the system in the pathogenesis and maintenance of hypertensive vascular disease. Figure 1 summarizes the common inhibitors of the prostanoid tetrad and their postulated sites of action.

As stated above, one can evaluate the role of the individual members of the prostanoid tetrad by selectively inhibiting the synthesis of prostacyclin, thromboxane, prostaglandins, or leucotrienes. With the exception of ibuprofen and eicosatetraynoic acid (ETA), which can inhibit the leucotriene system, most inhibitors of prostaglandin cyclooxygenase do not inhibit the formation of the lipoxygenase pathway, recently discovered by Samuelsson et al. (26). This pathway is believed to be involved in the production of slow-reacting substance of anaphylaxis (SRS-A) and other lipid peroxide compounds which may be important in the pathophysiology of myocardial infarction, pulmonary edema, and atherosclerosis (26). These are beyond the scope of this discussion. Nevertheless, the reader should bear in mind that these lipid peroxides may potentially play a role in hypertensive vascular disease, as well. The use of inhibitors other than ETA and ibuprofen leave this system intact, when the prostaglandins, thromboxanes, and prostacyclin may no longer be generated due to inhibition of prostaglandin cyclooxygenase. Moreover, with a reduction in the entry of arachidonic acid into the prostanoid triad pathway, the fatty acid may be shifted into the leucotriene pathway, with a resultant increase in the formation of these lipid peroxide compounds. Moreover, each of the "selective" inhibitors of prostaglandin-synthesizing enzymes have been found to inhibit a wide variety of non-prostanoid-related enzymes. Therefore, with the exception of some of the newer prostaglandin-analog-type inhibitors, the ability of prostaglandin synthetase, prostacyclin synthetase, or thromboxane synthetase inhibitors to modify the hypertensive process is not evidence per se that prostanoids are involved in the pathogenesis or maintenance of hypertension (9,10). Furthermore, inhibitors of prostaglandin-synthesizing enzymes such as indomethacin and meclofenamate may directly affect vascular smooth muscle function and structure by directly, through prostanoid independent mechanisms, altering vascular smooth muscle calcium metabolism, intracellular pH, or the enzymes involved in agonist activation or inactivation (for references, see Ref. 27). Therefore, in the study of the role of prostanoids in the pathogenesis of hypertension, it cannot be overemphasized that the data obtained from studies with inhibitors should be considered as suggestive, but not conclusive evidence of prostanoid participation in this disease process.

HEMODYNAMICS OF EXPERIMENTAL AND HUMAN HYPERTENSION

Hypertension, or the symptom of elevated blood pressure, is characterized by three distinct phases, as summarized in Table 1. In phase I, designated as the prehypertensive or labile hypertensive stage, the increase in arterial pressure is associated with an increase in cardiac output and a normal or decreased total peripheral resistance. Thus the increased flow appears to maintain the increased arterial pressure. In phase II, or established hypertension, the increased arterial pressure appears to be characterized by a normal cardiac output with an elevated total peripheral resistance, suggesting that vasoconstriction, rather than increased flow, maintains the elevated arterial pressure of this stage of the hypertension. In phase III, or accelerated hypertension, the increased arterial pressure is maintained by a grossly increased total peripheral resistance, or vasoconstriction. The cardiac output appears to be diminished as a result of the deleterious effects of the increased after load (arterial resistance) on the myocardium. The finding of

TABLE 1 Hemodynamics of Hypertension

Type of hypertension	B.P.	C.O.	TPR
Prehypertensive	↑	↑	NC, ↓
Established	↑	NC	↑
Accelerated	↑	↓	↑

[a]Blood pressure (B.P.) = cardiac output (C.O.) × total peripheral resistance (TPR).

an increased cardiac output in the early stages of hypertension has resulted in new insights into the pathogenesis of this disease process (for references, see Refs. 28-33).

Cardiac Output in Hypertension

Cardiac output is determined by the heart rate, stroke volume, intrinsic myocardial factors, and venous return to the heart. Venous return is modulated by the blood volume and vascular capacity of, primarily, the venous system. Intrinsic myocardial factors, heart rate, and myocardial derangements may not contribute to the increased cardiac output of hypertension. Studies measuring total blood volume and plasma volume demonstrate that, in spontaneous and renal hypertension, changes in these parameters cannot account for the increased cardiac output of associated with the hypertensive state (32-45). In fact, it has been shown that a decreased venous compliance secondary to venoconstriction, structural changes, or both factors may account for the increased cardiac output that precedes the increased arterial resistance of various forms of hypertension (46-58).

Relationship of Cardiac Output to Elevated Pressure. The increased cardiac output of most forms of hypertension appears to precede the increased total peripheral resistance, and returns to normal values as the arterial pressure and total peripheral resistance begins to rise. These findings are similar to the transient increased cardiac output of labile, juvenile hypertension and confirm the supposition that elevated cardiac output occurs early in the genesis of hypertension. However, the importance of the increased cardiac output remains undefined (59-65).

Myogenic Response of Bayliss. Passive stretch applied to a blood vessel causes an increase in VSM tone and subsequent contraction of the blood vessel (66). This phenomenon, described as the myogenic response of Bayliss, may be related to the oxygen requirements of the blood vessel, so that a vascular bed having normal oxygen requirements may, upon sensing the increased

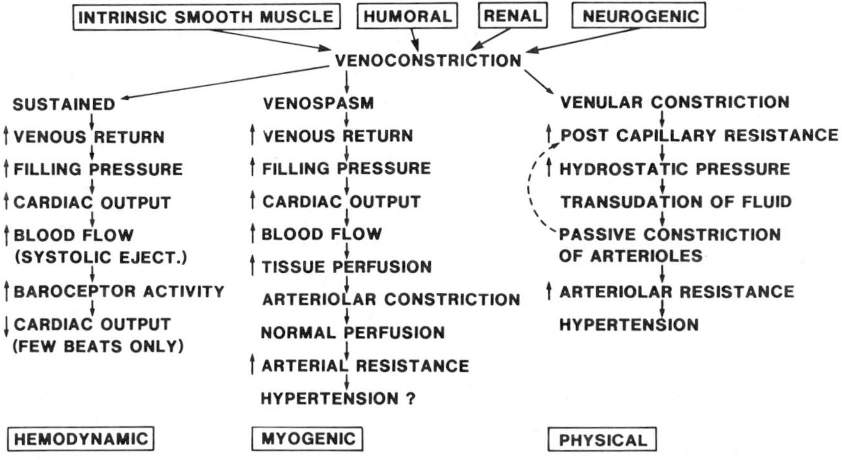

FIG. 4. Postulated role of the veins in the pathogenesis of hypertension.

oxygen delivery resulting from the increased blood flow, constrict and reduce blood flow and oxygen delivery to the levels required. Alternatively, the myogenic response of Bayliss may be related to the concentration of vasodilator and vasoconstrictor metabolites produced by the VSM cells or the surrounding tissues, in response to the increased pulse or tissue pressure. These metabolites may affect the active and passive properties of the blood vessels, resulting in constriction in response to the increased flow. Moreover, recent studies seem to suggest that local tissue or VSM production of prostanoids, in response to the membrane and cellular distortion produced by the increased pulatile flow, may play a modulatory role in the myogenic responses of renal, coronary, and skeletal muscle vasculature (67, 68). Although the exact nature of the myogenic response is as yet undefined, Guyton and coworkers have summarized the evidence which supports the concept that the increased arterial pressure of hypertension represents a whole-body autoregulatory response (or myogenic response) to the increased cardiac output of the labile hypertensive state (69-76). This concept is summarized in Fig. 4.

Theoretical and experimental support have been provided for the arguments that (1) changes in total peripheral resistance per se play little or no role in long-term regulation of arterial pressure, and (2) some change in fluid volume must occur, as a result of a change in renal function, for long-term hypertension to develop (69-76). The arguments are based on the hypothesis that the normal kidney will correct an abnormal fluid volume by excreting or retaining sodium and water until any imbalance is corrected and the hemodynamic abnormality controlled (see Fig. 5). In individuals or animals with impaired renal function, an increased blood volume would lead to an increased

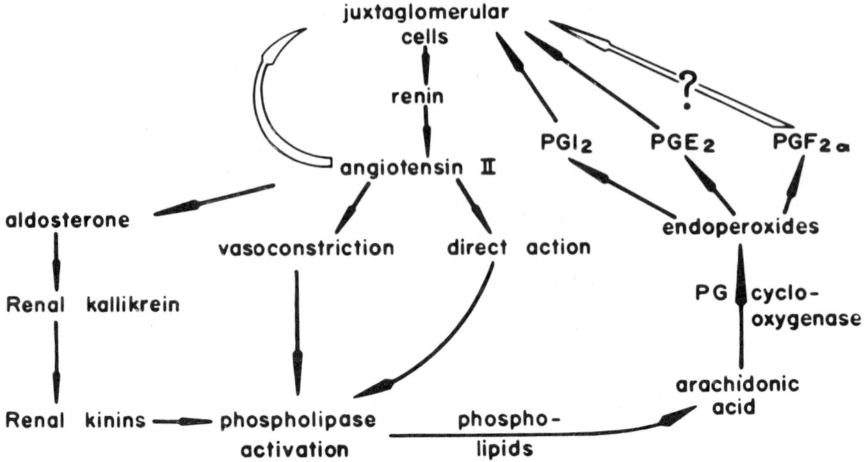

FIG. 5. Schema for the interaction of prostaglandins-renin-angiotensin-kinin systems in the regulation of blood pressure. (From Ref. 206.)

venous return and elevated cardiac output. Baroreceptor reflexes would initially maintain a normal arterial pressure, but this would eventually give way to the autoregulation of the peripheral circulation in response to the increased vascular perfusion. The increased total peripheral resistance and arterial pressure would increase the after load to the myocardium and thereby cause a return of cardiac output to normal values. The arteriolar constriction will cause water loss from the tissues so that the only residual change in the established hypertensive state would be the elevated total peripheral vascular resistance. Whole-body autoregulation occurs in animals deprived of their central nervous system (71). However, when baroceptor mechanisms are intact, withdrawal of sympathetic tone to the heart and vasculature prevents the increased arterial pressure in response to an increased cardiac output.

Although baroceptor mechanisms appear to be depressed in various models of hypertension, and the increased cardiac output of hypertension does not appear to be dependent on aberrant sympathetic or parasympathetic nervous activity to the myocardium, it is difficult to reconcile an increased cardiac output with hypertension unless factors other than baroceptor mechanisms are involved. Many patients with arteriovenous shunts and elevated cardiac outputs do not develop hypertension. Recent studies by Pfeffer et al. (59-61) demonstrate that chronic administration of β-adrenergic blocking agents to newborn spontaneously hypertensive rats prevents the increased cardiac output of this form of hypertension but does not prevent the sustained rise in arterial pressure or total peripheral resistance in the spontaneously hypertensive rat. It can be argued that a nonselective mixed β-adrenergic receptor antagonist, such as sotalol or propranolol, blocks peripheral vascular β-receptors which offset the decreased cardiac output with vasoconstriction. However, studies with a wide variety of β-blocking agents suggest that this is not the case. Moreover, recent studies demonstrated that occlusion of the vena cavae and reduction of the increased cardiac output of renal hypertensive animals failed to prevent the elevated arterial pressure and total peripheral resistance of the hypertension (43). Therefore, while the cardiac output of the hypertensive patient and animal may increase prior to the increased pressure and arterial resistance of the hypertension, it appears to reflect an increased venous return rather than being causal to the elevated intraarterial pressure. This would suggest that changes in venous smooth muscle structure and function may occur prior to, or simultaneously with, the changes that occur on the arterial side of the circulation in hypertensive vascular disease. The significance of this observation may reside in the possibilities that (1) changes in the vascular smooth muscle may precede, and be causal to, the increased arterial resistance of hypertension; and (2) since these changes may occur both in arteries and veins, circulating or locally produced factors may be responsible for the early vascular smooth muscle changes in hypertensive vascular disease (see below).

STRUCTURAL AND FUNCTIONAL CHANGES IN VASCULAR SMOOTH MUSCLE IN EXPERIMENTAL AND HUMAN HYPERTENSION

The pressor responses of intact animals and humans to vasoactive stimuli are enhanced in many forms of hypertension. This subject has been recently reviewed in detail (77-94). The factors that can influence the responses of the vasculature to vasoactive stimuli are summarized in Table 2. Vascular geometry, intrinsic properties of the VSM cell, and the effects of pressure are the three most important factors which influence the in vivo assessment of vascular function in hypertension, and are the subject of major controversy.

The increased responsiveness of vascular smooth muscle to many vasoactive agonists appears to be manifest as an enhancement of the concentration of agonist required to produce 50% of maximal activation of the blood vessel (ED_{50}+) to the agonist, independent of the actual magnitude of contraction. This is referred to as the reactivity of VSM. Alternatively, the ED_{50} for an agonist may not differ between the same blood vessel obtained from a normotensive or hypertensive animal, but rather the minimal concentration of agonist, just necessary to elicit a measurable biologic response, may differ. This is known as the threshold of activation. An enhanced reactivity or enhanced threshold to vasoactive stimuli may reflect alterations in the mechanisms regulating VSM excitation, excitation contraction coupling, or in the binding of the agonist with its receptor in or on the VSM cell membrane (93). These derangements could result from alterations in the abilities of divalent ions to stabilize the excitability of the VSM, to the presence or

TABLE 2 Factors That Influence Responses of the Vasculature to Neurogenic and Humoral Stimuli

1. Vascular geometry—medial hypertrophy; water-logging
2. Long-term effects of increased intravascular pressure
3. Circulating humoral factors: prostaglandins, steroids, renin
4. Intrinsic production of humoral factors within the vascular smooth muscle cell
5. Long-term effects of disturbed neurotransmission
6. Alterations in receptor-transduction mechanisms
7. Properties of elastic and collagenous elements in the vascular wall
8. Intrinsic malfunction in the vascular smooth muscle cell
9. Platelet or plasma cell growth factors
10. Production of factors within endothelium

absence of endogenously produced substances which are essential for maintenance of normal membrane perturbations following the interaction of the agonist with its receptor on the VSM cell membrane, the number and integrity of the receptors themselves, the composition of the proteolipids and mucopolysaccharides that make comprise the receptor complex, and/or as yet undefined defects in the VSM cell membrane (93).

The ability of a blood vessel to develop pressure or to contract in vitro and the magnitude of the resultant pressure or tension is the contractility of the muscle. Maximal pressure development appears to be increased in the intact and perfused vasculature of hypertensive humans and animals, respectively (95-101). However, when the geometric pattern of the blood vessel is interrupted and in vitro studies performed in the absence of geometric influences, contractility of the arterial vasculature appears actually to be depressed (96-104). Contractility of VSM is dependent on the energy supply available to support the contractile machinery; the subcellular organelles involved in the active sequestration and extrusion of activator calcium ion; the integrity, composition, and adenosinetriphosphatase (ATPase) activity of the contractile protein complex actomyosin; and the integrity and composition of the modulatory proteins troponin, tropomyosin, and calmodulin. In addition, the passive properties of the connective tissues such as elastin and collagen, as well as the compliance of the series elastic component (SEC) of the muscle and the parallel elastic component (PEC) of the muscle could indirectly influence the magnitude of vascular smooth muscle contraction. A stiffer or less compliant SEC may result in a greater amount of tension output, with the same degree of shortening of the muscle (93).

Another prime determinant of VSM contractility is the concentration of ionized calcium ion in the region of the contractile proteins. Depending on the source of activator calcium ion, i.e., extracellular versus tightly bound or intracellular calcium ion, alterations in membrane permeability to calcium ion or in the lability of the intracellular or tightly bound compartment of calcium ion could limit the quantity of calcium ion made available for contraction. Similarly, impaired mechanisms for calcium sequestration within the VSM cell, or calcium extrusion from the cell, could result in a higher intracellular concentration of free, ionized calcium ion to the contractile proteins. These defects in calcium metabolism could be influenced by altered levels of cyclic nucleotides resulting from changes in the levels of prostanoids within the VSM cell (89-94). However, this would appear unlikely, since recent studies demonstrate that the altered contractility of the VSM in hypertension cannot be normalized by altering the levels of calcium ion in the extracellular fluid, nor by acute treatment of hypertensive animals with inhibitors of prostaglandin synthesis (see "Potential Significance of Venous Changes and Role of Prostanoids").

ROLE OF ALTERED VASCULAR REACTIVITY IN HYPERTENSION

Current concepts regarding the role of enhanced vascular reactivity in experimental hypertension indicate that the early vascular changes in reactivity, and perhaps structure, may occur prior to, and independent of, the increased intraarterial pressure of hypertension. Support for this concept arises from the study of veins in hypertension, where it has been found that the venous smooth muscle is less compliant, hypertrophied, and exhibits enhanced contractility (105-117). Nevertheless, three major theories predominate to explain the role and significance of the enhanced vascular reactivity of hypertensive vascular disease.

Geometry Theory

Folkow and coworkers have presented evidence indicating that most, if not all, of the enhanced vascular reactivity and increased total peripheral resistance of the established phase of hypertension is caused by the increased arterial smooth muscle medial thickness (95-104, 106-108). In a hollow tube, such as a perfused or intact blood vessel, the arterial pressure is determined by the fourth power of the radius of the blood vessel. Hypertrophy of the arterial smooth muscle cells and increased thickness of the medial smooth muscle layer occurs in hypertensive vascular disease with an increase in the ratio of the wall thickness to lumen size. The law of Laplace would predict that a smaller amount of tension development would be required to produce shortening of the hypertrophied vasculature, consistent with an apparent enhanced reactivity and pressure development in response to a specific concentration of agonist (95). The concentration-response curves of renal and spontaneously hypertensive rats to norepinephrine differs from those of normotensive animals in the same manner as do calculated concentration effect curves of a mathematical model with normal wall thickness, in which it is assumed that the medial wall thickness was increased by approximately 30%, and the increase in wall thickness encroached on the lumen when the smooth muscle was completely relaxed to maximal dilation (95-99). Similar conclusions were derived by the studies of Conway (63,65), who observed that maximal dilation of the human forearm vasculature with acetylcholine results in a greater resistance in the forearm of hypertensive humans than in normotensive humans. These findings led to the suggestion that structural vascular changes may be responsible for the increased vascular resistance and enhanced vascular reactivity of the established phase of hypertension. Tobian (102) suggested that the increased wall/lumen ratio and enhanced vascular reactivity may be due, in part, to the water-logging (increased sodium and water) of the vascular wall rather than solely due to hypertrophy. However, according to Folkow et al. (103), water-logging does not occur, at least in the rat, until late in the hypertensive process, although water-logging has recently been found in dog veins of perinephritic hypertensive dogs and renal hypertensive rats (49,53).

Pressure Influences and Vascular Reactivity

The increased vascular reactivity and altered ion and water permeability may occur prior to the increased arterial pressure and resistance of hypertension (77-93). However, the experiments of Hansen and Bohr (91) and Weiderheim (104) also showed that a reduction in pressure itself, similar to the reduction in pressure used in studies to protect the vasculature from the elevated pressure of the hypertension, was a sufficient stimulus to alter vascular reactivity in both normotensive and hypertensive animals. Therefore, as suggested by the investigators themselves (91,104), the intervention used to assess the influences of pressure on vascular reactivity in hypertension may have direct effects on the vascular parameters under investigation. This possibility has also been suggested by the studies of Bevan et al. (81,82) employing rings of rabbit ear and saphenous artery, and veins from the high- and low-pressure regions of rabbits with aortic coarctation hypertension. These investigators demonstrated that the increased intravascular pressure of this form of hypertension was associated with an increased tension development of the arteries and veins obtained from high-pressure sites above the coarctation. This was not observed in blood vessels obtained from the low-pressure sites below the coarctation. The increased tension development was directly correlated with the magnitude of the rise in arterial pressure. Thus intrinsic changes in vascular smooth muscle function may be masked or modified by the hypertension itself. This conclusion was supported and reinforced by the studies in dogs with renal (two-kidney, one-clip Goldblatt) hypertension (77,78).

These studies evaluated whether changes in arterial and venous smooth muscle contractility and extensibility preceded from the elevated arterial pressure and total peripheral resistance of two-kidney one-clip Goldblatt hypertension (2-KGH). The experiments measured the in situ characteristic of the perfused mesenteric vasculature of dogs days 1 and 32 postocclusion of the renal artery and compared the responses with those obtained in dogs with sham renal artery occlusion and prior to renal artery occlusion. Moreover, the experiments also measured the contractile and extensibility properties of rings of canine mesenteric, cutaneous, gracilis, and pulmonary arteries and veins (0.4-1.0 mm O.D.), prior to, and days 1 and 32 after 2-KGH produced by unilateral occlusion of the renal artery (URAC). The reactivity (ED_{50}) and tension development to norepinephrine (NE), angiotensin II (AII), potassium chloride (KCl), serotonin (5-HT), $9\alpha,11\alpha$-epoxymethanoprostaglandin H_2 (EMP), prostaglandin B_2 (PGB_2), and $CaCl_2$ were determined. Mean blood pressure (MAP) and peripheral resistance (TPR) were unchanged from pre-URAC values 24 hr post-URAC, but were significantly elevated 32 days post-URAC. The ED_{50} values for 5-HT, AII, EMP, and PGB_2 were decreased in each of the arteries and veins obtained from dogs with 2-KGH, within 24 hr post-URAC, and either became more pronounced (PGB_2, EMP, and 5-HT) or returned to pre-URAC values, by day 32 post-URAC. The ED_{50} values for NE, KCl, and $CaCl_2$ were unchanged from pre-URAC values. Maximal tension development of the arteries and veins to each of the agonists increased within 24 hr post-URAC, prior to an increase in MAP or TPR. Within 32 days post-URAC, maximal tension development of the veins obtained from 2-HGH was increased from pre-URAC values, whereas tension development by the arteries was decreased. Extensibility decreased in each of the arteries and veins obtained from dogs with 2-KGH, 24 hr post-URAC. The extensibility decreased further, by day 32 post-URAC, as the arterial resistance increased. These data support the postulate that altered venous and arterial smooth muscle contractility and extensibility precede the elevated MAP and TPR of 2-KGH in dogs. Moreover, since these changes occur in both artery and vein, they must reflect the action of circulating humoral or intrinsic vascular or neural substances. Finally, the decrease in arterial contractility suggests that the enhanced vascular responses in vivo and in situ may reflect the greater mechanical advantage of the hypertrophied blood vessel, and not an arterial vasculature with enhanced contractility or reactivity (77,78).

MECHANISM OF VSM DERANGEMENTS IN HYPERTENSION

As stated above, three major hypotheses can explain the changes in VSM structure and function in 2-KGH. The first hypothesis suggests the primary changes in hypertensive vascular disease occur in the small resistance vessels, which constrict and increase pressure and wall stress upstream. This initiates the functional and hypertrophic changes of the VSM. The intraluminal pressure downstream from the constriction would not be elevated, because of the constriction, thereby sparing vessels smaller than 100 μm

O.D. from the functional, structural, and hypertrophic sequellae of an elevated intravascular pressure. The increased reactivity of hypertension then results from the hypertrophic state of the vasculature (95-103).

A second major hypothesis suggests that changes in VSM reactivity and contractility precede, and may be causal to, the increased MAP and TPR of hypertension. This hypothesis is based on the findings that the arterial VSM responses to vasoactive agents are enhanced, in vivo and in situ in many forms of hypertension (77-94, 105, 106, 110-117). The decreased compliance, hypertrophy, and permeability changes of the arteries are believed to be secondary to the deleterious effects of an elevated intravascular pressure (106-108). However, cerebral and mesenteric arteries obtained from stroke-prone spontaneously hypertensive rats exhibit structural changes indicative of hypertrophy and a decreased compliance, prior to an increased systemic or cerebral pressure (109). Moreover, veins obtained from renal and spontaneously hypertensive rats undergo hypertrophy and are less extensible than veins obtained from normotensive rats, despite normal venous pressures (112, 114). These data suggest that the structural and functional derangements of VSM from hypertensive animals may occur prior to the elevated pressure of the disease. This postulate is supported by experiments which demonstrated that the increased vascular reactivity and permeability of the arterial smooth muscle occurred prior to, and early in the development of spontaneous and deoxycorticosterone acetate (Doca) hypertension (77-94). Moreover, arterial pressor responses to many agonists, in situ and in vivo, are enhanced within 2-7 days after the initiation of Doca, Grollman, and aortic coarctation hypertension (77-94). However, as stated previously, hypertrophy of VSM may occur prior to the increased pressure and resistance of hypertension and the altered vascular geometry may then result in exaggerated pressor responses to vasoactive agents (77). This possibility is supported by the studies presented herein and elsewhere (77, 78) and by studies showing decreased arterial VSM contractility at a time when in situ pressor responses were enhanced in renal hypertension. The postulate that the elevated pressure subsequently modifies the pressure independent changes of the arterial VSM is supported by the studies in rabbits with aortic coarctation hypertension (84), which show that a rise in MAP is associated with an increased contractility of rabbit arteries, whereas the arteries obtained from sites below the coarctation do not exhibit any change in contractility. Moreover, Hansen and Bohr (91) demonstrated that a reduction in pressure in vascular beds of hypertensive rats modifies the contractile and extensibility properties of arteries.

The third hypothesis supports the tenet that the vasculature is not the site of the primary defect(s) in hypertension, but that the vascular smooth muscle responds to circulating, humoral, or neural factor(s), the concentration of which are altered in hypertension. Studies of parabiosis of normotensive salt-resistant with salt-sensitive Dahl strain rats (118, 119) and renal hypertensive with normotensive rats (73, 119) demonstrated the transmission of blood pressure from the hypertensive to the normotensive animals. Moreover, studies with sera extracts from normotensive and hypertensive humans have demonstrated the existence of substances present in the sera from the hypertensives, which enhance the responses of the vasculature from normotensive animals to vasoactive agents (120-124). Similarly, injections of extracts of kidneys from hypertensive animals, when administered to normotensive animals, elevates blood pressure and vascular permeability to proteins (120,121). The effects are similar to those obtained with ligation of the carotid artery, aortic coarctation, and injections of phenylephrine or AII (120,121). Grollman and colleagues (120,124) demonstrated the existence of a pressor substance in the renal venous effluent of Grollman hypertensive dogs. This substance was a proteinlike material but differed from both renin and AII. Moreover, it affected vascular reactivity in normotensive dogs, similar to the effects of the extracts from hypertensive humans (123). Recently, Sen et al. (125) described the effects of a urinary protein, excreted from hypertensive humans, which both raised blood pressure and stimulated adrenal cortical hypertrophy in dogs. Moreover, Simon (126) showed that sera obtained from dogs with perinephritic hypertension increased the permeability of the smooth muscle cells from canine aorta, in culture, to electrolytes. This effect could not be explained by the presence of renin, creatinine, or catecholamines in the sera. These data all support the conclusion that circulating factors, other than renin, AII, and catecholamines, may modulate or initiate the functional and structural derangements of the vasculature in hypertension (127). Parabiosis of Wistar-Kyoto normotensive rats (WKYs) with age- and sex-matched spontaneously hypertensive rats (SHRs) results in the decreased extensibility and enhanced contractility of the portal veing of the WKYs (128). In view of these, and the aforementioned studies cited (see abovc), the following modified hypothesis on the role of altered VSM function in hypertension appears to be justified.

In various forms of hypertension, circulating factors or neural factors are released from or activated by the kidney. These substances act on the VSM to modify the receptors for some vasoactive substances, alter the contractile apparatus, and decrease vascular compliance. On the arterial side of the circulation arterial constriction begins to occur, then MAP increases and subsequently damages the contractile apparatus of the arteries. In the established form of hypertension the enhanced pressor responses are maintained by the altered geometry of the hypertrophied arteries rather than by a VSM with a greater contractile tension output. On the venous side of the circulation, the enhanced venous contractility and decreased extensibility may result in a decrease in venous capacity and a shift in blood volume from the peripheral to the cardiopulmonary circulation, thereby accounting for the increased cardiac output of this form of hypertension. Since venous and PA pressures do not increase, the changes in contractility, extensibility and structure may reflect the levels of the circulating humoral or trophic factors released from, or activated by, the kidney, and may serve as a monitor of the progression or the severity of the disease process.

VENOUS STRUCTURE AND FUNCTION IN HYPERTENSION

Changes in the Veins in Hypertension

Recent studies from this laboratory (77-79, 111-115, 127, 128) and by others (49-56, 81, 82, 110, 115-117, 129-141) demonstrated that venous smooth muscle contractility, extensibility, compliance, and structure differ between normotensive and hypertensive animals and humans. The decreased extensibility and the enhanced contractile response of the veins from animals with aortic coarctation hypertension, as well as the decreased venous compliance of humans with essential hypertension appear to be maintained, in part, by enhanced sympathetic tone to the veins and pressure-induced changes in the α-adrenergic receptor. However, a large component of the increased stiffness of the veins appears to result from structural changes, similar to those that occur on the arterial side of the circulation. The functional and structural changes in the veins appear to be dependent both on the form of hypertension and the species of animal since Doca hypertension in Long-Evans rats does not produce any change in venous smooth muscle reactivity or contractility, yet Doca hypertension in dogs alters the venous smooth muscle reactivity and compliance.

The SHR is used as a model for human essential hypertension. Contractility, extensibility, prostanoid synthesis, and the protein content of portal veins (PV), vena cavae, and pulmonary arteries (PA) were found to differ between the SHR and the WKY. Moreover, the veins and PA obtained from SHRs exhibited hypertrophy and the functional and structural changes of the veins obtained from SHRs could be found in the veins of age- and sex-matched WKYs parabiosed to SHRs. These findings implied that a circulating or trophic factor may be responsible for the changes in venous smooth muscle structure and function in SHRs. Alternatively, these findings could have reflected the action of substances present in the SHRs, which is unique to this form of hypertension. Thus other studies were made to evaluate the existence of functional and biochemical changes in the veins and PA obtained from rats with two forms of renal hypertension and to compare these derangements with those found in the veins and PA obtained from the SHRs. The data supported the conclusion that alterations in venous smooth muscle structure and function are not genetic derangements specific to the SHRs, but can be induced in the veins obtained from rats with one-kidney (1-KGH) and two-kidney (2-KGH) Goldblatt hypertension.

ABNORMALITIES IN PROTEIN SYNTHESIS IN HYPERTENSION

The results of many studies demonstrate that veins obtained from hypertensive animals weigh more than veins obtained from corresponding normotensive animals in many forms of experimental hypertension. The increase in weight is not accompanied by an increase in water or fat, but rather by an increase in cellular protein. Moreover, the concentration of DNA decreases, because the amount of DNA does not increase in proportion to the amount of protein. This supports the concept that the veins from hypertensive animals undergo hypertrophy, not hyperplasia. The hypertrophy does not result from water-logging because the content of water only increases in the veins obtained from animals with 1-KGH, which is insufficient to account for the increase in dry-defatted weight and protein in these blood vessels. The increase in cell weight cannot result from an elevated intravascular pressure, because the venous and right ventricular pressures are not increased and the fat contents of the veins and PA are not elevated when obtained from the hypertensive animals. Therefore, the increase in cell protein must reflect an increase in cell protein synthesis or a decrease in cell protein degradation. A previous study demonstrated that the rate of decline of radiolabeled leucine by the PV obtained from SHRs and WKYs was similar. The increased content of the precursors of cell protein and glycosaminoglycan, at a time period reflecting the incorporation of these substances into cell protein, rather than the uptake mechanism into the cell (79), supports the concept that cell protein synthesis is increased in the veins and PA obtained from hypertensive animals. The degree of increase in protein content of the blood vessels appears to be related both to the duration and severity of the hypertension. The mechanisms remains to be examined. However, some limited conclusions may be drawn based upon published findings in the literature.

The experiments of Crane (142) support the conclusion that glycosaminoglycan synthesis may be modulated by factors normally released by the kidney, which act on the blood vessel wall. A similar conclusion was made concerning the mechanism of compensatory renal hypertrophy to unilateral nephrectomy and volume loading. It has been suggested that a factor of renal origin may decrease the level of cyclic AMP within the renal and smooth muscle cells which leads to a subsequent derepression of an inhibitory effect of cyclic AMP on the processes controlling cell growth. The hypertrophic arterial smooth muscle exhibits an increase in membrane glycosaminoglycans as well as in cellular proteins. Veins obtained from hypertensive animals exhibit all the changes in cellular composition and cyclic AMP as do the artery and kidney undergoing hypertrophy (for references, see Refs. 143-179). Therefore, it is speculatively possible that the changes in venous and PA chemical composition reflect the actions of a circulating humoral factor which increases in hypertension and acts on the veins and arteries to initiate these derangements (143-179).

DISCREPANCIES IN LITERATURE

The studies of Bostrom and Fryklund (146), Altman and Simon (52), and Mulvany et al. (184) differ from each other and from the data cited above.

Altman and Simon (52) found that an increased hexosamine content was present in the veins obtained from renal hypertensive rats, but not from SHRs. They concluded that the increased hexosamine content reflected the increased synthesis of glycosaminoglycans by the veins from renal hypertensive rats, but that the increased hexosamine content could not explain the decreased extensibility of the veins. Moreover, veins from SHRs contained a lower protein content than did veins obtained from WKYs. They concluded that a shorter, but thicker, vein was responsible for the decreased venous compliance in SHRs. Their data are not mutually exclusive from the findings reported herein. For equal lengths of vein, the amount of protein of a thicker venous wall should be increased. Bostrom and Fryklund (146) reported that veins from SHRs had a lower protein content per gram of rat. This normalization procedure has dubious significance. Greenberg (79) reported that veins from SHRs and 1-KGHs contained a greater content of protein and DNA, and an increased concentration of protein and decreased concentration of DNA, than did veins from corresponding WKYs. Therefore, the data are also not mutually exclusive.

The study of Mulvany et al. (184) provides the most critical challenge to the concept that veins change in hypertension. The discrepancies between the studies may be more apparent than real. The study of Mulvany et al. (184) found no differences existed in the structure, extensibility, or function of PV obtained from 4-month-old SHRs and WKYs. The SHRs in their study weighed more than the WKYs and exhibited only slight changes in myocardial structure. This is different from any study with SHRs and age- and sex-matched WKYs (for references, see Ref. 79). Therefore, the use of proper strains of rat is questionable. Extensibility was measured with an initial length obtained at the optimal portion of the length-tension curve, and the stress-strain (SS) curve prepared with incremental strains from this inappropriate L_i. This procedure would normalize any differences in initial extensibility, with little resultant differences betweeen the veins from SHRs and WKYs. Structural studies were performed on contracted muscle preparations without the use of any vasodilator or relaxant to eliminate differences in the initial states of contraction. The studies of Greenberg et al. (112) were performed on muscles that were completely relaxed with nitroglycerin prior to fixation. Therefore, methodological and perhaps differences in the WKYs, SHRs, or both can explain the discrepancies between the Mulvany study and these findings.

Veins do not see the increased intravascular pressure of hypertension. Intrinsic changes in venous smooth muscle function and structure occur in hypertension prior to the rise in arterial pressure. Therefore, the following postulates may be made: (1) hypertrophy and altered VSM function may have both pressure-dependent (arteries) and pressure-independent (veins) components; (2) vascular changes may precede, and be causal to, the increased arterial pressure and resistance of hypertension; and (3) circulating or humoral factors may promote or initiate the vascular derangements in hypertension.

POTENTIAL SIGNIFICANCE OF VENOUS CHANGES AND ROLE OF PROSTANOIDS

Veins from spontaneously hypertensive rats are less sensitive to the vasodilator agonists isoproterenol, papaverine, and acetylcholine than are veins obtained from normotensive animals. Ramananthan and Shibata (92) concluded that the enhanced contractility of veins from hypertensive animals may be related to, or result from, the decreased ability of the veins to relax to vasodilators, and this decreased ability to relax may result from a deficit of cyclic AMP in the veins. Subsequently, these investigators showed that the veins obtained from SHR exhibited a decreased adenylate cyclase activity and an increased type II phosphodiesterase activity (92). The severity of the changes were linked to the hypertension since cross-breeding of hypertensive and normotensive rats resulted in a rat with intermediate pressures and levels of cyclic AMP and of the synthetic and degradative enzymes for cyclic AMP. Greenberg and Curro (see Ref. 79) confirmed the changes in cyclic nucleotides but could not relate them to the level of tension development or relaxation by the veins. Evidence was also presented that the decreased adenylate cyclase activity, as reflected by the levels of cyclic AMP, may be related to an enhanced release of prostaglandins by the venous smooth muscle. This finding was confirmed by the studies of Limas and Limas (190), who showed that prostaglandin synthetase activity was enhanced in the veins obtained from spontaneously hypertensive and renal hypertensive rats. However, no relationship among the prostanoids, cyclic nucleotides, and contractile tension development was elucidated (191-195). Greenberg et al. (111-114) speculated that enhanced contractility of the veins may reflect synthesis of an altered protein(s) within the venous smooth muscle, and this synthetic process may be altered by the levels of prostanoid and cyclic nucleotides within the VSM cells.

Speculatively, the mechanisms for hypertrophy may reflect altered levels of cyclic AMP within the cells of the arteries and veins (see above). The changes in cyclic nucleotide could result from an altered prostanoid system. PGI_2, PGE_2, and PGE_1 stimulate increases in cyclic AMP within VSM. Thromboxanes, PGD, PGB, and $PGF_{2\alpha}$ decrease arterial and venous as well as platelet cyclic AMP and stimulate cell growth (155, 159, 172, and references therein). A more rapidly growing cell has lower cyclic AMP levels than do more slowly growing cells. Stimulation of cell growth will decrease cyclic AMP and decreases in cyclic AMP will stimulate cell growth (155, 159). Veins from spontaneously hypertensive rats have a decreased cyclic AMP content and an increased synthesis of $PGF_{2\alpha}$ and thromboxane B_2 (TxB_2), with either no change or a decrease in PGI_2 (79, 191-195). This would be consistent with a sufficient stimulus for hypertrophy, which in and of itself, may alter VSM contractility. Although prostacyclin synthesis does increase in arterial smooth muscle in hypertension, the rise appears to be a compensatory response to the elevated intravascular pressure, in an apparent attempt to restore pressure to normal values or to try to limit the rise in pressure and thereby protect the vascular smooth muscle (191-195, 79).

The results cited earlier indicate support for the theory that circulating humoral or trophic factors may be responsible for the increased arterial resistance of hypertension, through their effects on the vascular smooth muscle. The putative humoral factors purported responsible for the increased ion permeability, vascular reactivity, decreased extensibility, and altered VSM structure may or may not be prostanoids released from the VSM and/or kidney or platelets (see the section "Platelets, Prostaglandins, and Hypertension"). However, the independence of these changes from that of pressure suggests that if prostanoids do play a role in the vascular changes of hypertension, they are not initially responding to a pressure-mediated stimulus, but may also respond to other circulating factors. The potential sites and significance of these changes are the subject of the next portion of this chapter.

RENAL PROSTAGLANDINS AND HYPERTENSION

Extensive interest exists in the potential role of renal prostaglandins as mediators or modulators of essential hypertension. The actions of the renal prostaglandins include (1) release of renin within the cortical nephrons by prostacyclin; (2) a natriuetic effect of prostaglandins E_2 and PGI_2; (3) intrarenal vasodilation by prostaglandins D, E, and I_2; (4) vasoconstrictor effects of TxA_2; (5) prostaglandin I_2- and E_2-mediated modulation of sympathetic nerve activity to the vasculature and juxtaglomerular cells within the kidney; and (6) prostanoid-induced alterations in the responses of the kidney and vasculature to bradykinin and angiotensin II (191-210). The actions of these prostanoids elaborated from the kidney would most likely be intrarenal in nature, since most of the prostanoids are rapidly cleared by the lung (211). Although Vane et al. (212, 213) suggest that PGI_2 may act as a circulating hormone, the fine and rapid control exerted by locally produced renal prostaglandins would tend to support the postulate that renal prostaglandins would tend to exert their action within the parenchyma and vasculature of the kidneys in hypertension.

As stated previously, the Guytonian-Ledingham-Borst concept of hypertension suggests that the inability of the kidney to excrete a given load of sodium and fluid may be associated with the increased arterial resistance of hypertension. If this concept is accepted, then the kidney, and thereby the intrarenal prostanoids, are assigned a primary role in hypertensive vascular disease. Since most intrarenal prostanoids are vasodepressor and natriuretic in nature (214, 215), it has been suggested that a deficiency in renal prostanoid production could account for the aberrant renal function of hypertension (214-243). Measurement of the release of renal prostaglandins from the kidneys, renal medulla and papilla, and renal vasculature of animals with various forms of experimental hypertension, and measurement of the urinary excretion of prostaglandin E and the metabolites of prostacyclin metabolism

(6-keto-$PGF_{1\alpha}$) from normotensive and hypertensive humans, demonstrated a decrease in the synthesis of both prostaglandin E and I_2 (220-245). Moreover, lower urinary excretions of immunologically reactive prostaglandin E were found in patients with low-renin hypertension (230) and in patients in which renin was artificially elevated by volume depletion with furosemide (230, 234). Thus the initial evidence supported the conclusion that deficiencies in vasodilator, intrarenal prostanoids may account for the altered sodium excretion, renin release, and intravascular pressure of hypertension (214-246; see "Prostaglandins and the Renin-Angiotensin-Aldosterone Axis").

This conclusion was challenged by the studies of Dunn (244, 245), who, utilizing the kidneys of the SHR, showed that renal prostaglandin E production within the medulla was consistently elevated compared with the rates of PGE synthesis by medullary tissue from WKYs. Armstrong et al. (220) and Pace-Asciak and colleagues (192, 193) reported that renal prostaglandin E production was diminished in the kidneys of New Zealand genetically hypertensive rats and SHRs, respectively. Therefore, Dunn (245) simultaneously measured the urinary excretion and renal venous concentrations of PGE_2 and $PGF_{2\alpha}$. He postulated that with an increase in PGE metabolism and a decrease in PGE catabolism an increased urinary synthesis of PGE should be found, since urinary PGE is believed to reflect intrarenal rather than circulating PGE (206). However, these investigators did not find any difference in the urinary excretion of PGE or metabolites or in the renal venous concentrations of PGE in the SHR and WKY. These results were difficult to understand since Limas and Limas (190), utilizing the same model of hypertension, found enhanced renal synthesis of PGE_2 in the SHR compared with renal prostanoid synthesis in the WKY control. The findings of Dunn (244, 245) are difficult to interpret in view of the increases in enzymatic synthesis of prostaglandin E and its decreased degradation (220). Recent studies also demonstrated that prostacyclin synthesis is increased in the kidneys obtained from SHRs. Because PGE and PGI_2 are vasodilator and natriuretic, it is difficult to attribute a prohypertensive action to these prostanoids. However, it is possible that the increase in the levels of these substances, if they do in fact increase, are secondary to the elevated intrarenal pressure, which could act as a stimulus for prostanoid synthesis and release. Recent studies by Pace-Asciak and colleagues (192, 193), Skidgel and Printz (194, 195), and Greenberg (18) demonstrated that PGI_2 synthesis increases in the vasculature of rats with spontaneous hypertension and dogs with 2-KGH in response to, and parallel with, the rise in arterial pressure. The veins did not show a rise in prostacyclin synthesis, but rather an increase in TxB_2 and $PGF_{2\alpha}$ was found. Therefore, as the hypertension progresses, the elevated intraarterial pressure may stimulate the synthesis and release of intraarterial and intrarenal PGI_2 and PGE as a compensatory mechanism in an attempt to protect the vasculature and kidney against the elevated intravascular and intrarenal pressure and to promote sodium and water excretion. This postulate is more complex than it seems.

Dunn (244, 245) examined the possibility that an increased synthesis of renal prostaglandins (PGE) would be associated with a redistribution of intrarenal blood flow from the medulla to the cortex, with a predominant increase in blood flood to the juxtaglomerular cells of the kidney, of the SHR. They measured the inner and outer cortical distribution of blood flow with the microsphere technique. They demonstrated that the fractional blood flow to the outer cortical areas of the kidney was increased in spontaneously hypertensive rats. Moreover, Dunn and Hood concluded that PGE synthesis was unimpaired in the medulla of these animals, but that prostacyclin synthesis may be enhanced in the glomeruli (214). Since glomerular blood flow and capillary pressure increase in the rat with spontaneous hypertension, it was possible that the increased glomerular synthesis of prostacyclin mediated these changes in renal hemodynamics. The report of Azar et al. (236-238) disagreed with these speculations. Azar et al. (236-238) found that glomerular blood flow was reduced, and both afferent and efferent arteriolar resistances were elevated in the kidneys obtained from 18-week-old SHRs. Similar results were obtained by Dibona and Rios (247). However, when they utilized single-nephron micropuncture techniques, they found only an elevated afferent arteriolar resistance without any change in efferent arteriolar resistance.

The discrepancies between the in vivo, in situ, and in vitro biochemical studies are difficult to interpret. It is possible that the age of the SHRs, the severity and duration of the hypertension, or even the hypertensive model and the techniques utilized for the measurements of the hemodynamic and biochemical parameters can explain the discrepancies in the results reported above. However, the almost consistent failure to demonstrate a decrease in intrarenal PGI_2 or PGE within the kidney of hypertensive animals does not allow for the conclusion that deficiency of intrarenal prostanoids plays a pathogenetic role in the genesis of hypertensive vascular disease.

The hypothesis of Lee et al. (248-250) suggests that a deficiency of PGA_2 in hypertensive patients may account for the increased arterial resistance of the disease. These authors present evidence to support the postulate that a decrease in PGA_2 within the kidney results in a shift of blood from salt-losing to salt-retaining nephrons, with a resultant decrease in sodium excretion and accumulation of sodium and fluid within the vascular tree. In addition, they postulated that a decrease in circulating levels of PGA_2, which is poorly metabolized by the lung, added to the increased arterial resistance and elevation of arterial pressure. The difficulty with this hypothesis is that the synthesis of prostaglandin A_2 in the kidney, in sufficient concentrations to modulate renal function or VSM tone, has been questioned or refuted. The possibility that PGE_2 may serve the function of PGA_2 is also in doubt because of the studies of Dunn (244, 245), Azar et al. (236-238), and those studies cited above. Thus the postulate that a deficiency in circulating prostanoids or intrarenal prostanoids may contribute to the elevated vascular resistance and pressure of hypertension is far from established.

EFFECT OF INHIBITORS OF PROSTANOID SYNTHESIS

Were the prostanoids to play a role in elevating the arterial pressure of hypertensive vascular disease by altering sodium excretion or directly modulating VSM tone, then inhibition of prostaglandin synthesis should reverse, to some degree, the severity of the hypertension. These studies have been performed and the results are inconclusive. Inhibition of the entire prostanoid cascade (i.e., prostaglandins, thromboxanes, and PGI_2) with indomethacin, meclofenamic acid, ibuprofen, and/or naproxen results in a mild to moderate elevation of pressure in both normotensive and hypertensive subjects. The magnitude of pressure rise depends on the route of inhibitor administration (intravenously versus orally), the presence or absence of anesthesia, the degree of vasoconstriction prior to administration of inhibitor, the levels of angiotensin AII and kinins, and the condition of the animal (intact or surgically modified), to name but a few factors. The finding that inhibition of prostaglandin synthesis results in an increased arterial pressure is consistent with the postulate that a decrease in the levels of intrarenal or vascular prostanoids may contribute to the elevations in arterial pressure in hypertension. Moreover, increases in vasodilator prostanoids, in response to the increased pressure, would also be consistent with a pathophysiologic compensatory mechanism attempting to reduce the magnitude of the rise in pressure. Intrarenal prostaglandins also modulate the responses of the end organ to norepinephrine (which releases renin from the juxtaglomerular cells of the kidney), AII, and bradykinin. In vitro, in vivo, and in situ, inhibitors of prostanoid synthesis enhance the vascular and renal actions of AII and inhibit the vascular and renal responses to bradykinin. AII and bradykinin stimulate the synthesis and release of prostaglandins within the VSM and the kidney. Tachyphylaxis of VSM to AII and bradykinin may be mediated by the prostanoids generated locally by these two peptide-stimulant substances. The prostanoid compounds formed appear to oppose the vasoconstrictor action of AII and mediate the vasodilator and venoconstrictor action of bradykinin. Inhibitors of prostanoid synthesis enhance the magnitude and duration of the pressor and contractile responses to AII and abolish the vasodilator and venoconstrictor responses to bradykinin. An increase in the intrarenal or intravascular synthesis of prostanoids in hypertension could inhibit the intrarenal actions of AII and enhance the salt-losing and vasodilating effects of bradykinin. A deficit of intrarenal or VSM prostanoids could have the opposite effect (Fig. 6). However, this conclusion too must be challenged (251-282).

Anesthetized animals demonstrate an increase in arterial pressure after the administration of the inhibitors of prostaglandin synthesis. Similarly, the responses of perfused preparations in situ to vasoactive agents are enhanced, as is perfusion pressure, after inhibition of prostaglandin synthetase. However, when conscious, undisturbed, or nontraumatized anesthetized animals are utilized for study, inhibition of prostaglandin synthesis does not affect renal blood flow, arterial pressure, or any major

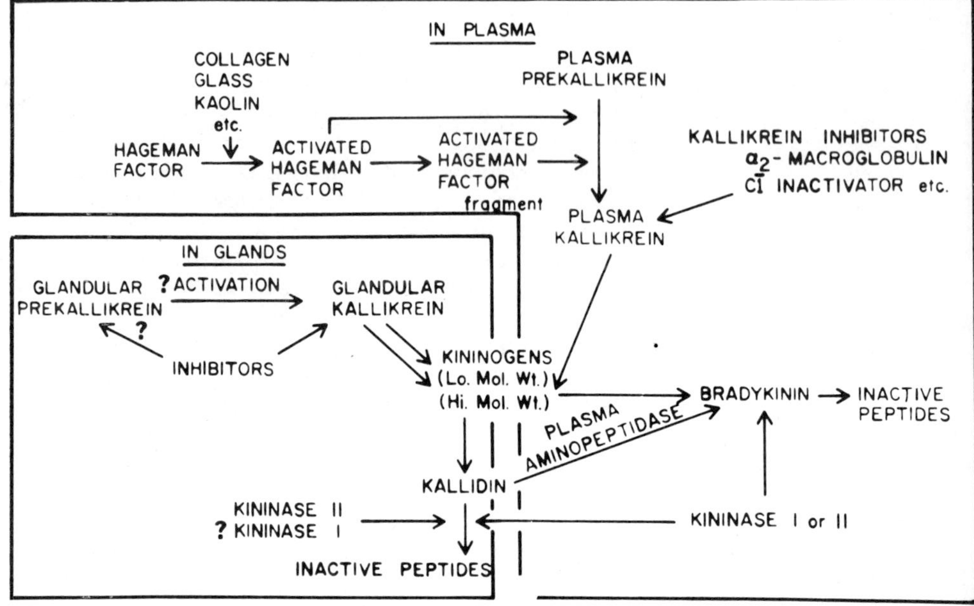

FIG. 6. The renal kallekrein-kinin system. (Modified from Ref. 301.)

hemodynamic parameter (282). These findings suggest that manipulation of the experimental animal may activate, artificially, phospholipase A_2 activity, with a subsequent aberrant rate of synthesis of prostaglandins. Upon inhibition of prostaglandin synthesis, an anomalous increase in pressure and resistance may occur. Zimmerman et al. (283,284) demonstrated that indomethacin and meclofenamate increased renal vascular resistance in an acutely instrumented dog kidney, while the resistance of the contralateral kidney, instrumented a few weeks prior to the experiment, was essentially unchanged. In chronically instrumented dogs, indomethacin reduces renal prostaglandin synthesis by 75% without any effects on renal vascular resistance. Therefore, the possibility that intrarenal prostaglandins mediate the vascular resistance changes in hypertension must still be critically examined (283-295).

PROSTAGLANDINS AND THE RENIN-ANGIOTENSIN-ALDOSTERONE AXIS

Angiotensin II stimulates the synthesis of prostaglandins E and I within the kidney and VSM by two major mechanisms. AII-induced stimulation of prostanoid synthesis may be due to vasoconstriction, local ischemia, and activation of phospholipase A_2 activity as a result of the perturbational changes produced in the cell membrane. AII may also directly stimulate the deacylation of phospholipids, thereby providing an increased source or substrate, arachidonic acid, to the cyclooxygenase within the kidney cell membranes. Thus in renal hypertension or in conditions where elevated renin levels result in the increased generation of AII, an increase in intrarenal prostaglandins may represent a compensatory increase to both the vasoconstrictor effects of the AII and the direct actions of AII on phospholipids.

In contrast to the expected inhibitory feedback loop between the prostanoids-renin-AII and aldosterone, inhibition of prostaglandin synthesis in normotensive and hypertensive animals and humans results in a decrease in the peripheral venous renin activity. Similarly, infusions of PGE_2 and PGI_2 into the kidneys of experimental animals results in elevations in the peripheral plasma renin activity. This is not due to the vasodilator effects of the prostanoids, resulting in reflex increases in renin release because prostaglandin D_2, an intrarenal vasodilator, does not promote renal renin release. The effects of PGE and prostacyclin on renal renin release appear to result from direct action of these prostanoids on the juxtaglomerular apparatus within the kidneys (the site of renin production). The effects of PGE and prostacyclin appear to occur despite inhibition of sympathetic nervous activity to the vasculature with propranolol as well as after inhibition of endogenous prostanoid synthesis with indomethacin. Thus in high-renin hypertension, elevated renin may occur as a result of the actions of elevated levels of PGE_2 or PGI_2. The prostanoids may be stimulated by the elevated levels of arterial pressure as well as by the elevated levels of AII, in a positive feedback cycle. However, this remains speculative at the present time. A question that must be asked, however, is the following: If elevated levels of AII stimulate prostanoids, which subsequently increase the synthesis or release of renin from juxtaglomerular cells, thereby accounting for the high-renin hypertension, should intrarenal prostanoid levels be decreased in low-renin hypertension? Similarly, can the differences in sodium and fluid excretion in low- and high-renin hypertension be explained by the natriuretic effects of the intrarenal prostanoids? In addition, are the increases in intrarenal prostanoids a deleterious mechanism, in as much as they increase renin, or do the prostanoids increase as a compensatory mechanism to aid in sodium and volume excretion, thereby attempting to reduce pressure in a compensatory manner?

To further complicate matters, recent studies seem to suggest that prostaglandins of the E series and prostacyclin may inhibit the conversion of angiotensinogen to angiotensin I, a renin-dependent action. This would tend to limit the formation of AII, and thereby act to decrease the magnitude of AII-induced constriction as well as angiotensin-induced stimulation of prostanoid synthesis. Moreover, prostacyclin and PGE_2 seem to oppose and limit the magnitude of AII-induced vasoconstriction and may be responsible for the lack of sustained vasoconstriction by maintained concentrations of AII (fade) as well as for the tachyphylaxis to AII. Therefore, the relationship among intrarenal prostanoids, angiotensin, and renin is difficult to unravel at the present time. Nevertheless, the data do suggest that the renin-angiotensin-aldosterone axis has diametrically opposed actions to that of the primary intrarenal prostanoids. The positive feedback loop between these two systems may aid in the regulation of blood pressure and electrolyte and fluid excretion. It is possible that a defect or imbalance between these two systems may result in sodium retention and an elevated blood pressure, despite an increase in the synthesis of the vasodilator prostanoids. The increase in prostanoids may be a compensatory attempt to correct the original imbalances, the origin of which may be far removed from the levels of the prostanoids themselves. This speculative postulate must await further investigation to validate or refute its potential significance (255-271, 274-281).

RENAL KALLEKREIN-KININ-PROSTAGLANDIN SYSTEM

In addition to vasoconstriction and stimulation of aldosterone and renal prostanoids, AII produces chronic changes in the renal kallekrein-kinin system, the products of which may also stimulate the synthesis of prostanoids within the kidney and vasculature.

Bradykinin, kallidin, and methionyl kallidin are biologically active, potent polypeptides found in plasma and tissues, which may also act as local hormones. These polypeptides are released from their precursor kininogens by the enzyme kallekrein, which occurs in high concentrations in various tissues, sweat glands, and the kidney. The urinary kallekreins arise mainly from the renal kallekrein-kinin system, originating within the kidney (Fig. 6).

The renal kallekrein-kinin system may play a role in various forms of experimental hypertension and in human hypertension. Excess mineralocorticoid activity or a sudden shift into positive sodium balance is believed to activate the renal kellekrein system, which then augments the urinary excretion of sodium and fluid. Aldosterone and other mineralocorticoids stimulate kellekrein production, whereas spironolactone, an aldosterone antagonist, reduces the excretion of urinary kallekrein. This system may also protect the kidney against the deleterious effects of an elevated intravascular pressure, or vasoconstriction by AII, since bradykinin is a potent renal vasodilator. In addition, the kallekreins also stimulate the synthesis and release of prostanoids from within the kidney by directly activating phospholipase A_2 activity and deacylating phospholipids to liberate arachidonic acid. Thus the kinins release prostanoids, which act to increase urinary excretion of sodium as well as producing vasodilation. Whether the actions of the kinins are mediated directly through the prostanoid system awaits further investigation (296-314).

ANTIHYPERTENSIVE NEUTRAL RENOMEDULLARY LIPID

Muirhead and coworkers (316, 317) examined the possibility that renal prostaglandins may play an important antihypertensive role by acting to reverse the increased arterial resistance of hypertension. These investigators attempted to reverse the hypertension of rabbits and rats with explants and products of the kidneys obtained from normotensive animals. Utilizing the techniques of transplanting normotensive kidneys into hypertensive animals as well as transplantation and implantation of renal medullary tissue obtained from normotensive animals into the hypertensives, Muirhead et al. (316, 317) demonstrated that cultures of renal medullary cells, and renal tissue itself, reduced the blood pressures of rabbits, dogs, and rats with various forms of hypertension. The antihypertensive activity resided in the medullary interstitial cells, was not reduced or inhibited after inhibition of prostaglandin synthesis, and did not appear to be a prostanoid-related compound. This compound was termed antihypertensive neutral renomedullary lipid (ANRL). Whether this substance is derived from the lipoxygenase pathway, which is not inhibited by the conventional inhibitors of prostaglandin synthesis, is as yet unknown. The role of this substance in the pathogenesis of hypertension must await further experimentation.

SUMMARY ON KIDNEY, PROSTANOIDS, AND HYPERTENSION

A mass of data exists supporting an in vitro and in situ modulatory role for prostanoids in the maintenance of renal function, blood pressure, and hypertension, as well as in regulation of VSM function and autoregulation and release of neurotransmitter to the VSM. However, studies in conscious animals seem to indicate that prostaglandins may not contribute to normal physiologic regulation of cardiovascular and renal function but may play a role in the pathophysiologic processes resulting in renal and vascular dysfunction. Thus it has been suggested that prostaglandin may function as both prohypertensive and antihypertensive substances during the development and maintenance of the hypertension. The principal role attributed to the prostanoids have been their ability to alter renal function, renin release, and blood flow distribution during the hypertensive process, and the possible role of prostaglandins E, A, I, and TxA_2 as natriuretic and vasoconstrictor hormones. This relegates the kidney to the backbone of the hypertensive process, as it appears to be in renal hypertension. However, the prostaglandins are ubiquitous substances. They affect aldosterone production, renin release, transmitter release, vascular reactivity, and other functions that modulate the hypertensive process. In hypertension of both renal and nonrenal origin, prostaglandin production by the blood vessels themselves, or circulating TxA_2 released by the platelets, may be more important in the regulation and modulation of total peripheral resistance and VSM function than the renal prostanoids. Thus it is possible that the renal prostaglandins may be essential for the modulation of renal dysfunction (renin and aldosterone, natriuresis, kaluresis), whereas vascular derangements result from the action of locally produced prostanoids by the VSM itself.

VSM, PROSTAGLANDINS, AND HYPERTENSION

Studies designed to evaluate VSM-prostaglandin interactions have provided some interesting information about the sensitivity of blood vessels to these fatty acids. Levy (318-322) demonstrated that the contractile responses of aortic strips obtained from spontaneously hypertensive rats to PGE_2 and $PGF_{2\alpha}$ were depressed, whereas the contractile responses to PGE_1 were enhanced compared with the responses of aortae from normotensive rats. Similar results were obtained by Altura and colleagues (323-325). Leach et al. (326) found that the vasodepressor responses of spontaneously hypertensive rats to prostaglandins A_2 and E_2 were enhanced in spontaneously hypertensive rats when compared with the vasodepressor responses of normotensive Wistar rats. Similar results were obtained by Simpson (327). Ellis and Hutchins (328), measuring mean arterial pressure, heart rate, and vascular diameter of the cremaster muscles of the spontaneously hypertensive rat, observed that the responses to $PGF_{2\alpha}$ were enhanced when compared with the responses obtained in Wistar-Kyoto controls. These findings all suggested that enhanced sensitivity to the vasodepressor and venopressor actions of prostanoids is characteristic of the spontaneously hypertensive rat. Recently, it was reported that the microcirculation of spontaneously hypertensive rats exhibited an enhanced sensitivity to prostacyclin at a time when the responses to arachidonic acid were depressed. These studies all suggest that the enhanced responses to prostaglandins in hypertensive animals may reflect a diminution of endogenous prostanoids at their receptor sites.

Inhibition of prostaglandin synthesis potentiates the vascular responses to exogenously administered prostaglandins (329, 330). Leary has shown that the kidneys of spontaneously hypertensive rats may synthesize up to 50% less prostaglandin E-like material than kidneys obtained from normotensive rats (270). However, the studies of Dunn and Azar (see "Renal Prostaglandins and Hypertension") cannot reproduce these findings. Moreover, the studies of Zusman and Keiser (265) demonstrate enhanced PGA and PGF_2, while those of Pace-Asciak et al. (192, 193), Skidgel and Printz (194, 195), and Greenberg (18, 79) all show an increase in PGI, $PGF_{2\alpha}$, PGE, and TxB_2, in the arterial and venous smooth muscle of spontaneously hypertensive rats and renal hypertensive dogs. Therefore, it is unlikely that a decreased endogenous synthesis of prostanoids can explain the enhanced responses of the vasculature to prostaglandins. Moreover, under conditions where local mechanisms for prostaglandin synthesis and metabolism are operant, rather than passage across the lung, arterial smooth muscle does not demonstrate an enhanced response to PGA, whereas veins contract to

PGA rather than relax (318,322,332). This would suggest that factors other than synthesis and metabolism of prostaglandins alter the response of the vasculature to exogenously administered prostaglandins. The recent studies of Altura et al. (323-325) and Greenberg et al. (333,334) suggest that the prostaglandin receptor may be a magnesium- and disulfide-dependent protein. Similar conclusions were obtained by Johnson et al. (see Ref. 332), who showed that the binding of prostaglandins E and F to uterine smooth muscle and red blood cell membranes was diminished by disulfide bond reduction with dithiothreiotol and dithiobisnotrobenzoic acid, disulfide bond-reducing agents. Magnesium ion is also essential for the binding of radiolabeled prostaglandins to the membranes of vascular smooth muscle. Magnesium ion is altered in the vascular smooth muscle obtained from SHRs (79). Moreover, measurement of membrane disulfide groups in the venous and arterial smooth muscle obtained from these rats is increased as well (79). It is possible that these changes can account for the altered sensitivity of the veins and arteries obtained from hypertensive animals to exogenously administered prostaglandins. Further studies must await verification or refutation of these postulates.

Prostacyclin (PGI_2) is a potent arterial vasodilator and inhibitor of platelet aggregation (see Chap. 10). PGI_2 is produced predominantly by the vascular endothelium, with some production occurring in the vascular smooth muscle. TxB_2, produced by platelets and VSM, is a potent constrictor of VSM as well as a humoral mediator of platelet aggregation (1,9-12,17). Recent studies demonstrated that platelet aggregability was enhanced in SHRs (185), despite the fact that aortic smooth muscle synthesis of PGI_2 is increased in spontaneous and renal hypertension (192-195). The increase in PGI_2 synthesis appeared to be specific for the arteries, since an increase in venous smooth muscle synthesis of PGI_2 or its metabolite 6-keto-$PGF_{1\alpha}$ could not be detected. Since the increase in arterial smooth muscle PGI_2 synthesis paralleled the increase in arterial pressure, it was suggested that the increase in PGI_2 synthesis resulted from, and to compensate for, the increased intravascular pressure of hypertension (191-195). The studies of Skidgel and Printz (194,195) also demonstrated that the veins obtained from hypertensive animals appear to synthesize more of a compound resembling $PGF_{2\alpha}$. Limas and Limas (190) also demonstrated that veins from SHRs and renal hypertensive rats, with established hypertension, appear to synthesize more of a prostaglandin E-like material compared with veins obtained from normotensive animals.

During the conduct of experiments evaluating vascular function in dogs with 2-KGH (18), it was observed that the mesenteric venous and arterial dilator responses to arachidonic acid (AA) were decreased during the early phase of the hypertension (unpublished observations). A decreased vasodilator response to AA could result from a decreased conversion to PGI_2 or other vasodilator prostanoids, or an increase in the conversion of AA to constrictor prostanoids such as TxB_2. In view of the results which demonstrate that platelet aggregability is enhanced in hypertension (185), despite the increased release of PGI_2 (192-195), the possibility existed that TxB_2 synthesis may also increase in hypertension (79).

A recent study (18) demonstrated that 2-KGH in dogs decreases in mesenteric vascular synthesis of PGI_2 and increases in mesenteric venous and platelet synthesis of TxB_2 precede the increased MAP and TPR of the hypertension. The changes in vascular responsiveness to AA cannot be accounted for by a decrease in the sensitivity of the vascular smooth muscle to the end products of AA metabolism, but rather reflect a decreased conversion of AA to PGI_2. As the hypertension progresses, arterial smooth muscle synthesis of PGI_2 increases, probably in response to, and to compensate for, the increased intravascular pressure. In addition, the increased venous pressure appears to be maintained by TxB_2 because inhibition of TxB_2 synthesis with imidazole restores mesenteric venous pressure, day 32 post-URAC, to pre-URAC values. These data support the concept that changes in mesenteric vascular and platelet prostanoid synthesis occur prior to, and may contribute to, the increased MAP and TPR of canine 2-KGH. In addition, altered platelet synthesis of TxB_2 may contribute to the altered platelet aggregability reported in hypertension. Finally, because the changes in prostanoid synthesis occur prior to any changes in pressure and resistance, they cannot reflect the effects of an elevated pressure but may result from the action of a circulating substance(s) released from the kidney as a result of URAC.

AA is the precursor for bisenoic prostaglandins, PGI_2, and TxA_2. PGI_2 is the major vasodilator metabolite formed by the vascular endothelium and smooth muscle, whereas TxA_2, a vasoconstrictor and potent stimulant of platelet aggregation, is produced by platelets, with some evidence for synthesis by vascular smooth muscle. The vascular responses to exogenously administered AA depend on the algebraic sum of the effects of all the prostanoid compounds released in response to the fatty acid.

The mesenteric arterial smooth muscle responses to AA are mediated by PGI_2 and, to a small extent, some prostaglandins, since the vasodilator responses are abolished after treatment of the dogs with tranylcypromine, an inhibitor of PGI_2 synthetase. The responses to AA are accompanied by an increase in the concentration of 6-keto-$PGF_{1\alpha}$ in mesenteric venous effluent, and concentrations of tranylcypromine and ibuprofen that abolish the responses to AA decrease or abolish AA-induced release of 6-keto-$PGF_{1\alpha}$. The venoconstrictor responses to AA are probably mediated by TxA_2 since they are accompanied by release of TxB_2, the metabolite of TxA_2, from platelet and smooth muscle and are abolished by imidazole, an inhibitor of thromboxane synthetase. It is difficult to determine, however, whether TxB_2 produced by the mesenteric veins or TxB_2 generated by platelets is responsible for the venoconstriction produced by the administration of AA day 32 post-URAC.

The venous and arterial smooth muscle responses to AA are depressed day 1 post-URAC, prior to an increase in arterial pressure. The decrease in response to this fatty acid may result from (1) the passive constriction of the blood vessels, overcoming the vasodilation, as a result of the enhanced intestinal response to AA; (2) a decreased sensitivity to the PGI_2 formed from AA; (3) an increased production of vasoconstrictor prostanoids by the platelets and vasculature; (4) a decreased production of PGI_2; or (5) any combination of these potential mechanisms.

Although these studies cannot definitively rule out the possibility that mesenteric compression, as a result of the enhanced intestinal response to AA, passively negates the vasodilator responses to this fatty acid, this possibility seems unlikely. The temporal responses of the veins and intestine to AA differ (77), in that the maximum response of the veins to AA occurs prior to the response of the intestine. In addition, a previous study has shown that contractile and relaxant responses to serotonin and other constrictor substances are not significantly affected by the response of the intestinal smooth muscle, under the present experimental conditions (77). It is also unlikely that a decreased responsiveness of the vasculature to the PGI_2, formed in response to AA, can account for the decreased responses to AA day 1 or 32 post-URAC, because the responses of the vasculature to PGI_2 are enhanced rather than inhibited at these time periods.

The decreased vascular responses to AA, day 1 post-URAC, are associated with a decreased release of 6-keto-$PGF_{1\alpha}$, both in situ and in vitro. Moreover, the decrease in response to AA and the decrease in the synthesis of 6-keto-$PGF_{1\alpha}$ occurs without an increase in venous or arterial pressure. These data support the conclusion that the synthesis of PGI_2 is initially decreased in the incipient stages of 2-KGH and that this cannot result from, or occur in response to, an elevated intravenous or intraarterial pressure. In addition, it is possible that a portion of the decrease in the responses to AA results from an increased release of thromboxanes or endoperoxides by the platelets. Endoperoxide intermediates are vasoconstrictor substances, as are thromboxanes. Platelet reactivity is enhanced in SHRs (185). Thromboxane B_2 levels are increased in the mesenteric venous effluent, day 1 post-URAC. Therefore, the data support the conclusion that the decreased vasodilator responses to AA may be mediated, in part, by vasoconstrictor prostanoids, released from the platelets. In view of the findings that neither arterial nor venous pressure increases day 1, post-URAC, the data are consistent with the postulate that the increased release of TxB_2 also cannot result from an elevated intravascular pressure. Speculatively, the changes in prostanoid synthesis in the early stages of 2-KGH, and in the veins, may result from the action of circulating humoral or neural trophic factors, released from the constricted kidney, on the vascular and platelet prostanoid system. Alternatively, the turbulent flow within the constricted kidney may modify platelet release of TxB_2, endoperoxides, and other substances which affect the vascular smooth muscle and endothelial synthesis of PGI_2.

This may relate to, or result from, the altered acylation and deacylation of the phospholipids, which has been reported in the spontaneously hypertensive rat (269,276).

The increased responsiveness to AA day 32 post-URAC probably reflects the increased synthesis of PGI_2 by the mesenteric arterial vasculature. These findings are in agreement with those of other investigators (192-195). However, since tranylcypromine did not abolish the responses to AA day 32 post-URAC, it is possible that substances other than PGI_2 may be increased in the vasculature of dogs with 2-KGH.

AA-induced venodilation is converted to venoconstriction by day 32 post-URAC, coincident with an increased synthesis of TxB_2 and a decreased synthesis of PGI_2 by the mesenteric veins and platelets. Since the venoconstrictor responses to AA day 32 post-URAC were enhanced after inhibition of PGI_2 synthesis with tranylcypromine, and inhibited after inhibition of TxB_2 synthesis with imidazole and ibuprofen, an inhibitor of the entire prostanoid cascade, the data support the conclusion that the venoconstrictor responses to AA were mediated by release of TxB_2. However, as stated previously, it is uncertain whether the in vivo venoconstriction, similar to the contractile responses of the mesenteric veins in vitro, were due solely to TxB_2 released by the vasculature or whether the platelets also contributed to the response of the veins to AA. Moreover, the venoconstrictor responses to AA may also reflect an enhanced sensitivity of the veins to TxB_2, superimposed on an enhanced production and release of this prostanoid by the veins and platelets. Mesenteric veins obtained from dogs with 2-KGH exhibit an enhanced contractile response to a thromboxane A_2 receptor stimulant when evaluated days 1 and 32 post-URAC. These possibilities probably all contribute to the venoconstrictor responses of the veins, and possibly the arteries (day 32 post-URAC) to AA.

Despite the fact that VSM synthesis of prostanoids is altered in hypertension, the experiments of many investigators cannot attribute a role of the altered prostanoids to the altered vascular reactivity to any agonist other than arachidonic acid. Moreover, except perhaps for the altered venomotor tone of hypertension, and this too is far from proven, a direct role of the altered prostanoids to the hemodynamic changes of hypertension is far from established. However, some insight into the role of prostaglandins in hypertension can be gleaned from the recent studies with antihypertensive agents.

ANTIHYPERTENSIVE DRUGS AND PROSTAGLANDINS

Thiazide diuretics are the first-line drugs of choice in the treatment of mild to moderate essential hypertension. This mechanism of action remains unknown. However, their antihypertensive action appears to be divorced from their diuretic activity (332). The effects of the diuretic are slow to occur and, while being due to a decrease in vascular tone, are not due to direct arterial vasodilation. A recent study suggests that benzofluomethiazide may act on the vascular wall to stimulate prostacyclin synthesis (336). Recent studies also suggest that the antihypertensive action of hydralazine may be dependent on its ability to inhibit platelet thromboxane synthesis (337, 338) as well as thromboxane synthesis by the vascular smooth muscle (339). The ability of hydralazine to depress vascular smooth muscle function does not appear to be related to its direct antihypertensive action (340). Since arterial smooth muscle synthesis of prostacyclin is increased in the established phase of hypertension, whereas thromboxane synthesis by the platelets and vasculature may be increased, the ability of benzofluomethiazide to increase further prostacyclin synthesis and hydralazine to decrease thromboxane synthesis may result in altered arterial pressure and resistance. Moreover, these changes may also promote a reversal of the structural vascular changes associated with the hypertensive state (see below).

PROSTAGLANDINS, CYCLIC NUCLEOTIDES, AND HYPERTENSION

Cyclic nucleotides may modulate both the level of vascular smooth muscle tone as well as the hypertrophic process within the vasculature. The cyclic nucleotide system is altered by the members of the prostaglandin-thromboxane-prostacyclin triad. The changes in cyclic nucleotides are dependent on the specific prostanoids themselves and on the ratio of the individual prostanoids that act on the vascular smooth muscle. Cyclic nucleotides are decreased and prostaglandins are increased in the arterial and venous smooth muscles obtained from hypertensive animals (180; see above). The data in the literature have consistently failed to correlate these changes with altered vascular reactivity or tone, but have attempted to relate the changes in cyclic nucleotides to the blood pressure itself. Moreover, few studies have attempted to relate the changes in VSM cyclic nucleotide and prostaglandin levels to the hypertrophic process in hypertensive animals.

There is increasing evidence that cyclic nucleotides may play a role in inhibiting cell growth. For many types of cells, basal cyclic AMP levels appear to be elevated in slowly growing cells and decrease in more rapidly growing cells. The growth of cultured fibroblasts appear to be inhibited by dibutyryl cyclic AMP or prostaglandin E_1, which stimulates the formation of cyclic AMP. Cyclic AMP and epinephrine inhibit the growth of lens epithelial cells. The effects of epinephrine were associated with a twofold increase in the concentration of cyclic AMP within the epithelium. The levels of cyclic AMP are not only associated with their levels of synthesis, but also by their levels of degradation. Type II phosphodiesterase activity is increased in the vascular smooth muscle of spontaneously hypertensive and renal hypertensive rats, while the levels of cyclic AMP are diminished (92). Some evidence supports the concept that the synthesis of cyclic AMP may be decreased in the vasculature of hypertensive animals in vivo, despite the fact that in vitro studies fail to find this (92, 180). Calcium ion modulates the activity of

TABLE 3 Determinants of Vascular Smooth Muscle Reactivity and Contractility

Reactivity	Contractility
1. Membrane properties	1. Energy supply: ATP, creatinine, PO_4
2. Receptor characteristics	2. Integrity of contractile proteins
3. Calcium stabilization of membrane excitation	3. Integrity of modulating proteins—calcium sensitivity
4. Magnesium modulation of membrane excitation	4. Availability of ionized calcium
5. Presence or absence of endogenous receptor antagonists	5. Presence or absence of messengers modulating the storage of calcium within the cell
6. Endothelial inactivation or production of prostacyclin	6. Compliance of passive-elastic components of blood vessel
	7. Endothelial inactivation or production of prostacyclin
	8. Activity of actomyosin ATPase
	9. Orientation of muscle fibers in vitro

adenylate cyclase. Calcium binding and content may be altered in the vasculature obtained from hypertensive animals (93,341). In vivo studies may minimize this by placing blood vessel strips or rings in PSS and studying their adenylate cyclase activity at a time when the calcium gradients within the cell has not returned to the levels which it has reached in vivo. Thus it is possible that both synthesis and degradation are altered (see Tables 3-5). The increase in vasoconstrictor prostanoids, such as thromboxanes and $PGF_{2\alpha}$, may promote a decrease in cyclic AMP, which then leads to cellular

TABLE 4 Actions of Prostaglandins on Vascular Smooth Muscle

1. Contracts arteries and veins
2. Responses inhibited by ouabain
3. Responses inhibited in magnesium-free medium
4. Stimulates sodium-, potassium-, magnesium-dependent ATPase
5. Increases sodium and decreases potassium content of blood vessel
6. Increases calcium turnover
7. Decreases calcium binding
8. Decreases sulfhydryl groups
9. Decreases cyclic AMP/GMP ratio
10. Sensitivity enhanced by synthetase inhibition
11. Responses dependent on metabolic and oxygen state of the blood vessel

TABLE 5 Summary of Changes in Venous Smooth Muscle in Hypertension

Alterations

1. Enhanced contractility
2. Decreased extensibility and compliance
3. Decreased sensitivity to vasodilators
4. Enhanced reactivity to vasoconstrictor agents
5. Decreased cyclic AMP
6. Decreased sensitivity to angiotensin II
7. Enhanced prostaglandin synthesis
8. Hypertrophy
9. Increased membrane glycoprotein synthesis
10. Diminished prostacyclin synthesis
11. Enhanced pulmonary responses to sympathetic nerve stimulation

Hypertensive models

1. Human essential hypertension
2. Spontaneously hypertensive rats
3. Renal hypertensive rats
4. Doca hypertensive rats
5. Aortic coarctation hypertension in rats and rabbits
6. Perinphritic hypertension in dogs
7. Renal hypertension in dogs
8. Hypertensive humans

Veins affected

1. Portal vein
2. Femoral vein
3. Mesenteric vein
4. Forearm vein
5. Saphenous vein
6. Vena cavae vein
7. Pulmonary artery
8. Vena venorum

Potential significance

1. Changes in venous smooth muscle function, not secondary increased intravascular pressure or altered vascular geometry.
2. An increase in venular pressure may further aggravate the hypertension by affecting, actively or passively, precapillary arteriolar resistance.
3. Since these changes are found in venules and major veins, they could explain the increased cardiac output during the labile phase of hypertension.
4. Prostaglandins may play a role in cellular mechanisms modulating membrane structural changes in hypertension.
5. Antihypertensive therapy may chronically modulate venous function in hypertension by modulating protein synthesis.
6. Veins may provide a model for the study of defects intrinsic in smooth muscle in hypertension.

protein synthesis and hypertrophy. The process of hypertrophy may, in and of itself, alter the vascular responses to vasoactive agents.

Preliminary studies from this laboratory and by other investigators (see 79) demonstrated that chronic treatment of hypertensive animals with clonidine and α-methyldopa reverses arterial and venous smooth muscle hypertrophy, stimulates the formation of prostacyclin, inhibits the formation of thromboxane, and results in an increase in cyclic AMP. Whether these actions are related or separate events remains to be determined. However, the cyclic nucleotides and prostanoids appear to be an important link in the relationship between altered vascular function and structure in hypertension.

Although an underlying, unifying hypothesis to link prostaglandins to vascular smooth muscle function, structure, and the elevation in arterial pressure in hypertension cannot be formulated, one must raise the question as to whether or not prostanoids derived from other than the vascular smooth muscle can account for the vascular changes of hypertension. The studies of Terragno et al. (196) suggest that an intrarenal inhibitor of prostaglandin synthesis may exist which could influence vascular prostaglandin synthesis. Similarly, other factors produced by the kidney or present in plasma may alter vascular prostaglandin production. In addition, the platelets serve as a vast potential source of prostaglandins (thromboxanes and endoperoxides) which can profoundly influence the vascular smooth muscle.

PLATELETS, PROSTAGLANDINS, AND HYPERTENSION

Platelets are believed to play a critical role in the vascular changes in atherosclerosis. Hypertension is the leading, predisposing factor to the development of atherosclerotic changes in the vascular smooth muscle and endothelium of experimental animals and humans. Platelets release endoperoxides, thromboxanes, serotonin, and growth factors (PGDF) which can modulate cyclic nucleotides within the vascular smooth muscle and endothelium, possibly altering the control mechanisms regulating cell growth and contractile function. Moreover, PGDF can stimulate both cellular hypertrophy in vivo and in cells in culture and hyperplasia in situ. The principal cell types involved in the action of PDGF are endothelial and smooth muscle cells. Endothelial cells are induced to proliferate and migrate in vivo and in culture, whereas smooth muscle cells are induced to proliferate and increase the synthesis of connective tissue, proteins collagen, elastin, and proteoglycans. Elimination of platelets or inhibition of platelet function eliminates atherosclerotic lesion formation. Antiplatelet antibodies administered to dogs decreases arterial pressure and, if administered slowly over a prolonged period of time, results in a stable blood pressure but with a decreased susceptibility to vasoconstrictor stimuli. The hypertrophic changes of the vasculature in hypertension as well as the altered pressure and vascular reactivity are similar to those caused by PDGF as well as thromboxanes and prostaglandins. However, a detailed investigation into

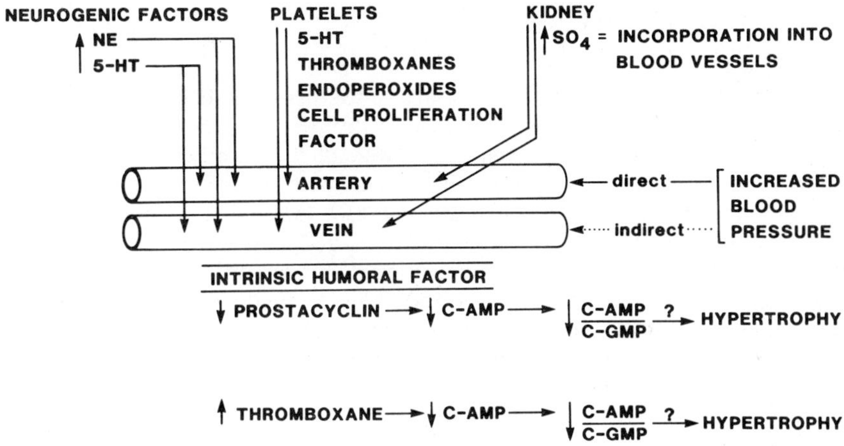

FIG. 7. Potential role of prostanoids and platelets in vascular and pressure changes in hypertension.

the role of platelets in hypertension has not been forthcoming (for references, see Refs. 79 and 182).

In view of the potential importance of platelets as a stimulator of arterial and venous smooth muscle hypertrophy, the finding that venous smooth muscle changes in hypertension by undergoing changes in cyclic nucleotides and hypertrophy is important. It is possible, albeit this is speculative at the present time, that the platelet is a critical link as a circulating prohypertensive factor in this disease process.

As summarized in Fig. 7, the kidney may activate the vascular smooth muscle or platelet thromboxane-prostanoid system. The platelets may liberate substances such as TxA_2, 5-HT, endoperoxides, or PDGF, which act directly on the vasculature or stimulate TxA_2 synthesis within the vascular smooth muscle and vascular endothelium. This could lead to a decrease in cyclic AMP, altered vascular reactivity, and the beginnings of pressure-independent hypertrophy. In the arterial side of the circulation, small changes in arterial wall thickness will lead to an increase in pressure, which then acts as a further stimulus to hypertrophy and also masks the initial changes seen in the arterial smooth muscle. The veins, on the other hand, continue to reflect the actions of the circulating humoral factors which were initially responsible for the incipient hemodynamic and vascular changes within the arterial and venous vasculature (Fig. 7, Table 5). To reiterate, this is speculative. However, it is one postulate that can explain the altered vascular function as well as the structural changes in both the high- and low-pressure systems of the vascular tree in hypertension.

SUMMARY AND CONCLUSIONS

This chapter has attempted to summarize the bases for the hemodynamic and vascular derangements as they relate to the prostanoid system and hypertension. Obviously, this review is biased in favor of the humoral theory of vascular derangements in hypertension. Although in vitro studies report biochemical alterations in the intrarenal prostanoid system in hypertension, the in vivo evidence seems to contradict the biochemical findings. Similarly, vascular smooth muscle prostanoid synthesis is also altered in hypertension. Attempts to relate this to the acute vascular derangements have met with little success. Studies that inhibit the individual components of the prostaglandin triad prior to the induction of the hypertensive stimulus will shed light on the role of the prostaglandin system in the altered vascular reactivity and elevated arterial pressure of hypertension. Finally, it has been postulated that the platelet prostanoid system, which is altered in hypertension, may account for the altered vascular structure, function, and pressures of this disease process. Further studies are necessary to evaluate the role of the prostanoid system in hypertensive vascular disease.

ACKNOWLEDGMENTS

This research was supported in part by U.S. Public Health Service Grants HL-22216, 22177, and RCDAHL7KO4-00428-04, National Heart Lung and Blood Institute, NIH; a grant from Boehringer Ingelheim, Ingelheim, Germany; and AHA 75-929. The author was also a recipient of Research Career Development Award 7-KO4 HL-00428-04 from the Hypertension Branch of the National Institutes of Health during these studies.

The author gratefully acknowledges Dr. W. Blackburn of the Department ment of Pathology, College of Medicine, University of South Alabama, for performing the histological analysis of the blood vessels. The author also expresses his deepest appreciation to the following individuals, without whose effort the studies cited herein could not have been completed: David Sweatt, Krista Gaines, Claude McGowan, Monica Gaida, Frederick Curro, Eugene C. Palmer, and Walter Wilborn.

REFERENCES

1. Kurzrok, R., and Leib, C. Biochemical studies of human semen: II. The action of semen on the human uterus. Proc. Soc. Exp. Biol. Med. 28:268-272, 1930.
2. Moncada, S. R., Gryglewski, J., Bunting, S., and Vane, J. R. An enzyme isolated from arteries transforms prostaglandin endoperoxides to an unstable substance that inhibits platelet aggregation. Nature (Lond.) 263:663-665, 1976.

3. Hamberg, M., Svensson, J., and Samuelsson, B. Thromboxanes: a new group of biologically active compounds derived from prostaglandin endoperoxides. Proc. Natl. Acad. Sci. USA 72:2994-2998, 1976.
4. Hamberg, M., Svensson, J., and Samuelsson, B. Prostaglandin endoperoxides: a new concept concerning the mode of action and release of prostaglandins. Proc. Natl. Acad. Sci. USA 71:3824-3828, 1974.
5. Pace-Asciak, C. R., and Rangaraj, G. Distribution of prostaglandin biosynthetic pathways in several rat tissues. Formation of 6-keto-prostaglandin $F_{1\alpha}$. Biochim. Biophys. Acta 486:579-582, 1977.
6. Lands, W. E. M., Lee, R., and Smith, W. Factors regulating the biosynthesis of various prostaglandins. Ann. N.Y. Acad. Sci. 180:107-122, 1971.
7. Needleman, P., Raz, A., Minkes, M. S., Ferrendelli, J. A., and Sprecher, H. Triene prostaglandins: prostacyclin and thromboxane biosynthesis and unique biological properties. Proc. Natl. Acad. Sci. USA 76:944-948, 1979.
8. Lefer, A. M. Role of the prostaglandin-thromboxane system in vascular homeostasis during shock. Circ. Shock 6:297-303, 1979.
9. Moncada, S., and Vane, J. R. The role of prostacyclin in vascular tissue. Fed. Proc. 38:66-71, 1979.
10. Gryglewski, R. J. Prostaglandins and the vascular wall. In Prostaglandins and Thromboxanes, F. Berti, B. Samuelsson, and G. P. Velo (Eds.). Plenum Press, New York, pp. 265-274, 1977.
11. Hamberg, M., and Samuelsson, B. Detection and isolation of the endoperoxide intermediate in prostaglandin biosynthesis. Proc. Natl. Acad. Sci. USA 70:899-903, 1973.
12. Morrison, A. R., and Needleman, P. Biochemistry and pharmacology of the renal prostaglandins. In Contemporary Issues in Nephrology, Vol. 4, B. M. Brenner and J. M. Stein (Eds.). Churchill-Livingstone, New York, pp. 68-88, 1979.
13. Ellis, E. F., Oelz, O., Roberts, L. G., Payne, M. A., Sweetman, B. J., Nies, A. S., and Oates, J. A. Coronary arterial smooth muscle contraction by a substance released from platelets: evidence that it is thromboxane A_2. Science 193:1135-1137, 1976.
14. Gryglewski, R. J., Zmuda, A., Korbut, R., Krecioch, E., and Beiron, K. Selective inhibition of TxA_2 biosynthesis in blood platelets. Nature (Lond.) 267:627-628, 1977.
15. Needleman, P., Moncada, S., Bunting, S., Vane, J. R., Hamberg, M., and Samuelsson, B. Identification of an enzyme in platelet microsomes which generates TxA_2 from prostaglandin endoperoxides. Nature (Lond.) 261:558-560, 1976.
16. Needleman, P., Moncada, S., Bunting, S., and Vane, J. R. Identification of an enzyme in platelet microsomes which generates thromboxane A_2 from prostaglandin endoperoxides. Nature (Lond.) 261:558-560, 1976.

17. Greenberg, S., McGowan, C., and Glenn, T. M. Pulmonary vascular smooth muscle in porcine sphlanchnic arterial occlusion shock. Am. J. Physiol. 241[Heart and Circ. Physiol. 10]: H35-H45, 1981.
18. Greenberg, S. Mesenteric prostanoid synthesis in canine two-kidney, one-clip Goldblatt hypertension. In Prostanoids in Cardiovascular and Cardiopulmonary Function, S. Greenberg and T. M. Glenn (Eds.). Academic Press, New York, 1982, in press.
19. Hagen, A. A., White, R. P., and Robertson, J. T. Synthesis of prostaglandins and thromboxane B_2 by cerebral arteries. Stroke 10:306-309, 1979.
20. White, R. P. Prostaglandins and cerebral vasospasm. In Prostaglandins: Organ Specific Actions, S. Greenberg, P. J. Kadowitz, and T. F. Burks (Eds.). Marcel Dekker, New York, Chap. 14, 1981.
21. Salzman, P. M., Salmon, J. A., and Moncada, S. Prostacyclin and thromboxane A_2 synthesis by rabbit pulmonary artery. J. Pharmacol. Exp. Ther. 215:240-247, 1980.
22. Hanszen, F. H. A., and Nugteren, D. H. Histochemical localization of prostaglandin synthetase. Histochemie 27:159-164, 1971.
23. Frolich, J. C., Sweetman, B. J., Carr, K., Splawinski, J., Watson, J. T., Anggard, E., and Oates, J. A. Occurrence of prostaglandins in human urine. Ad. Biosci. 9:321-330, 1973.
24. Anggard, E., and Samuelsson, B. Metabolism of prostaglandin E_1 in guinea pig lung. the structure of two metabolites. J. Biol. Chem. 239: 4097-4102, 1964.
25. McGiff, J. C., and Wong, K. C. Cardiovascular actions of 6-keto-prostaglandin E_2. Eur. J. Pharmacol. 22:317-320, 1978.
26. Samuelsson, B., Borgeat, P., Hammerstrom, S., and Murphy, R. C. Leukotrienes: a new group of biologically active compounds. Adv. Prostaglandin Thromboxane Res. 6:1-18, 1980.
27. Robinson, H. J., and Vane, J. R. Prostaglandin Synthetase Inhibitors. Raven Press, New York, 1974.
28. Hawthorne, E. W., Hinds, J. E., Crawford, W. J., and Tearney, R. J. Left ventricular myocardial contractility during the first week of renal hypertension in conscious dogs. Circ. Res. 34/35(Suppl. I):223-234, 1974.
29. Frohlich, E. D., Ulrych, M., Tarazi, R. C., Dustan, H. P., and Page, I. H. A hemodynamic comparison of essential and renovascular hypertension. Circ. Res. 35:289-297, 1967.
30. Bello, C. T., Sevy, R. W., and Harakal, C. Varying hemodynamic patterns in essential hypertension. Am. J. Med. 250:24-35, 1965.
31. Frohlich, E. D., Tarazi, R. C., and Dustan, H. P. Re-examination of the hemodynamics of hypertension. Am. J. Med. Sci. 257:70-79, 1969.
32. Holman, D. V., and Page, I. H. The cardiac output in arterial hypertension: Part II. A study of arterial hypertension produced by constricting

the renal arteries in unanesthetized and anesthetized (pentobarbital) dogs. Am. Heart J. 16:321-328, 1938.

33. Widimsky, J., Fejfarova, M. H., and Fejfar, A. Changes of cardiac output in hypertensive disease. Cardiologica 31:381-389, 1957.
34. Lucas, J. A., and Floyer, M. A. Renal control of changes in the compliance of the interstitial space: a factor in the aetiology of renoprival hypertension. Clin. Sci. 44:397-416, 1973.
35. Lucas, J. A., and Floyer, M. A. Changes in body fluid distribution and interstitial tissue compliance during the development and reversal of experimental and renal hypertension. Clin. Sci. Mol. Med. 47:1-11, 1974.
36. Ulrych, M., Frohlich, E. D., Tarazi, R. C., Dustan, H. P., and Page, I. H. Cardiac output and distribution of blood volume in central and peripheral circulations in hypertensive and normotensive man. Br. Heart J. 31:570-574, 1969.
37. Ulrych, M. The role of vascular capacitance in the genesis of essential hypertension. Clin. Sci. Mol. Med. 51:203-205, 1976.
38. Ulrych, M. Pathogenesis of essential hypertension. Angiology 30:104-116, 1979.
39. Ulrych, M., and Ulrych, Z. Significance of increase in labelled albumin disappearance rate in arterial hypertension. Clin. Sci. Mol. Med. 51:211-213, 1976.
40. Liard, J. F., and Peters, G. Role of retention of water and sodium in two types of experimental renovascular hypertension in the rat. Pfluegers Arch. 344:93-108, 1973.
41. Bianchi, G., Tilda-Tenconi, L., and Lucca, R. Effect in the conscious dog of constriction of the renal artery to a sole remaining kidney on heamodynamics, sodium balance, body fluid volume, plasma renin concentration and pressor responsiveness to angiotensin. Clin. Sci. 38: 741-766, 1970.
42. Ferrario, C. M. Contribution of cardiac output and peripheral resistance to experimental renal hypertension. Am. J. Physiol. 226:711-717, 1974.
43. Ferrario, C. M., and Page, I. H. Current views concerning cardiac output in the genesis of experimental hypertension. Circ. Res. 43:821-831, 1976.
44. Bianchi, G., Baldoni, E., Lucca, R., and Barbin, P. Pathogenesis of arterial hypertension after the constriction of the renal artery leaving the opposite kidney intact both in the anesthetized and conscious dog. Clin. Sci. 42:651-664, 1972.
45. Ferrario, C. M., Page, I. H., and McCubbin, J. W. Increased cardiac output as a contributory factor in experimental renal hypertension in dogs. Circ. Res. 27:799-810, 1970.
46. Richardson, T. Q., Fermoso, J. D., and Guyton, A. C. Increase in mean circulatory filling pressure in Goldblatt hypertension. Am. J. Physiol. 207:751-754, 1964.

47. Overbeck, H. W. Hemodynamics of early experimental renal hypertension in dogs: normal limb blood flow, elevated vascular resistance and decreased venous compliance. Circ. Res. 31:653-663, 1972.
48. Averill, D. B., Ferrario, C. M., Tarazi, R. C., Sen, S., and Bajbus, R. Cardiac performance in rats with renal hypertension. Circ. Res. 38:280-288, 1976.
49. Simon, G. Altered venous function in hypertensive rats. Circ. Res. 38:412-418, 1976.
50. Walsh, J. C., Hyman, C., and Maronde, R. Venous distensibility in essential hypertension. Cardiovasc. Res. 3:338-341, 1969.
51. Wood, J. E. Peripheral venous arteriolar responses to infusions of angiotensin in normal and hypertensive subjects. Circ. Res. 9:768-774, 1961.
52. Altman, S., and Simon, G. Abnormal venous wall composition in spontaneously hypertensive rats. Proc. Soc. Exp. Biol. Med. 165:13-21, 1980.
53. Simon, G., Panmani, M. G., Dunkel, J. F., and Overbeck, H. W. Mesenteric hemodynamics in early experimental renal hypertension in dogs. Circ. Res. 36:791-798, 1975.
54. Takeshita, A., and Mark, A. Decreased venous distensibility in hemodynamics in early experimental renal hypertension in dogs. Circ. Res. 36:791-798, 1975.
55. Simon, G., Pamnani, B., and Overbeck, H. W. Decreased venous compliance in dogs with chronic renal hypertension. Proc. Soc. Exp. Biol. Med. 152:1221-1225, 1976.
56. Simon, G., Franciosa, J., and Cohn, J. Decreased venous distensibility in essential hypertension: lack of systemic hemodynamic correlates. Angiology 30:147-159, 1979.
57. Greenberg, S., McGowan, C., and Gaida, M. M. Hemodynamics and vascular responses of conscious dogs to vasoactive agents during the development of Goldblatt hypertension. Am. J. Physiol. [Heart Circ. Physiol.], 1981, in review.
58. Greenberg, S., McGowan, C., and Gaida, M. M. Effect of caval occlusion on the arterial resistance and vascular reactivity of two-kidney, two-clip Goldblatt hypertension in dogs. Clin. Exp. Hypertension 3, 1981, in review.
59. Pfeffer, M. A., and Frohlich, E. D. Hemodynamic and myocardial function in young and old spontaneously hypertensive rats. Circ. Res. 32/33(Suppl. I):28-35, 1973.
60. Pfeffer, M. A., Pfeffer, J. M., and Frohlich, E. D. Hemodynamics of the spontaneously hypertensive rat: effects of isoproterenol. Proc. Soc. Exp. Biol. Med. 145:1025-1030, 1974.
61. Pfeffer, M. A., Frohlich, E. D., Pfeffer, J. M., and Weiss, A. K. Pathophysiologic implications of the increased cardiac output of young spontaneously hypertensive rats. Circ. Res. 34/35(Suppl I):235-242, 1974.

62. Olmstead, F., and Page, I. H. Hemodynamic changes in trained dogs during experimental renal hypertension. Circ. Res. 16:134-139, 1965.
63. Conway, J. A vascular abnormality in hypertension. Circulation 27: 520-529, 1963.
64. Conway, J. Blood flow and peripheral resistance in normotensive and hypertensive dogs. Circ. Res. 18:273-277, 1966.
65. Conway, J. Changes in sodium balance and hemodynamics during development of experimental renal hypertension in dogs. Circ. Res. 22:763-767, 1968.
66. Bayliss, W. M. On the local reactions of the arterial wall to changes in internal pressure. J. Physiol. (Lond.) 28:220-232, 1902.
67. Moncada, S., and Vane, J. R. The role of prostacyclin in vascular tissue. Fed. Proc. 38:66-71, 1979.
68. Vane, J. R., and McGiff, J. C. Possible contribution of endogenous prostaglandins to the control of blood pressure. Circ. Res.
69. Guyton, A. C., Coleman, T. G., Bower, J. D., and Granger, H. D. Circulatory control in hypertension. Circ. Res. 26/27(Suppl. II):135-147, 1970.
70. Guyton, A. C., Granger, H. J., and Coleman, T. G. Autoregulation of the total system circulation and its relation to the control of cardiac output and arterial pressure. Circ. Res. 28/29(Suppl. I):93-97, 1971.
71. Granger, H. J., and Guyton, A. C. Autoregulation of the total systemic circulation following destruction of the central nervous system in the dog. Circ. Res. 25:379-388, 1969.
72. Guyton, A. C., Coleman, T. G., Cowley, A. W., Manning, R. D., Norman, R. A., and Ferguson, J. D. A systems analysis approach to understanding long-range arterial blood pressure control and hypertension. Circ. Res. 35:159-176, 1974.
73. Ledingham, J. M. Mechanisms in renal hypertension. Proc. R. Soc. Med. 64:409-418, 1971.
74. Ledingham, J. M., and Cohen, R. D. Role of the heart in the pathogenesis of renal hypertension. Lancet 2:979-982, 1963.
75. Borst, J. G. G., and Borst-de-Geus, A. Hypertension explained by Starling's theory of circulatory homeostasis. Lancet 1:677-682, 1963.
76. Ledingham, J. M., and Pelling, D. Hemodynamic and other studies in the renoprival hypertensive rat. J. Physiol. (Lond.) 210:230-253, 1970.
77. Greenberg, S. Segmental vascular responses to vasoactive agents during the development of two-kidney, one-clip Goldblatt hypertension in dogs. Circ. Res., 49:484-495, 1981.
78. Greenberg, S. Contractile properties of vascular smooth muscle from dogs with two-kidney, one-clip Goldblatt hypertension. Am. J. Physiol. 241[Heart Circ. Physiol. 10]: H525-H540, 1981.
79. Greenberg, S. Venous smooth muscle structure and function in experimental and human hypertension. Methods Findings Exp. Clin. Pharmacol. 3:233-254, 1981.

80. Dietz, R., Schomig, A., Haebara, H., Mann, F., Rascher, W., Luth, J., Grunherz, J., and Gross, F. Studies on the pathogenesis of spontaneous hypertension of rats. Circ. Res. 43:98-106, 1978.
81. Bevan, J. A., Bevan, R. D., Chang, P. C., Pegram, B. L., Purdy, R. E., and Su, C. Changes in the responses of arteries and veins from hypertensive rabbits to sympathetic nerve activity: assessment of some post-synaptic influences. Blood Vessels 13:167-180, 1976.
82. Bevan, J. A., Bevan, R. D., Chang, P. C., Pegram, B. L., Purdy, R. E., and Su, C. Analysis of activity of rabbit arteries and veins two weeks after induction of hypertension by coarctation of the abdominal aorta. Circ. Res. 37:183-198, 1975.
83. Bevan, R. D., Van Marthens, E., and Bevan, J. A. Hyperplasia in experimental hypertension in the rabbit. Circ. Res. 38(Suppl. II):58-62, 1976.
84. Floyer, M. A., Cantab, M. D., and Richardson, P. C. Mechanisms of arterial hypertension. Lancet 1:253-255, 1961.
85. Berecek, K. H., and Bohr, D. F. Whole body vascular reactivity during the development of desoxycorticosterone acetate hypertension in the pig. Circ. Res. 42:764-771, 1978.
86. Berecek, K. H., Stocker, M., and Gross, F. Changes in renal vascular reactivity at various stages of deoxycorticosterone hypertension in rats. Circ. Res. 46:619-624, 1980.
87. Ichikawa, S., Johnson, J. A., Fowler, W. L., Jr., Payne, C. G., Jurz, K., and Keitzer, W. F. Pressor responses to norepinephrine in rabbits with 3 day and 30 day renal artery stenosis. Circ. Res. 43:437-446, 1979.
88. Click, R. L., Gilmore, J. P., and Joiner, W. L. Differential response of hamster cheek pouch microvessels to vasoactive stimuli during the early development of hypertension. Circ. Res. 44:512-517, 1979.
89. Collis, M. G., and Alps, B. J. Vascular reactivity to noradrenaline, potassium chloride and angiotensin II in the rat perfused mesenteric vasculature preparation during the development of renal hypertension. Cardiovasc. Res. 9:118-126, 1975.
90. Haeusler, G., and Finch, L. Vascular reactivity to 5-hydroxy-tryptamine and hypertension in the rat. Arch. Exp. Pathol. Pharmacol. 272:101-116, 1972.
91. Hansen, T. R., and Bohr, D. F. Hypertension, transmural pressure, and vascular smooth muscle response in rats. Circ. Res. 36:590-598, 1975.
92. Ramananthan, S., and Shibata, S. Cyclic AMP blood vessels of spontaneously hypertensive rats. Blood Vessels 11:312-318, 1974.
93. Bohr, D. F. Reactivity of smooth muscle from normal and hypertensive rats. Fed. Proc. 33:127-132, 1974.
94. Shibata, S., Kurahushi, K., and Kuchii, M. Possible etiology of contractility impairment of vascular smooth muscle from spontaneously hypertensive rats. J. Pharmacol. Exp. Ther. 185:406-417, 1973.

95. Folkow, B. Cardiovascular structural adaptation: its role in the initiation and maintenance of primary hypertension. Clin. Sci. 55(Suppl.): s3-s22, 1978.
96. Friedman, S. M. Arterial contractibility and reactivity. In Hypertension, J. Genest, E. Kiow, and O. Kuchel (Eds.). McGraw-Hill, New York, pp. 470-475, 1977.
97. Folkow, B., Hallback, M., Lundgren, Y., and Weiss, L. Structurally based increase in flow resistance in spontaneously hypertensive rats. Acta Physiol. Scand. 79:373-386, 1970.
98. Folkow, B., Hallback, M., Lundgren, Y., Sivertsson, R., and Weiss, L. Importance of adaptive changes in vascular design for establishment of primary hypertension, studied in man and spontaneously hypertensive rats. Circ. Res. 32/33(Suppl. I):2-13, 1973.
99. Lundgren, Y. Adaptive changes of cardiovascular design in spontaneous and renal hypertension. Acta Physiol. Scand. 59(Suppl. 408):1-123, 1974.
100. Guyton, A. C. Control of the circulation in hypertension. Sci. Mol. Med. 55(Suppl.):s3-s21, 1978.
101. Guyton, A. C., and Jones, C. E. (Eds.). Cardiovascular Physiology. University Park Press, Baltimore, pp. 259-368, 1974.
102. Tobian, L. How sodium and kidney relate to the hypertensive arteriole. Fed. Proc. 33:138-142, 1974.
103. Folkow, B., Hallback, M., Lundgren, Y., and Weiss, L. The effects of immunosympathectomy on blood pressure and vascular reactivity in normal and spontaneously hypertensive rats. Acta Physiol. Scand. 84: 512-523, 1972.
104. Weiderheim, C. A. Effects of transmural pressure on vascular smooth muscle. Bibl. Anat. 3:62-66, 1967.
105. Panmami, M., and Overbeck, H. Abnormal ion and water composition of veins and normotensive arteries in coarctation hypertension in rats. Circ. Res. 38:375-378, 1976.
106. Giacomelli, F., Rooney, J., and Weiner, J. Cerebrovascular ultrastructure and permeability after carotid artery constriction in experimental hypertension. Exp. Mol. Pathol. 28:309-321, 1978.
107. Friedman, S. M., Scott, G. H., and Nakashima, M. Vascular morphology in hypertensive states in the rat. Anat. Rec. 171:529-551, 1971.
108. Frith, C. H., McMurtry, F., Alexander, A. F., and Will, D. G. Influence of hypertension and hypoxemia on arterial biochemistry and morphology in swine. Atherosclerosis 20:189-206, 1974.
109. Nordborg, C., and Johansson, B. The ratio between thickness of media and internal radius in cerebral, mesenteric and renal arterial vessels in spontaneously hypertensive rats. Clin. Sci. 57:s27-s29, 1979.
110. Peiper, U. P., Klempt, P., and Popov, R. The contractility of venous

vascular smooth muscle in spontaneously hypertensive or renal hypertensive rats. Basic Res. Cardiol. 74:21-34, 1979.
111. Greenberg, S., and Bohr, D. F. Venous smooth muscle in hypertension: enhanced contractility of portal veins from spontaneously hypertensive rats. Circ. Res. 36(Suppl. I):208-214, 1975.
112. Greenberg, S., Palmer, E. C., and Wilborn, W. M. Pressure-independent hypertrophy of veins and pulmonary arteries of spontaneously hypertensive rats. Clin. Sci. Mol. Med. 55(Suppl.):s31-s36, 1978.
113. Greenberg, S., Palmer, E. C., and Wilborn, W. M. Venous smooth muscle structure and function in spontaneously hypertensive rats. Arch. Int. Pharmacodyn., 1982, in press.
114. Greenberg, S., and Wilborn, W. M. Effect of clonidine and propranolol on the veins of spontaneously hypertensive rats. Arch. Int. Pharmacodyn., 1982, in press.
115. Pang, C. C. Y., and Sutter, M. C. Contractile responses of aortic portal vein strips during the development of Doca-salt hypertension. Blood Vessels 17:281-292, 1980.
116. Pang, C. C. Y., and Sutter, M. C. Hydralazine prevents changes in the contractile response of aortic but not portal vein strips in hypertensive rats. Blood Vessels 17:293-301, 1980.
117. Sutter, M. C., and Lungt, B. Contractility, muscle mass and agonist sensitivity of isolated portal veins from normo and hypertensive rats. Acta Physiol. Scand. 99:484-495, 1977.
118. Dahl, L. K., Knudson, K. D., Heine, M., and Leitl, G. Effect of chronic excess salt ingestion. Genetic influence on the development of salt hypertension in parabiotic rats; evidence for a humoral factor. J. Exp. Med. 126:687-699, 1967.
119. Dahl, L. K., Knudsen, K. D., and Iwai, J. Genetic influence of the kidney in hypertension-prone rats. Circ. Res. 26/27(Suppl. I):277-289, 1970.
120. Edihara, A., and Grollman, A. Evidence for a pressor substance in renal venous blood from hypertensive dogs. Am. J. Physiol. 214:1-5, 1968.
121. Eto, T., Onidi, H., Onoyama, K., Omae, T., and Yamato, T. Increased permeability of arteriolar wall caused by renal extract in nephrectomized rats. Jap. Heart J. 18:473-481, 1977.
122. Eto, T., Onoyama, K., Tanaka, K., Omae, T., and Yamamoto, T. Early vascular changes in the intestine of bilaterally nephrectomized rats. J. Pathol. 124:141-148, 1978.
123. Greenberg, S., Goldstein, B. M., and Wilson, W. R. Effect of plasma from human hypertensives on the responses of the perfused canine paw to vasoactive agents. Clin. Pharmacol. Ther. 15:337-343, 1974.
124. Grollman, A., and Krishnamurty, V. S. R. Further studies on a pressor substance in hypertension. Am. J. Physiol. 221:1499-1505, 1971.

125. Sen, S., Bravo, E. L., and Bumpus, F. M. Isolation of a hypertension producing compound from normal human serum. Circ. Res. 40(Suppl. I):5-10, 1977.
126. Simon, G. Angiopathic serum factor in perinephritic hypertensive dogs. Hypertension 1:197-200, 1979.
127. Greenberg, S. Effect of chronic administration of clonidine, propranolol, and alphamethyldopa on venous structure and function in experimental hypertension. J. Pharmacol. Exp. Ther. 218:779-792, 1981.
128. Greenberg, S., Gaines, K., and Sweatt, D. Evidence for circulatory humoral factors as a cause of venous hypertension in parabiosed SHR. Am. J. Physiol. 241[Heart Circ. Physiol. 10]:421-432, 1981.
129. Cohen, M., and Batemen, S. Decreased relaxation of venous smooth muscle in spontaneously hypertensive rats. J. Pharmacol. Exp. Ther. 205:258-469, 1977.
130. Safar, M., Chau, N., Weiss, Y., London, G., and Milliez, P. Control of cardiac output in essential hypertension. Studies in hypertension. Am. J. Cardiol. 38:332-336, 1976.
131. Safar, M. E., London, G., Weiss, Y., and Milliez, P. Vascular reactivity to norepinephrine and hemodynamic parameters in borderline hypertension. Am. Heart J. 89:480-486, 1975.
132. Safar, M. E., Chau, N., Weiss, Y., London, G., Simon, A., and Milliez, P. The pressure volume relationship in normotensive and permanent essential hypertensive patients. Clin. Sci. Mol. Med. 50: 207-212, 1976.
133. Rippe, B., and Folkow, B. Capillary permeability to albumin in normotensive and spontaneously hypertensive rats. Acta Physiol. Scand. 101:72-83, 1977.
134. Samar, R. A., and Coleman, T. G. Mean circulatory filling pressure and vascular capacitance in the rat. Am. J. Physiol. 234 [Heart Circ. Physiol. 5]:H94-H100, 1978.
135. Suzuki, T., Oyama, K., and Nakamura, T. Observations on microcirculation in the mesentery of Doca hypertensive rats. Microvasc. Res. 5:20-33, 1973.
136. Weigman, D., Joshua, I., Morff, R., Harris, P., and Miller, F. Microvascular responses to norepinephrine in renovascular and spontaneously hypertensive rats. Am. J. Physiol. 236[Heart Circ. Physiol. 7]:H45-H49, 1979.
137. Caliva, F., Napadano, R., Stafford, R., Loftus, W., and Lyons, R. Digital hemodynamics in the normotensive and hypertensive states: II. Studies in hypertension. Circ. Res. 28:415-425, 1963.
138. Brown, W., Brown, F., and Krishan, I. Stabilized venous distensibility of normotensive and hypertensive humans on high and low sodium intake. Circulation 43:433-442, 1978.
139. Bohlen, H., Gore, R., and Hutchins, P. Comparison of microvascular pressure in normal and spontaneously hypertensive rats. Microvasc. Res. 13:125-130, 1977.

140. Edwards, T., and Diana, J. Effect of exercise on pre- and post-capillary resistance in the spontaneously hypertensive rat. Am. J. Physiol. 234:H439-H446, 1979.
141. Brock, R., and Diana, J. Effect of Doca-NaCl hypertension on pre- and post-capillary resistance in isolated hindlimbs of dogs. Am. J. Physiol. 236:H586-H589, 1979.
142. Crane, W. A. J. Sulphate utilization and mucopolysaccharide synthesis by the mesenteric arteries of rats with experimental hypertension. J. Pathol. Bacteriol. 84:113-122, 1962.
143. Culvenor, A., and Jarrott, B. Effect of alphasympatholytics on synthesis of glycosaminoglycans. Molecular Pharmacol. 15:86-100, 1979.
144. Haeusler, G. Cardiovascular regulation by central adrenergic mechanisms and its alteration by hypotensive drugs. Circ. Res. 36:223-238, 1975.
145. Yamori, Y., and Ohta, K. Chemical analysis of vascular collagen in stroke prone spontaneously hypertensive rats. Jap. Circ. J. 44:173-176, 1980.
146. Bostrom, S. L., and Fryklund, J. Protein synthesis and composition of cardia and vascular tissue in spontaneously hypertensive rats and the effects of B-adrenergic antagonist treatment. Clin. Sci. 57(Suppl.): s39-s41, 1979.
147. Iwatsuki, K., Cardinale, G., Spector, S., and Udenfriend, S. Hypertension: increase of collagen biosynthesis in arteries, but not veins of spontaneously hypertensive rats. Science 162:403-404, 1977.
148. Malt, R. A. Macromolecular metabolism in compensatory renal hypertrophy. Yale J. Biol. Med. 51:419-428, 1978.
149. Martel-Pelletier, J., and Bergeron, M. Compensatory renal hypertrophy: I. Evidence for a factor of renal origin inhibiting DNA synthesis. Can. J. Physiol. Pharmacol. 55:839-847, 1977.
150. Murphy, R.A. Relationship of actomyosin content and ATPase activity to tension generation in vascular smooth muscle. J. Gen. Physiol. 55:473-482, 1978.
151. Nakashima, Y., Okamoto, S., Torii, S., Arakawa, K., and Nakamura, M. Changes of glycosaminoglucuronoglycans in the aortic wall of SHR. Jap. J. Const. Med. 34:51-52, 1970.
152. Ooshima, O., Fuller, G. C., Cardinale, G. J., Spector, S., and Udenfriend, S. Collagen synthesis in blood vessels of hypertensive rats and reversal by antihypertensive agents. Proc. Natl. Acad. Sci. USA 71:3019-3022, 1974.
153. Ooshima, A., Yamori, Y., Ohta, K., Nara, Y., and Horie, R. Biochemical alterations of connective tissue metabolism in the arterial walls of stroke-prone spontaneously hypertensive rats. Clin. Sci. 57(Suppl.):s35-s37, 1979.
154. Ouellette, A. J. Messenger RNA in compensatory renal hypertrophy. Yale J. Biol. Med. 51:413-418, 1978.

155. Solomon, S., Wise, P. M., Sanborn, C., and Ratner, A. Cyclic nucleotide concentrations in relation to renal growth and hypertrophy. Yale J. Biol. Med. 51:373-379, 1978.
156. Wolinsky, H. Effects of hypertension and its reversal on the thoracic aorta of male and female rats. Circ. Res. 28:622-631, 1971.
157. Bostrum, S. L., and Fryklund, J. Protein synthesis and composition of cardiac and vascular tissue in spontaneously hypertensive rats and the effects of B-adrenergic antagonist treatment. Clin. Sci. 57(Suppl.): s39-s41, 1979.
158. Dyson, R. D. Cell Biology: A Molecular Approach. Allyn and Bacon, Boston, pp. 70-134, 1978.
159. Hollander, W., Kramsch, D. M., Farmelant, M., and Madoff, J. M. Arterial wall metabolism in experimental hypertension of coarctation of the aorta of short duration. J. Clin. Invest. 47:1221-1228, 1968.
160. Jung, M. S., Palfreyman, M. G., Wanger, J., Bey Ribereau Gayon, G., Zraka, M., and Koch-Weser, J. Influence of alphamethyldopa and alpha sympatholytics on protein synthesis. Life Sci. 24:1037-1044, 1979.
161. Kallfelt, B. J., Hjalmarsson, A. C., and Isaksson, O. G. In vitro effects of catecholamines on protein synthesis in perfused rat heart. J. Cell. Mol. Cardiol. 8:787-801, 1976.
162. Mankine, C., Costan, M., Sipes, G., and Haddock-Russell, D. Further evidence of cyclic-AMP mediated hypertrophy as a prerequisite of drug-specific enzyme induction. Biochem. Pharmacol. 27: 219-234, 1978.
163. Maragoudakis, M. E., Kalinsky, H. J., and Wasvari, J. Effects of clonidine on renal basement membrane synthesis. J. Pharmacol. Exp. Ther. 204:372-383, 1978.
164. Nakada, T., and Lovenberg, W. Lysine incorporation in vessels of spontaneously hypertensive rats; effects of adrenergic drugs. Eur. J. Pharmacol. 48:87-96, 1978.
165. Nakashima, Y., Okamoto, S., Torii, S., Arakawa, K., and Nakamura, M. Changes of glycosaminoglucuronoglycans in the aortic wall of SHR. Jap. J. Const. Med. 34:51-52, 1970.
166. Ooshima, O., Fuller, G. C., Cardinale, G. J., Spector, S., and Udenfriend, S. Collagen biosynthesis in blood vessels of hypertensive rats and its reversal by antihypertensive agents. Proc. Natl. Acad. UA 71:3019-3022, 1974.
167. Ooshima, O., Yamori, Y., Ohta, K., and Horie, R. Biochemical alterations of connective tissue metabolism in the arterial walls of stroke prone spontaneously hypertensive rats. Clin. Sci. 57(Suppl.): s35-s37, 1980.
168. Weiner, J., Loud, A., Giacomelli, F., and Anversa, P. Morpho metric analysis of hypertension-induced hypertrophy of rat thoracic aorta. Am. J. Pathol. 88:619-634, 1977.

169. Solomon, S., Hathaway, S., and Curb, D. Evidence that a renal response to volume expansion involves a blood borne factor. Biol. Neonate 35:113-120, 1979.
170. Preuss, H. G., Goldin, H., and Shivers, M. Further studies on a renotropic system in rats. Yale J. Biol. Med. 51:403-412, 1978.
171. Preuss, K., Grant, K., Parris, R., Zmudka, M., and Slotkoff, L. Effect of sera and sera fractions from spontaneously hypertensive rats on renal organic ion transport. Proc. Soc. Exp. Biol. Med. 145:397-402, 1974.
172. Mandal, A. K., Bell, R., Parker, D., Nordquist, J., and Lindeman, R. D. An analysis of the relationship of malignant lesions of the kidney to hypertension. Microvasc. Res. 14:279-292, 1977.
173. Lund, D. D., and Tomanek, R. J. Myocardial morphology in spontaneously hypertensive and aortic constricted rats. Am. J. Anat. 152:141-151, 1978.
174. Kaufman, O. Mitoses in hypertrophied smooth muscle tissue of the rat posterior vena cavae. Exp. Biol. Med. (USSR) 81:485-487, 1976.
175. Karmali, R. A., Horrobin, D. F., and Patel, P. The relationship between concentrations of prostaglandin A_1, E_1, E_2 and F_{2a} and rates of cell proliferation. Pharmacol. Res. Commun. 11:69-75, 1979.
176. Hochman, G., Bozner, A., Lackovic, V., Ciznar, I., and Hostacka, H. Urinary proteins inhibit fibroblast formation. Gen. Pharmacol. 10:153-155, 1979.
177. Guyton, J. R., and Karnovsky, M. J. Smooth muscle proliferation in the occluded rat carotid artery. Am. J. Pathol. 94:586-596, 1979.
178. Giacomelli, F., and Wiener, J. The cellular pathology of experimental hypertension. Am. J. Pathol. 72:221-240, 1973.
179. Diezi, J., Hausel, M., and Buxel, N. N. Studies on the possible mechanisms of early functional compensatory adaptation in the remaining kidney following nephrectomy. Yale J. Biol. Med. 51:265-270, 1978.
180. Amer, M. S., Doba, M., and Reis, D. J. Changes in cyclic nucleotide metabolism in aorta and heart of neurogenically hypertensive rats. Possible trigger mechanism. Proc. Natl. Acad. Sci. USA 72:2135-2139, 1974.
181. Schmitt, H., and Schmitt, H. Localization of the hypotensive effect of (2,6-dichlorophenylamino)-2-imidazoline hydrochloride (ST-155—Catapressan). Eur. J. Pharmacol. 6:8-12, 1969.
182. Sen, S, Tarazi, R. C., and Bumpus, M. Reversal of cardiac hypertrophy in renal hypertensive rats. Fed. Proc. (abstr.) 37: 849, 1978.
183. Rabinowitz, M. Overview on the pathogenesis of myocardial hypertrophy. Circ. Res. 35(Suppl. 2):3-14, 1974.
184. Mulvany, M. J., Ljung, B., Stoltze, M., and Kjellstadt, A. Contractile and morphological properties of the portal vein in spontaneously hypertensive rats. Blood Vessels 17:202-215, 1980.
185. Hamet, P. Cyclic nucleotides and aggregation of platelets of spontaneously hypertensive rats. Circ. Res. 43:583-591, 1978.

186. Bunting, S., Gryglewski, R., Moncada, S., and Vane, J. R. Arterial walls generate from prostaglandin endoperoxides a substance (prostaglandin X) which relaxes strips of mesenteric and coeliac arteries and inhibits platelet aggregation. Prostaglandins 12:897-913, 1976.
187. Cottee, F., Flower, R. J., Moncada, S., Salmon, J. A., and Vane, J. R. Synthesis of 6-keto PGF_{1a} by ram seminal vesicles. Prostaglandins 14:413-423, 1977.
188. Greenberg, S., and Kadowitz, P. J. Difference in prostaglandin modulation of arterial and venous smooth muscle responses to bradykinin and norepinephrine. J. Lab. Methods Exp. Clin. Pharmacol. 3:000-000, 1981, in press.
189. Herman, A. G. Distribution of prostacyclin across the arterial wall. Arch. Int. Pharmacodyn. Ther. 232:342-343, 1978.
190. Limas, C. J., and Limas, C. Vascular prostaglandin synthesis in the spontaneously hypertensive rat. Am. J. Physiol. 233[Heart Circ. Physiol. 2]:H493-H499, 1977.
191. Moncada, S., and Vane, J. R. Prostacyclin in perspective. In Prostacyclin, J. R. Vane and S. Bergstrom (Eds.). Raven Press, New York, pp. 5-16, 1979.
192. Pace-Asciak, C. R., Carrara, M. C., Rangaraj, G., and Nicolau, K. C. Enhanced formation of PGI_2, a potent hypotensive substance, by aortic rings and homogenates of the spontaneously hypertensive rat. Prostaglandins 15:1005-1016, 1978.
193. Pace-Asciak, C. R., and Carrara, M. C. Ontogeny of aortic PGI_2 formation in the developing spontaneously hypertensive rat: correlations with elevations in blood pressure. Adv. Prostaglandin Thromboxane Res. 7:797-802, 1980.
194. Skidgel, R. A., and Printz, M. P. PGI_2 production by rat blood vessels: diminished prostacyclin formation in veins compared to arteries. Prostaglandins 16:1-10, 1978.
195. Skidgel, R. A., and Printz, M. P. Vascular PG synthesis in hypertensive and normotensive rats. Adv. Prostaglandin Thromboxane Res. 4:803-808, 1980.
196. Terragno, N. A., McGiff, J. C., and Terragno, A. Prostacyclin (PGI_2) production by renal blood vessels: relationship to an endogenous prostaglandin synthesis inhibitor. Clin. Res. (abstr.) 26:546A, 1978.
197. Muirhead, E. E. Renal prostaglandins. In The Prostaglandins: Pharmacological and Therapeutic Advances, M. F. Cuthbert (Ed.). Lippincott, Philadelphia, pp. 201-254, 1973.
198. Bergstrom, S., Carlsson, L. A., and Weeks, J. R. The prostaglandins: a family of biologically active lipids. Pharmacol. Rev. 20: 11-63, 1968.
199. Nakano, J. Cardiovascular actions. In The Prostaglandins, Vol. 1, P. W. Ramwell (Ed.). Plenum Press, New York, pp. 239-268, 1973.
200. Lee, J. B. Renal homeostasis and the hypertensive state: a unifying

hypothesis. In The Prostaglandins, Vol. 1, P. W. Ramwell (Ed.). Plenum Press, New York, pp. 133-239, 1973.

201. McGiff, J. C., Crowshaw, K., and Itskowitz, H. D. Prostaglandins and renal function. Fed. Proc. 33:39-47, 1974.

202. Oates, J. A., Whorton, A. R., Gerkens, J. F., Branch, R. A., Hollifield, J. W., and Frohlich, J. C. The participation of prosta glandins in the control of renin release. Fed. Proc. 38:72-74, 1979.

203. Hedquist, P. Prostaglandins as modulators of autonomic neuroeffector transmission. In Prostaglandin Synthetase Inhibitors, H. J. Robinson and J. R. Vane (Eds.). Raven Press, New York, pp. 303-309, 1974.

204. Hedquist, P. Prostaglandins as modulators of autonomic neuroeffector transmission. In Prostaglandins and Thromboxanes, F. Berti, B. Samuelsson, and G. P. Velo (Eds.). Plenum Press, New York, pp. 423-432, 1977.

205. Moncada, S., and Vane, J. R. Pharmacology and endogenous roles of prostaglandin endoperoxides, thromboxane A_{2+} and prostacyclin. Pharmacol. Rev. 30:293-331, 1978.

206. Dunn, M. J. Renal prostaglandins: influences on excretion of sodium and water, the renin angiotensin system renal blood flow and hypertension. In Contemporary Issues in Nephrology, B. M. Brenner and J. H. Stein (Eds.), Churchill Livingstone Press, New York, pp. 238-309, 1978.

207. Fitzpatrick, T. M., Alter, I., Corey, E. J., Ramwell, P., Rose, J. C., and Kot, P. A. Cardiovascular responses to PGI_2 (prostacyclin) in the dog. Circ. Res. 42:192-194, 1978.

208. Friesinger, G. C., Oelz, O., Sweetman, B., Nies, A. S., and Oates, J. Prostaglandin D_2, another renal prostaglandin. Prostaglandins 15: 969-977, 1978.

209. Gerber, J. G., Branch, R. A., Nies, A. S., Gerkens, J. F., Shand, D. G., Hollifield, J., and Oates, J. A. Prostaglandins and renin release: II. Assessment of renin secretion following infusions of PGI_2, E_2 and D_2 into the renal artery of anesthetized dogs. Prostaglandins 15:81-88, 1978.

210. Frohlich, J. C., Hollifield, J. W., Dormois, J. C., Frohlich, B. L., Seyberth, H., Michelakis, A. M., and Oates, J. A. Suppression of plasma renin activity by indomethacin in man. Circ. Res. 39:447-452, 1976.

211. Gerkens, J. J., Friesinger, G. C., Branch, R. A., Shand, P. G., Gerber, J. G., and Oates, J. C. Pulmonary, renal and hepatic extraction of PGI_2—a potential circulating hormone. Clin. Res. (abstr.) 26:13A, 1978.

212. Moncada, S., Korbut, R., Bunting, S., and Vane, J. R. Prostacyclin is a circulating hormone. Nature (Lond.) 273:767-768, 1978.

213. Dusting, G. J., Moncada, S., and Vane, J. R. Recirculation of prostacyclin in the dog. Br. J. Pharmacol. 64:315-320, 1978.

214. Dunn, M. J., and Hood, V. L. Prostaglandins and the kidney. Am. J. Physiol. 233[Renal Electrolyte Physiol. 3]:F169-178, 1977.
215. Kadowitz, P. J., Chapnick, B. M., Feigen, L. P., Hyman, A. L., Nelson, P. K., and Spannhake, E. W. Pulmonary and systemic vasodilator effects of the newly discovered prostaglandin, PGI_2. J. Appl. Physiol. 45:408-413, 1978.
216. Speckart, P., Zia, P., Zipser, R., and Horton, R. The effect of sodium restriction and prostaglandin inhibition on the renin-angiotensin system in man. J. Clin. Endocrinol. Metab. 44:832-839, 1977.
217. Herbaczynska-Cedro, K., and Vane, J. R. Contribution of intrarenal generation of prostaglandin to autoregulation of renal blood flow in the dog. Circ. Res. 33:428-432, 1973.
218. Bayliss, C., and Brenner, B. M. Evidence for a functional role for endogenous prostaglandins (PG) on the superficial renal cortex. Kidney Int. 12:550-562, 1978.
219. Bayliss, C., Dean, W. M., Myers, B. D., and Brenner, B. M. Effect of some vasodilator drugs on transcapillary fluid exchange in renal cortex. Am. J. Physiol. 230:1148-1153, 1976.
220. Armstrong, J. M., Blackwell, G. J., Flower, R. J., McGiff, J. C., Mullane, K. M., and Vane, J. R. Genetic hypertension in rats is accompanied by a defect in renal prostaglandin catabolism. Nature (Lond.) 260:582-584, 1976.
221. Armstrong, J. M., Lattimer, N., Moncada, S., and Vane, J. R. Comparison of the vasodepressor effects of prostacyclin, 6-oxo-prostaglandin $F_{1\alpha}$, with those of prostaglandin E_2 in rats and rabbits. Br. J. Pharmacol. 62:125-130, 1978.
222. Armstrong, J. M., Boura, A. L. A., Hamberg, M., and Samuelsson, B. A. A comparison of the vasodepressor effects of the cyclic endoperoxide PGG_2 and PGH_2, with those of PGD_2 and PGE_2 in hypertensive and normotensive rats. Eur. J. Pharmacol. 39:251-258, 1976.
223. Edwards, W. G., Strong, C. G., and Hunt, J. C. A vasodepressor lipid resembling prostaglandin E_2 (PGE_2) in the renal venous blood of hypertensive patients. J. Lab. Clin. Med. 74:389-396, 1969.
224. Daniels, E. G., Hinman, J. W., Leach, B. E., and Muirhead, E. E. Identification of a prostaglandin E_2 as the principal vasodepressor lipid of rabbit renal medulla. Nature (Lond.) 215:1298-1300, 1967.
225. Sirois, P., and Guignon, D. J. Vasodepressor response of arachidonic acid in spontaneously hypertensive rats. Experientia 30:1418-1419, 1974.
226. Nekrasova, A. A., and Lantsberg, L. A. Role of renal prostaglandins in the pathogenesis of hypertension. Kardiologiya 9:86-93, 1969.
227. Nekrasova, A. A., Paleseva, F. M., and Khundadze, S. S. Content of depressor prostaglandin-like substances and renin activity in the kidneys of patients with renovascular hypertension. Kardiologiya 10:88-97, 1970.

228. Nishikawa, K., Morrison, A., and Needleman, P. Exaggerated prostaglandin biosynthesis and its influence on renal resistance in the isolated hydronephrotic rabbit kidney. J. Clin. Invest. 59:1143, 1977.
229. Tan, S. Y., and Mulrow, P. J. Inhibition of renin and aldosterone response to furosemide by indomethacin. J. Clin. Endocrinol. Metab. 45:174, 1977.
230. Tan, S. Y., Sweet, P., and Mulrow, P. Impaired renal production of prostaglandin E_2: a newly identified lesion in human essential hypertension. Prostaglandins 14:139, 1977.
231. Terragno, D. A., Crowshaw, K., Terragno, N. A., and McGiff, J. C. Prostaglandin synthesis by bovine mesenteric arteries and veins. Circ. Res. 36/37(Suppl. I):76-80, 1975.
232. Terragno, N. A., Terragno, D. A., Early, J. A., Roberts, M. A., and McGiff, J. C. Endogenous prostaglandin synthesis inhibitor in the renal cortex: effects on production of prostacyclin by renal blood vessels. Clin. Sci. Mol. Med. 55:s199-s202, 1978.
233. Terragno, N. A., Terragno, D. A., and McGiff, J. C. Contribution of prostaglandin to the renal circulation in the conscious, unanesthetized and laparotomized dog. Circ. Res. 40:590-598, 1977.
234. Tobian, L., and Azar, S. Antihypertensive and other functions of the renal papilla. Trans. Assoc. Am. Physicians 84:281-291, 1971.
235. Tobian, L., and O'Donnell, M. Renal prostaglandins in relation to sodium regulation and hypertension. Fed. Proc. 35:2388-2395, 1975.
236. Azar, S., Johnson, M. A., and Hertel, B. Single nephron pressures, flows and resistances in hypertensive kidneys with nephrosclerosis. Kidney Int. 12:28-33, 1977.
237. Azar, S., Johnson, M. A., Iwai, J., Bruno, L., and Tobian, L. Single nephron dynamics in post-salt rats with chronic hypertension. J. Lab. Clin. Med. 91:156-163, 1978.
238. Azar, S., Johnson, M. A., Bruno, L., and Tobian, L. Single nephron dynamics in the Kyoto hypertensive and normotensive rat. In Spontaneous Hypertension: Its Pathogenesis and Complications, Department of Health, Education, and Welfare, Washington, D.C., pp. 294-301, 1977.
239. Bailie, M. D., Crossland, K., and Jook, J. R. Natriuretic effect of furosemide after inhibition of prostaglandin synthesis. J. Pharmacol. Exp. Ther. 199:469-477, 1976.
240. Needleman, P., Douglas, J. R., Jakschik, B., Stoechlein, P. B., and Johnson, E. M. Release of renal prostaglandins by catecholamines: relationship to renal endocrine function. J. Pharmacol. Exp. Ther. 188:453-465, 1974.
241. Needleman, P., Bronson, S. D., Wyche, A., Sivakoff, M., and Nichalou, K. C. Cardiac and renal prostaglandin I_2: biosynthesis and biological effects in isolated perfused rabbit tissues. J. Clin. Invest. 61:839-846, 1978.

242. Hornych, A., Bedrossian, J., Bariety, J., Menard, J., Corcovol, P., Safar, M., Fontalrian, F., and Milliez, P. Prostaglandins and hypertension in chronic renal disease. Clin. Nephrol. 4:144-162, 1975.
243. Hornych, A., Weiss, Y., Safar, M., Menard, J., Corcovol, P., Fontalrian, F., Bariety, J., and Milliez, P. Prostaglandins A and B in the peripheral blood of hypertensive patients. Eur. J. Clin. Invest. 6:314-321, 1976.
244. Dunn, M. J. Renal prostaglandin synthesis in the spontaneously hypertensive rat. J. Clin. Invest. 58:862-871, 1976.
245. Dunn, M. J. Renal prostaglandin synthesis in the spontaneously hypertensive rat. In Spontaneous Hypertension: Its Pathogenesis and Complications (Proc. 2nd Int. Symp. SHR). DHEW Publ. 77-1179, Washington, D.C., pp. 359-365, 1977.
246. Ahnfelt-Ronne, I., and Arrigoni-Martinelli, E. Degradation of renal prostaglandins. Biochem. Pharmacol. 26:485-488, 1977.
247. Dibona, D. F., and Rios, L. L. Mechanism of the exaggerated diuresis in the spontaneously hypertensive rat. Am. J. Physiol. 235[Renal Electrolyte Physiol. 6]:342-347, 1978.
248. Lee, J. B., Covino, B. G., Takman, B. H., and Smith, E. R. Renomedullary vasodepressor substance, medullin: isolation, chemical characterization, and its physiological properties. Circ. Res. 17:57-66, 1965.
249. Lee, J. B., Crowshaw, K., Takman, B. H. Attrep, K. A., and Gougoutas, J. Z. The identification of prostaglandin E_2, $F_{2\alpha}$ and A_2 from rabbit kidney medulla. Biochem. J. 105:1251-1258, 1967.
250. Lee, J. B., Kannegiesser, H., O'Toole, J., and Westura, E. Hypertension and the renomedullary prostaglandins: a human study of the hypotensive effects of PGE_1. Ann. N.Y. Acad. Sci. 180:218-233, 1971.
251. Higgs, G. A., Moncada, S., and Vane, J. R. Prostacyclin as a dilator of arterioles in the hamster cheek pouch. J. Physiol. (Lond.) 280: 30-31P, 1978.
252. Higgs, G. A., Moncada, S., and Vane, J. R. Prostacyclin (PGI_2) reduces the number of slow moving leucocytes in hamster cheek pouch venules. J. Physiol. (Lond.) 280:55-56P, 1978.
253. Hill, T. W. K., and Moncada, S. The renal hemodynamic and excretory actions of prostacyclin and 6-oxoPGF in anesthetized dogs. Prostaglandins 17:87-98, 1979.
254. Hintze, T. H., Kaley, G., Martin, E. G., and Messina, E. PGI_2 induces bradycardia in the dog. Prostaglandins 15:12-13, 1978.
254a. Messina, E., Hintze, T. H., and Kaley, G. Responses to prostacyclin and arachidonic acid in the spontaneously hypertensive rat. Hypertension 2:412-421, 1980.
255. Aiken, J. W., and Vane, J. R. Angiotensin II induced renal vasoconstriction is opposed by the intrarenal generation of prostaglandins. J. Pharmacol. Exp. Ther. 184:678-687, 1973.

256. Aiken, J. W. Effects of prostaglandin synthesis inhibitors on angiotensin tachyphylaxis on the isolated coeliac and mesenteric arteries of the rabbit. Pol. J. Pharmacol. Pharm. 26:217-227, 1974.
257. Negus, P., Jones, R. L., and Dunn, M. J. Indomethacin potentiates the vasoconstrictor actions of angiotensin II in normal man. Prostaglandins 12:75-80, 1976.
258. McGiff, J. C., Crowshaw, K., Terragno, N. A., and Lonigro, A. Release of a prostaglandin-like substance into renal venous blood in response to angiotensin II. Circ. Res. 26/27(Suppl. I):121-129, 1970.
259. Douglas, J. R., Johnson, E. M., Marshal, G. R., Jaffe, B. M., and Needleman, P. Stimulation of splenic prostaglandin release by angiotensin and specific inhibition by cysteine-8-AII. Prostaglandins 3:67-78, 1973.
260. Gimbrone, M. A., and Alexander, R. W. Angiotensin II stimulation of prostaglandin production in cultured human vascular endothelium. Science 189:219-221, 1975.
261. Pugsley, D. J., Beilin, L. J., and Peto, R. Renal prostaglandin synthesis in the Goldblatt hypertensive rat. Circ. Res. 36/37(Suppl. I): 81-87, 1975.
262. Romero, J. D., Aguilo, J. J., and Strong, C. G. Effects of indomethacin blockade of prostaglandin synthesis in the Goldblatt hypertensive rat. Circulation 51/52(Suppl.):124, 1975.
263. Scholkens, B. A., and Steinbach, R. Increase of experimental hypertension following inhibition of prostaglandin biosynthesis. Arch. Int. Pharmacodyn. Ther. 214:328-341, 1975.
264. Levy, J. V. Changes in systolic arterial blood pressure in normal and spontaneously hypertensive rats produced by acute administration of inhibitors of prostaglandin biosynthesis. Prostaglandins 13:153-162, 1977.
265. Zusman, R. M., and Keiser, H. R. Prostaglandin biosynthesis by rabbit renomedullary interstitial cells in tissue culture: stimulation by vasoactive peptides. J. Clin. Invest. 60:215-223, 1977.
266. Kirschenbaum, M. A., and Stein, J. H. The effect of inhibition of urinary prostaglandin synthesis on urinary sodium excretion in the conscious dog. J. Clin. Invest. 57:517-525, 1976.
267. Finn, W. F., and Arendshorst, W. J. Effect of prostaglandin synthetase inhibitors on renal blood flow in the rat. Am. J. Physiol. 231: 1541-1547, 1976.
268. Larsson, C., Weber, P., and Anngard, E. Arachidonic acid increases and indomethacin decreases plasma renin activity in the rabbit. Eur. J. Pharmacol. 28:391-394, 1974.
269. Larsson, C., and Anngard, E. Arachidonic acid lowers and indomethacin increases the blood pressure of the rabbit. J. Pharm. Pharmacol. 25:653-655, 1973.
270. Leary, W. P., Ledingham, J. E., and Vane, J. R. Impaired prosta-

glandin release from the kidneys of salt loaded rats. Prostaglandins 7:425–434, 1974.
271. Lee, J. B. Antihypertensive activity of the kidneys: the renomedullary prostaglandins. N. Engl. J. Med. 277:1073-1081, 1976.
272. Davis, H. A., and Horton, E. W. Output of prostaglandins from the rabbit kidney: its increase on renal nerve stimulation and inhibition by indomethacin. Br. J. Pharmacol. 46:658-665, 1972.
273. Feigen, L. P., Kaliner, E., Chapnick, B. M., and Kadowitz, P. J. The effect of indomethacin on renal function in pentobarbital-anesthetized dogs. J. Pharmacol. Exp. Ther. 198:457-468, 1976.
274. Franco, R., Tan, S. Y., and Mulrow, P. Renin release in an in vitro superfusion system of rat kidney slices: effects of prostaglandins. Clin. Res. 25:594A, 1977.
275. Abe, K., Yasujima, M., Chiba, S., Irakawa, N., Ito, T., and Yoshinaga, K. Effect of furosemide on urinary excretion of prostaglandin E in normal volunteers and patients with essential hypertension. Prostaglandins 14:513-524, 1977.
276. Danon, A., Chang, L. C., Sweetman, A. S., Nies, A. S., and Oates, J. A. Synthesis of prostaglandins by the rat renal papilla in vitro, mechanism of stimulation by angiotensin II. Biochim. Biophys. Acta 388:71-81, 1975.
277. Werning, C., Vetter, W., Weichmann, P., Schweikert, H. U., Steil, D., and Siegenthaler, W. Effect of prostaglandin E_1 on renin in the dog. Am. J. Physiol. 220:852-858, 1971.
278. Whorton, A. R., Misono, K., Hollifield, J., Frolich, J. C., Inagami, T., and Oates, J. A. Prostaglandins and renin release: I. Stimulation of renin release from rabbit cortical slices by PGI_2. Prostaglandins 14:1095-1104, 1977.
279. Zenser, T. V., Herman, C. A., Gorman, R. R., and Davis, B. B. Metabolism and action of prostaglandin endoperoxide PGH_2 in the rat kidney. Biochem. Biophys. Res. Commun. 79:357-363, 1977.
280. Weber, P. C., Larsson, C., Anggard, E., Hamberg, M., Corey, E. J., Nicholau, K. C., and Samuelsson, B. Stimulation of renin release from rabbit renal cortex by arachidonic acid and prostaglandin endoperoxides. Circ. Res. 39:863-874, 1976.
281. Weber, P. C., Larsson, C., and Scherer, B. Prostaglandin E_2-9-ketoreductase as a mediator of salt intake-related prostaglandin renin interaction. Nature (Lond.) 266:67-69, 1977.
282. Zins, G. R. Renal prostaglandins. Am. J. Med. 58:14-24, 1975.
283. Zimmerman, B. G., Ryan, M. J., Gomer, S., and Kraft, E. Effect of prostaglandin synthesis inhibitors indomethacin and eicosa-5,8,11, 14 tetraynoic acid on adrenergic respondes in dog cutaneous vasculature. J. Pharmacol. Exp. Ther. 187:315-323, 1973.
284. Zimmerman, B. G., Ryan, M. J., Gomer, S., and Kraft, E. Renal vascular actions of inhibitors of prostaglandin synthesis indomethacin and meclofenamic acid in the dog. Life Sci. 11:1104-1112, 1974.

285. Venuto, R. C., O'Dorisiao, T., Stein, J. H., and Ferris, T. F. Uterine prostaglandin E secretion and uterine blood flow in the pregnant rabbit. J. Clin. Invest. 55:193-197, 1975.
286. Swain, J. A., Heyndricks, G. R., Boetcher, D. A., and Vatner, S. F. Prostaglandin control of renal circulation in the unanesthetized dog and baboon. Am. J. Physiol. 229:826-830, 1975.
287. Dubocovich, M. L., and Langer, S. Z. Evidence against a physiologic role of prostaglandins in the regulation of noradrenaline release in the cat spleen. J. Physiol. (Lond.) 251:737-762, 1975.
288. Feigen, L. P., Chapnick, B. M., Flemming, J. E., and Kadowitz, P. J. Prostaglandins: renal vascular responses to bradykinin, histamine and nitroglycerine. Am. J. Physiol. 234[Heart Circ. Physiol. 7]: H495-H502, 1978.
289. Greenberg, S., and Kadowitz, P. J. Difference in prostaglandin modulation of arterial and venous smooth muscle tone in the dog. Methods Findings Clin. Exp. Pharmacol. 4:34-45, 1982.
290. Gorog, P., and Kovacs, I. B. Superprecipitation of vascular actomyosin: the effect of vasoactive compounds and anti-inflammatory agents on the process. Biochem. Pharmacol. 21:1713-1723, 1972.
291. Northover, B. J. The effect of anti-inflammatory drugs on vascular smooth muscle. Br. J. Pharmacol. Chemother. 31:483-493, 1967.
292. Northover, B. J. Effect of indomethacin on calcium, sodium, potassium and magnesium fluxes in various tissues of the guinea pig. Br. J. Pharmacol. 45:651-659, 1972.
293. Northover, B. J. Effect of anti-inflammatory drugs on the binding of calcium to cellular membranes in various human and guinea-pig tissues. Br. J. Pharmacol. 48:496-504, 1973.
294. Northover, B. J. Effect of anti-inflammatory drugs on the membrane potential of vascular endothelial cells in vitro. Br. J. Pharmacol. 53: 113-120, 1975.
295. Stein, J. H. Prostaglandins and renal function: II. The effect of prostaglandin inhibition on autoregulation of renal blood flow in the intact kidney of the dog. Prostaglandin 9:817-828, 1975.
296. Brecher, G. A., and Brobmann, G. F. Effect of kallekrein on the cardiovascular system. Handb. Pharmacol. 25:351-361, 1970.
297. Haddy, F. J., Emerson, T. E., Scott, J. B., and Daugherty, R. M. The effect of kinins on the cardiovascular system. Handb. Pharmacol. 25:362-384, 1970.
298. McGiff, J. C., Itskovitz, H. D., and Terragno, N. A. The action of bradykinin and eleidoisin in the canine isolated kidney: relationships to prostaglandins. Clin. Sci. Mol. Med. 49:125-128, 1975.
299. McGiff, J. C., Itskovitz, H. D., Terragno, N. A., and Wong, P. K. Y. Modulation and mediation of the action of the renal kallekrein-kinin system by prostaglandins. Fed. Proc. 35:175-180, 1976.
300. McGiff, J. C., Terragno, N. A., Malik, K. A., and Lonigro, A. J.

Release of a prostaglandin E-like substance from canine kidney by bradykinin: comparison with eledoisin. Circ. Res. 31:36-43, 1972.

301. Margolius, H. S., and Buse, J. B. The renal kallekrein-kinin system. In Contemporary Issues in Nephrology, Vol. 4, B. M. Brenner and J. H. Stein (Eds.). Churchill Livingston Press, New York, pp. 115-163, 1979.

302. Crowshaw, K., and McGiff, J. C. Prostaglandins and the kidney: a correlative study of their biochemistry and renal function. In Mechanisms of Hypertension, M. P. Sambhi (Ed.). Elsevier, New York, pp. 254-286, 1973.

303. Wong, P. K. Y., and McGiff, J. C. Enzymic regulation of prostaglandin levels in blood vessels: relationship to cyclic GMP. Fed. Proc. 36:673, 1977.

304. Wong, P. K. Y., Terragno, D. A., Terragno, N. A., and McGiff, J. C. Dual effect of bradykinin on prostaglandin metabolism: relationship to the dissimilar actions of kinins. Prostaglandins 13:1113-1125, 1977.

305. Tuvemo, T., Strandberg, K., Hamberg, M., and Samuelsson, B. Formation and action of prostaglandin endoperoxides in the isolated human umbilical artery. Acta Physiol. Scand. 96:145-149, 1976.

306. Terragno, D. A., Crowshaw, K., Terragno, N. A., and McGiff, J. C. Prostaglandin synthesis by bovine mesenteric arteries and veins. Circ. Res. 36/37(Suppl. I):76-80, 1975.

307. Needleman, P., Keys, S. L., Denny, S. E., Isakson, P. C.,, and Marshall, G. R. Coronary vasodilation mediated by bradykinin and prostaglandin. Proc. Natl. Acad. Sci. USA 72:2060-2063, 1975.

308. Needleman, P. The synthesis and function of prostaglandins in the heart. Fed. Proc. 35:2376-2383, 1976.

309. Messina, E. J., Weiner, R., and Kaley, G. Prostaglandins and local circulatory control. Fed. Proc. 35:2367-2375, 1976.

310. Messina, E. J., Weiner, R., and Kaley, G. Inhibition of bradykinin vasodilation and potentiation of norepinephrine and angiotensin vasoconstriction by inhibitors of prostaglandin synthesis in skeletal muscle of the rat. Circ. Res. 37:430-437, 1975.

311. Goldberg, M. R., Chapnick, B. M., Joiner, P. D., Hyman, A. L., and Kadowitz, P. J. Influence of inhibitors of prostaglandin synthesis on venoconstrictor responses to bradykinin. J. Pharmacol. Exp. Ther. 198:357-365, 1976.

312. Goldberg, M., Joiner, P. D., Greenberg, S., Hyman, A. L., and Kadowitz, P. J. Effects of indomethacin on venoconstrictor responses to bradykinin and norepinephrine. Prostaglandins 9:385-390, 1975.

313. Goldberg, S., Kadowitz, P. J., and Greenberg, S. Indomethacin-induced reversal of angiotensin tachyphylaxis: evidence for a non-prostaglandin mechanism. Pharmacologist 17:(abstr.):221, 1975.

314. Wong, P. K. Y., McGiff, J. C., and Terragno, A. Polypeptides: vascular actions as modified by prostaglandins. In Prostaglandins and Thromboxanes, F. Berti, B. Samuelsson, and G. P. Velo (Eds.). Plenum Pres, New York, pp. 251-264, 1977.
315. Muirhead, E. E., Germain, G., Leach, B. E., Pitcock, J. A., Stephenson, P., Brooks, B., Brosius, W. L., Daniels, E. G., and Hinman, J. W. Production of renomedullary prostaglandins by renomedullary interstitial cells grown in tissue culture. Circ. Res. 31/32 (Suppl. II):161-167, 1972.
316. Muirhead, E. E., Jones, F., and Stirman, J. A. Antihypertensive property in renoprival hypertension of extract from renal medulla. J. Lab. Clin. Med. 56:167-178, 1960.
317. Muirhead, E. E., Brown, G. B., Germain, G. S., and Leach, B. E. The renal medulla as an antihypertensive organ. J. Lab. Clin. Med. 75:641-651, 1970.
318. Levy, J. V. Inhibitory effects of anti-inflammatory drugs on PGE_2 induced contractions of human vein strips. Clin. Res. 20:211, 1972.
319. Levy, J. V. Chronotropic and inotropic effects of PGE_2 on isolated rat atria from normal and spontaneously hypertensive rats. Prostaglandins 4:731-743, 1973.
320. Levy, J. V. Papaverine antagonism of prostaglandin E_2 induced contraction of rabbit aortic strips. Res. Commun. Chem. Pathol. Pharmacol. 5:297-310, 1973.
321. Levy, J. V. Studies on the contractile effects of prostaglandins on aortic preparations from normotensive and spontaneously hypertensive rats. Res. Commun. Chem. Pathol. Pharmacol. 6:365-373, 1973.
322. Levy, J. V. Differences in papaverine inhibition of prostaglandin-induced contraction of aortic strips from normotensive and spontaneously hypertensive rats (SHR). Eur. J. Pharmacol. 25:117-120, 1974.
323. Altura, B. M., and Altura, B. T. Influence of magnesium on drug-induced contractions and ion content in rabbit thoracic aorta. Am. J. Physiol. 220:938-944, 1971.
324. Altura, B. M., and Altura, B. T. Magnesium and contraction of arterial smooth muscle. Microvasc. Res. 7:145-155, 1974.
325. Altura, B. M., Altura, B. T., and Waldemar, Y. Prostaglandin-induced relaxation and contraction of arterial smooth muscle: effects of magnesium ions. Artery, 2:326-336, 1976.
326. Leach, B. E., Armstrong, F. B., Germain, G. S., and Muirhead, E. E. Vasodepressor action of prostaglandin A_2 and E_2 in the spontaneously hypertensive rat (SH rat): evidence for an action mediated by the vagus. J. Pharmacol. Exp. Ther. 185:479-491, 1973.
327. Simpson, L. L. The effect of prostaglandin E_2 on arterial blood pressure of normotensive and spontaneously hypertensive rats. Br. J. Pharmacol. 51:559-563, 1974.
328. Ellis, E., and Hutchins, P. Cardiovascular responses to prostaglandin $F_{2\alpha}$ in spontaneously hypertensive rats. Prostaglandins 7:377-386, 1974.

329. Armstrong, J. M., Boura, A. L. A., Hamberg, M., and Samuelsson, B. A comparison of the vasodepressor effects of the cyclic endoperoxides PGG_2 and PGH_2 with those of PGE_2 and PGD_2 in hypertensive and normotensive rats. Eur. J. Pharmacol. 39:251-258, 1976.
330. Bunting, S., Gryglewski, R., Moncada, S., and Vane, J. R. Arterial walls generate from prostaglandin endoperoxides a substance (prostaglandin X) which relaxes strips of mesenteric and coeliac arteries and inhibits platelet aggregation. Prostaglandins 12:897-913, 1976.
331. Murphy, R. A. Contractile system function in mammalian smooth muscle. Blood Vessels 13:1-23, 1976.
332. Bohr, D. F., Greenberg, S., and Bonacorrsi, A. Mechanisms of action of vasoactive agents. In Microcirculation, Vol. 2, G. Kaley and B. Altura (Eds.). University Park Press, Baltimore, pp. 311-348, 1978.
333. Greenberg, S., Kadowitz, P. J., Long, J. P., and Wilson, W. R. Studies on the nature of a prostaglandin receptor in canine and rabbit vascular smooth muscle. Circ. Res. 39:66-76, 1976.
334. Greenberg, S., and McGowan, C. Interaction between divalent ions and the prostanoids in canine vascular smooth muscle. In Proceedings of the Symposium on the Prostaglandins in the Microcirculation, G. Kaley (Ed.). University Park Press, Baltimore, 1981, in press.
335. Bohr, D. F. Vascular smooth muscle: dual effect of calcium. Science 139:597-599, 1963.
336. Dollery, C. T. Prostacyclin may mediate the antihypertensive effect of benzofluomethiazide in hypertensive patients. Br. J. Clin. Pharmacol. 6:301-305, 1981.
337. Glenn, T. M., Sakane, Y., and Wooley, B. Effect of hydralazine and toxemia of pregnancy on platelet reactivity in human patients. Fed. Proc. 39:643, 1981.
338. Greenwald, J. E., Wong, L. K., Alexander, M., and Bianchine, J. R. In vivo inhibition of thromboxane biosynthesis by hydralazine. Adv. Prostaglandin Thromboxane Res. 6:293-296, 1980.
339. Greenberg, S., Gaines, K., and Glenn, T. M. Hydralazine may relax venous smooth muscle by inhibiting thromboxane synthesis. In Role of Hydroxamic Acids in Biology, H. Koehl (Ed.). Raven Press, New York, 1982, in press.
340. Greenberg, S. Effect of chronic administration of hydralazine and minoxidil to spontaneously hypertensive rats on vascular smooth muscle. J. Pharmacol. Exp. Ther. 214:283-292, 1980.
341. Kadowitz, P. J., Spannhake, E. W., Greenberg, S., Feigen, L. P., and Hyman, A. L. Comparative effects of arachidonic acid, bisenoic prostaglandins and an endoperoxide analog on the canine pulmonary vascular bed. Can. J. Physiol. Pharmacol. 55:1369-1377, 1977.
342. McNamara, D. B., Roulet, M. J., Gruetterm, C. A., Hyman, A. L., and Kadowitz, P. J. Correlation of prostaglandin-induced mitochondrial

calcium release with contraction in bovine intrapulmonary vein. Prostaglandins 20:311-320, 1980.
343. Palaty, V. Distribution of magnesium in the arterial wall. J. Physiol. (Lond.) 218:353-368, 1971.
344. Palaty, V. Regulation of cell magnesium in vascular smooth muscle. J. Physiol. (Lond.) 242:555-569, 1974.
345. Somlyo, A. P., and Somlyo, A. V. Vascular smooth muscle: I. Normal structure, pathology, biochemistry and biophysics. Pharmacol. Rev. 20:197-272, 1968.
346. Somlyo, A. V., and Somlyo, A. P. Vascular smooth muscle: II. Pharmacology of normal and hypertensive vessels. Pharmacol. Rev. 22: 249-353, 1970.
347. Somlyo, A. P., Somlyo, A. V., and Woo, C. Y. Neurohypophyseal peptide interaction with magnesium in avian vascular smooth muscle. J. Physiol. (Lond.) 192:657-668, 1967.
348. Turlapaty, P., and Altura, B. M. Extracellular magnesium ions control calcium exchange and content of vascular smooth muscle. Eur. J. Pharmacol. 52:421-423, 1978.
349. Van Breeman, C. Blockade of membrane calcium fluxes by lanthanum in relation to vascular smooth muscle contractility. Arch. Int. Physiol. Biochim. 77:710-716, 1968.
350. Van Breeman, C., Farinas, B. R., Gerba, P., and McNaughton, E. D. Excitation contraction coupling in rabbit aorta: studies by the lanthanum method measuring cellular calcium influx. Circ. Res. 30:44-56, 1971.
351. Weiss, G. B. Quantitative measurement of binding sites and washout components for calcium ion in vascular smooth muscle. In Calcium in Drug Action, G. B. Weiss (Ed.). Plenum Press, New York, pp. 57-74, 1978.

Part II
PROSTAGLANDINS AND THE CIRCULATION

4 Prostaglandins and the Cutaneous Vasculature

BEN G. ZIMMERMAN / EARL W. DUNHAM / University of Minnesota Medical School, Minneapolis, Minnesota

KAZUNOBU SUGAWARA* / Nagasaki University School of Medicine, Nagasaki, Japan

The ability to synthesize prostaglandins (PGs) is a characteristic of many tissues, including the skin. Dog (1,2), rat (3-5), and human skin (6-8) all have the capacity to generate PGE_2, a potent dilator of cutaneous vessels. For the most part PG synthesis by the skin appears to comprise the compensatory response to various types of cutaneous tissue injury (2,6,7,9). Changes in blood flow are integrally involved in the various responses to cutaneous injury. As a result, it is conceivable that PGE synthesized during trauma to the skin would aid, through its ability to increase blood flow, in the repair and healing process. The known major factor regulating cutaneous blood flow is the sympathetic nervous system, primarily via the adrenergic innervation. Skin vessels in the dog's paw have served as a useful model of the cutaneous circulation for many years (10-12). These vessels, especially the thick-walled arteriovenous anastamoses of the footpads, are extremely sensitive to adrenergic nerve stimulation (10,13). This marked sensitivity to vasoconstrictor stimuli appears to involve the responsiveness of the vascular smooth muscle, a postsynaptic characteristic rather than greater adrenergic transmitter release (14), a presynaptic effect. In addition, the canine cutaneous vessels can be vasodilated by means of the sympathetic innervation. A sustained vasodilator response can be evoked in the dog's paw by sympathetic nerve stimulation following adrenergic blockade (12). Local factors, such as autoregulatory control, apparently play a minor role in cutaneous blood flow regulation in the dog (15); however, in humans, cutaneous vessels appear to autoregulate more effectively (16). Anesthesia may suppress this phenomenon in the dog.

We became interested in the possible participation of PGs in the cutaneous circulation, both as a putative neurotransmitter of the sustained vasodilator system referred to above and as a modulator of myogenic vascular

---

*Present affiliation: Yamagata University Hospital, Yamagata, Japan

tone and cutaneous adrenergic responses. In order to examine the potential role of PGE as a vasodilator neurotransmitter, the effect of PG synthesis inhibitors (PGSIs) was tested on the sustained vasodilator response evoked in the pump perfused dog's paw by sympathetic stimulation. Neither indomethacin or eicosatetraynoic acid (ETA) alone caused any reduction in the vasodilator response with concentrations known to inhibit PG synthesis, whereas higher concentrations caused some decrease in the response, presumably by a nonspecific action (17). In other experiments we were unable to detect a PGE in the venous outflow of the paw during sympathetic nerve stimulation which also suggested that release of a PG probably does not mediate sustained vasodilatation in the dog's paw (unpublished results). During the course of the pump perfusion experiments in which PGSIs were employed in the canine paw we noted that both indomethacin and ETA caused a gradually developing vasoconstrictor effect, suggesting a vasodilator role of endogenous PGE in this vascular bed. A study was carried out to determine whether PGs synthesized and released in the paw perfused at constant flow modulated adrenergic responses (18). PGE_2 itself administered intraarterially in a low dose (110 ng/min) suppressed vasoconstrictor responses to norepinephrine (NE) and adrenergic nerve stimulation (18). Since PGSI caused augmentation of the response to NE as well as that to nerve stimulation, a postsynaptic modulating influence of endogenous PG was indicated in this vascular bed. Previous investigations by Hedqvist et al. (19,20) had emphasized a presynaptic action of PGE_2 and those of Kadowitz had pointed to both pre- and postsynaptic effects of PGs (21,22). In summary, the results of our study suggested primarily a postsynaptic influence on adrenergic function of a PGE generated either in the cutaneous vasculature or tissue or possibly in the blood perfusing this bed. To further investigate the modulating action of PGs on the skin vessels we carried out studies with exogenous arachidonic acid (AA), the precursor to PGE_2 and $PGF_{2\alpha}$, in the paw vasculature in vivo and on isolated canine paw veins.

Many investigations of the influence of PGs have been carried out on vascular beds perfused with an animal's blood or with an artificial medium. We considered it important to determine whether the generation of endogenous PG in the constant flow and normal flow preparation is equivalent. It is conceivable that pump perfusion of the paw cutaneous vasculature may stimulate the synthesis of PGs in a manner similar to that of mechanical stimulation (23) or, as we have shown (24), by the blood-bathed organ technique of Vane.

A preparation was designed in which the arterial supply of the paw was connected to the femoral artery via a shunt. Blood flow was maintained by the animal's systemic arterial pressure and measured in the cranial tibial artery supplying the paw with a noncannulating blood flow probe (6 mm, Carolina Medical Electronics) coupled to a Carolina blood flowmeter. The paw was denervated in these experiments by sectioning the tibial nerve. Drugs were administered intraarterially to the paw by injection or infusion into the shunt, and venous blood samples were withdrawn from the catheterized saphenous vein draining the paw.

RESULTS

Effect of Exogenous AA on Intact Paw Vasculature

Since PGE_2 exerts a marked depressant effect on responses to norepinephrine in the pump perfused paw, we utilized this effect as a means of approximating the quantity of PGE_2 synthesized from exogenously supplied AA in the pump-perfused paw and in the paw perfused naturally without a pump (vide infra). We examined the relative inhibitory effect of PGE_2 and AA on vasoconstrictor responses to intraarterially administered NE. In the pump-perfused preparation, AA infused at 110 μg/min intraarterially markedly depressed responses to NE (25), whereas in the normally perfused paw the vasoconstrictor responses to NE were reduced only slightly (unpublished observations). This concentration of AA in the arterial inflow of the normally perfused paw caused only a moderate increase in blood flow of approximately 23% during its infusion. PGE_2 itself, infused at a rate that established a concentration range of 2.0-5.1 ng/ml in these experiments, almost abolished the responses to NE. These concentrations of PGE_2 also markedly increased paw blood flow by approximately 100%. In the pump-perfused paw, PGE_2 in this concentration range caused a similar decrease in the NE response as that produced by AA (18). This disproportionality between the effects of AA and PGE_2 on responses to NE in the pump-perfused and normally perfused paw suggested to us that more PGE_2 or possibly other products are formed from AA in the pump-perfused preparation compared to that in the normal paw.

Estimation of Prostaglandin Synthesis from AA in Normal and Pump-Perfused Paw

AA, prepared as the sodium salt, was infused (75-200 μg/min) into the paw through the cranial tibial artery while the paw was perfused first normally and subsequently in the same experiment with a Sigmamotor pump. The saphenous venous outflow was shunted into the femoral vein using a catheter with a T tube for collection of blood samples. Four milliliters of arterial and saphenous vein samples were taken during a control period prior to the AA infusion and 10 min after beginning the infusion while the paw was perfused normally. The preparation was then converted from normal to pump perfusion, and 30-61 min allowed to pass before a second pair of control samples were taken. The infusion of AA was repeated under the conditions of constant flow and blood samples were withdrawn as during normal perfusion. Meclofenamate sodium (2 and 4 μg/ml) or indomethacin (2 μg/ml) were administered intraarterially for 20 min and blood sampling repeated immediately after the infusion. AA was then administered again after PG synthesis blockade and blood sampling repeated. Plasma was separated from the blood, the PGs in the samples were extracted, and PGE was separated from PGF on silicic acid columns as described previously (24). PGE was analyzed by using a PGE antiserum, 1/3000 or PGF antiserum, 1/800 and PGF was

TABLE 1 PELM (pg/ml in PGE_2 equivalents) in Arterial (A) and Saphenous Vein (V) Plasma During Normal and Pump Perfusion and the Effect of AA and PG Synthesis Inhibition

	Normal perfusion				Pump perfusion							
									PG synthesis inhibition[a]			
	Control		AA		Control		AA		Control		AA	
	A1	V1	A2	V2	A3	V3	A4	V4	A5	V5	A6	V6
Mean	210	223	193	803	222	404	200	1576	219	514	184	573
SEM	57	44	40	274	59	84	48	310	45	110	49	130
n	15		15		15		15		13		12	

[a]Indomethacin was infused for 20 min to achieve a concentration of 2 μg/ml of paw arterial blood in five experiments and meclofenamate was infused for 20 min at 2 or 4 μg/ml in eight experiments.

determined using a 1/5000 dilution of the PGF antiserum. By utilizing the cross-reactivity of the PGF antiserum with PGE, the analysis of PGE was accomplished using this antiserum. PGF antiserum in the dilution of 1/800 did not cross-react with PGA_2 or the 15-keto-PGE_2 metabolite. PGE antiserum did not cross react appreciably with PGA_2 or $PGF_{2\alpha}$ (0.7% and 1.7%, respectively) (personal communication, D. Van Orden). Determination of PGE using the PGE antiserum revealed no significant AV difference across the paw. PGE-like material (PELM), however, was present when measured with the PGF antiserum. The concentrations of PELM in arterial and venous plasma when measured in this manner are in Table 1. In the control period before infusion of AA into the normally perfused paw, the AV difference of PELM was -13 ± 33 SEM pg/ml, which was not statistically significant. During infusion of AA the venous PELM concentration increased, and although there was a marked degree of variability, the AV difference of -610 ± 275 achieved statistical significance ($p < 0.05$). After a period ranging from 30 to 61 min of pump perfusion, the control venous PELM level was increased compared to the control period during normal perfusion and the AV difference of -202 ± 78 pg/ml ($p < 0.05$) was attained. Infusion of AA during pump perfusion achieved the highest venous PELM level (1576 pg/ml) and an AV difference of -1375 ± 298 pg/ml ($p < 0.001$). This AV difference was greater than that found during normal perfusion. In order to determine whether the quantity of PELM synthesized from AA was greater during the pump perfusion than during normal perfusion, the control AV differences during normal and pump perfusion were subtracted from the corresponding values attained during infusion of AA. Because in 11 of 15 experiments the resulting difference was greater during pump perfusion than that found during normal perfusion but in 4 experiments it was not, statistical significance utilizing a conventional paired t test was not achieved. However, when Wilcoxon's rank test for paired differences was utilized, the difference was greater during pump perfusion ($p < 0.02$). After administration of a PGSI, either meclofenamate or indomethacin, the AV difference of PELM attained during pump perfusion still remained in 9 of 13 experiments. Infusion of AA did not, however, increase further the venous level of PELM or the AV difference, which is suggestive of effective inhibition of the synthetase enzyme. The quantity of PGF formed from AA which was determined using the PGF antiserum was generally less than that of PELM, but appeared to parallel PELM in the normal and pump-perfused paw.

Blood pressure, blood flow, perfusion pressure, and the changes in blood flow and perfusion pressure caused by AA during normal or pump perfusion, respectively, are listed in Table 2. AA caused variable changes in flow with little or no mean change. In nine experiments flow was increased, in three experiments it was decreased, and a biphasic change in flow occurred in two experiments. During pump perfusion there was a more consistent vasoconstrictor effect obtained with AA, which accounted for the increase in perfusion pressure of 55 ± 18 ($p < 0.01$). This vasoconstrictor effect of AA was not consistently altered following PGSI. Apparently, the vasoconstrictor response predominated and masked any vasodilator effect attributable to PELM. Because the PGSIs, indomethacin and meclofenamate, would be expected to block the vascular responses due to the PGs and other cyclooxygenase products formed from AA, this vasoconstrictor action of AA is attributable to another substance formed from AA or to AA itself. Since the lipoxygenase-like enzyme is not inhibited by these agents, it is possible that another substance obtained by the action of this enzyme on AA produced the vasoconstrictor response.

Effect of AA on Isolated Paw Veins

It is conceivable that the variable effects of AA on paw blood flow and its PGSI-resistant vasoconstrictor effect in the pump perfused paw could in part reflect effects of AA on the venous segment of the paw vasculature. Venous and arterial smooth muscle may respond differently to given AA products and/or synthesize different products from this fatty acid. Several investigators have suggested that an increased ratio of vasoconstrictor to vasodilator PGs synthesized by veins may participate in the venoconstrictor activity of various substances. For instance, bradykinin enhanced formation of PGF-like material by the bovine mesenteric veins (26), which would correlate with the venoconstrictor activity of this agent. However, the effect of PGSIs on canine vein responses to bradykinin suggested that endogenous vasodilator PGs tend to oppose bradykinin-induced venoconstriction (27,28).

TABLE 2 Systemic Blood Pressure (BP, mmHg), Paw Blood Flow (F, ml/min) and Perfusion Pressure (PP, mmHg), and Changes Elicited by AA

	Normal perfusion				Pump perfusion									
										PG synthesis inhibition				
	Control		AA		Control			AA		Control			AA	
	BP	F	F	ΔF	BP	F	PP	PP	ΔPP	BP	F	PP	PP	ΔPP
Mean	141	34.5	35.4	-0.3	132	34.0	90	90	55	133	33	122	120	51
SEM	4.5	3.0	2.7	4.8	6.9	2.2	7.3	7.0	18	7.4	2.6	12	13.4	15.8
n	15		15		15			15		13			13	

Our experiments were undertaken in an attempt to further clarify the overall influence of the PG system on the paw vasculature and to investigate the possible participation of paw veins in the response of the intact paw to AA. An isolated vascular preparation was employed for these experiments in order to eliminate complicating factors (e.g., possible synthesis by platelets of non-PG products from AA) which can occur in vivo. The isolated canine lateral saphenous vein (SV) was employed for several reasons. The canine SV contains a relatively large amount of smooth muscle (29) and is very responsive to PGs. Isolated strips of SV, when precontracted with phenylephrine, are relaxed by low concentrations of PGE_2 (30) just as small paw vessels respond in vivo and the SV contracts in response to $PGF_{2\alpha}$. The SV can produce PG from endogenous precursors (31) and it was suggested that this formation mediates in part the venoconstrictor effects of ergotamine and dihydroergotamine (31,32). These workers also reported differential effects of AA on isolated dog paw arteries (relaxation) and SV (contraction) (32).

Segments of SV were cleaned of loose connective tissue and cut helically into strips of approximately 2.5 × 30 mm. The strips were suspended under a 1-g load in a 2-ml organ bath containing Krebs solution at 37.5°C and gassed with 5% CO_2 in O_2. Changes in vein strip length were monitored with a Harvard isotonic transducer fitted with an "auxotonic" pendulum lever (33). PGE_2 and AA (sodium salts) and glyceryl trinitrate were added directly to the muscle bath by microsyringe in a noncumulative fashion, the tissue being washed by overflow after 1 min of dose contact and allowed to recover before subsequent doses. Phenylephrine HCl and PGSI (sodium salts) were added as required to a reservoir supplying (1 ml/min) the muscle bath. In some experiments the wash effluent (10 min collection) was collected for subsequent PG analysis by methods described previously (34,35).

Effect of AA on Precontracted SV Strips

Individual SV preparations were contracted with a concentration of phenylephrine (0.2-0.4 μM) sufficient to elicit a steady submaximal contraction of the SV (25 ± 4% of maximal phenylephrine contraction). The contracted SV responded to AA (0.5-50 μM) in a concentration-dependent biphasic manner. With the lowest concentrations tested (0.5 and 2.5 μM), AA typically caused a slowly developing relaxation of long duration (Fig. 1). In 1 of the 11 experiments in which these levels of AA were tested, these and higher concentrations caused only venoconstriction. Since the SV from this dog was also relatively unresponsive to the relaxant effect of PGE_2, this experiment was arbitrarily omitted from the summary calculations of the data (Fig. 2). Although relaxation was the only measurable response to these lower concentrations of AA, the response was typically delayed (Fig. 1) and in some experiments did not develop until the wash cycle was initiated. The character of the response might suggest the concomitant formation of labile venoconstrictor substance(s) which may oppose the relaxant effect. Intermediate

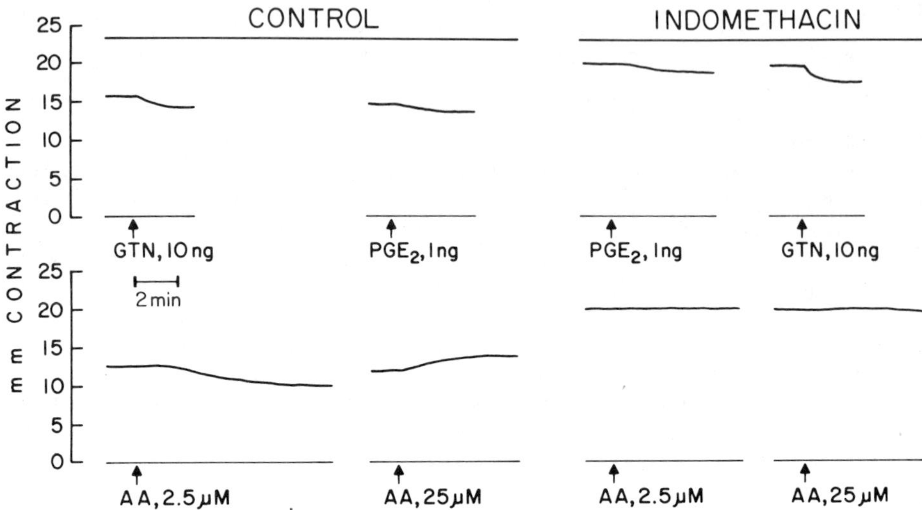

FIG. 1. Effects of arachidonic acid (AA), prostaglandin E_2 (PGE_2), and glyceryl trinitrate (GTN) on the isolated canine lateral saphenous vein before and during treatment with indomethacin (1.4 μM). Actual changes in muscle length are shown. The vein strip was submaximally contracted with phenylephrine (0.2 μM) from the resting length, indicated as 0 on the ordinate.

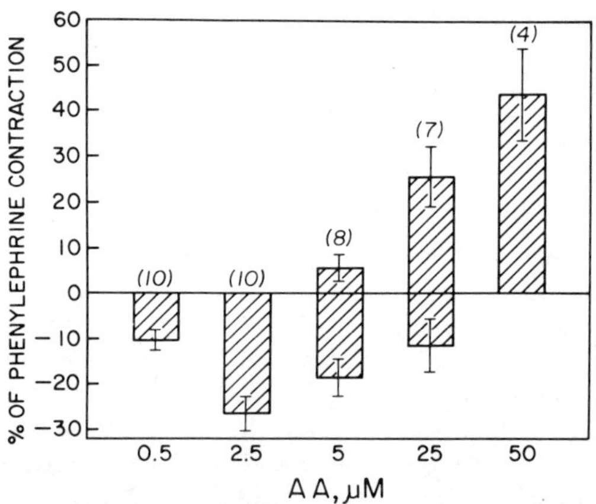

FIG. 2. Summary data of effect of arachidonic acid (AA) on saphenous vein contractility. Changes in muscle length induced by AA are depicted as a percentage of the phenylephrine-induced "tone" immediately preceding administration of AA. Numbers in parentheses indicate number of experiments in which the given AA concentrations are tested. Each experimental vein strip was obtained from a different dog. Contraction of the vein strip preceded relaxation when 5 and 25 μM concentrations of AA were administered.

concentrations of AA (5 and 25 μM) elicited biphasic responses, venoconstriction preceding relaxation (Fig. 2). Significant venorelaxation was observed in response to 5 μM AA, but the venorelaxation was quite delayed and was preceded by contraction of the SV in five of the eight experiments where this concentration of AA was employed. When the AA dose was increased further (25 μM, seven experiments), the dominant response was venoconstriction (Figs. 1 and 2). Four of the seven strips exhibited relaxation which was preceded by venoconstriction in six strips. In the four experiments where the highest concentration (50 μM) was tested, AA elicited venoconstriction only.

The AA product(s) mediating these effects were not identified in the present study. In preliminary experiments, we were unable to detect either basal or AA-stimulated release of a PGE-like substance into the bathing medium (10-min collection during the relaxant response) using either bioassay (34) or liquid chromatographic (35) methods. Radioimmunoassay or extraction of larger samples and/or pooling of samples may be required in future experiments. Moreover, since the magnitude of the relaxant response could usually be matched by very small (1-4 ng) quantities of PGE_2, the participation of this PG in the relaxant component of the AA response could not be ruled out. On the other hand, mediation of the contractile response by $PGF_{2\alpha}$ is unlikely, because the gerbil colon assay would easily have detected the amount of $PGF_{2\alpha}$ (25-50 ng) necessary to match the contractile response evoked by the higher AA concentrations unless a major fraction of the PG was metabolized by the SV strip.

Inhibition of SV Responses to AA by PGSI

The effects of the PGSIs, indomethacin and naproxen, on the AA-induced responses were examined in eight of the experiments described above. Indomethacin (four experiments, 1.4-14 μM) completely blocked both the relaxant and contractile components of the AA effect; however, in two experiments, PGE_2-induced relaxation was reduced by the higher concentrations (7 and 14 μM) of indomethacin. In four experiments 10 μM naproxen blocked AA effects without significantly affecting responses to PGE_2. Both PGSI caused substantial (approximately 25% of maximal) and sustained additional contraction of phenylephrine-contracted SV strips (Fig. 1, indomethacin). These experiments indicate that the biphasic effect of AA is probably due to the activity of cyclooxygenase product(s) rather than AA itself or products (HPETE, HETE) of the lipoxygenase-like enzyme. In some experiments a delayed relaxation of the SV strip was observed following administration of high concentrations of AA (25 and 50 μM) to PGSI-treated preparations, although the usual venoconstrictor effect was blocked. We cannot explain this effect at this time, although it may be due to a nonspecific depressant effect of high doses of the fatty acid which might have been masked in the control period by the venoconstrictor response. A depressant effect of non-PG precursor fatty acids on isolated strips of canine coronary artery which was not blocked by PGSIs has been described recently (36).

The present experiments provide additional information on the role of endogenous PGs as modulators of cutaneous vascular reactivity. Our data indicate the potential for opposing influences of endogenous products of PG synthetase on paw vein contractility. The findings supplement previous work by others, but differ in two respects. First, a depressant effect of low, perhaps more physiological, concentrations of AA on vein contractility was uncovered. This effect might have been masked in previous studies (31,32) due to the protocol these workers employed (cumulative concentration-effect curves). Since our work suggested that concomitant formation of venoconstrictor (perhaps labile) and relaxant material(s) followed AA administration, further elevation of AA levels before wash periods (31,32) may have masked expression of the depressant activity. The second major difference concerns the effect of PGSI on SV contractility. In our experiments indomethacin and naproxen invariably elicited additional contraction of SV strips precontracted with phenylephrine, whereas indomethacin antagonized SV contraction induced by ergotamine and dihydroergotamine (31,32) but did not affect responses to norepinephrine (27,31,32). We have no explanation for the differing effects of PGSI on vein contractility at this time, but collectively, these studies suggest that the PG system might modulate responses to different venoconstrictors by synthesis of different ratios of vasodilator and vasoconstrictor substances from AA.

DISCUSSION

A variety of factors can stimulate the in vivo synthesis of PGs. Renal ischemia, adrenergic and somatic nerve stimulation, mechanical stimulation of certain tissues, blood clotting, angiotensin II, bradykinin, norepinephrine, and other chemical agents as well as supplying exogenous precursor, AA, can cause increased generation of PGs in intact or artificially perfused organs. One mechanism proposed to account for accelerated PG synthesis by a drug is an increased availability of endogenous AA. It has been suggested that angiotensin stimulates PGE synthesis in rat renal papilla by freeing endogenous AA and making it available to the synthetase enzyme (37). Based on our in vivo data presented above there was no evidence of basal PG synthesis in the normally perfused cutaneous vasculature of the dog's paw. No significant AV differences of PELM existed when the vascular bed was normally perfused. However, although there was no measurable AV difference of PGE or PELM, synthesis may still be occurring in the cutaneous tissue without significant quantities reaching the venous outflow. This possibility is suggested by the finding of a decrease in blood flow caused by PGSI in the normally perfused paw (38) presumably due to the elimination of PGE. Supplying the substrate AA in vivo resulted in PG synthesis as reflected by the significant AV difference of PELM attained. Pump perfusion itself appeared not only to increase PG synthesis, but also increased the capacity for synthesis when substrate was provided. We consider this to be a very important finding. Heretofore, the limiting factor in PG synthesis was believed to be the quantity of substrate available to the PG synthetase enzyme. Bridenbaugh et al. (39) have also reported that the conditions of the experiment (i.e., the shock state), rather than the supply of AA alone, determined the quantity of PG synthetized in vivo. The exact identity of the PELM analyzed in our experiments by radioimmunoassay is not known. It is not likely to be PGE itself since it was not detectable by use of a PGE specific antiserum, but it was bound more readily by a PGF antiserum. It is conceivable that PELM is a PGE metabolite which is eluted with the PGE fraction from the silicic acid column we employ or which elutes with a portion of the PGA fraction which may not be completely separated from the PGE fraction.

The variable effects of exogenous AA on the intact paw vasculature are probably attributable to the variety of AA metabolites which might potentially be formed upon presentation of this fatty acid to the numerous cell types (e.g., platelets, endothelial cells, smooth muscle) present in an intact preparation. The presence in canine vasculature and platelets of enzyme systems which generate some of these products (e.g., thromboxane, HPETE, PGI) as well as definition of their effects on small vessels has not been documented, but it is likely that these or similar AA metabolites contribute to the complex response of the paw vasculature to exogenous AA. The effects of these substances on different dog paw vessels are yet to be defined.

DIRECTIONS OF FUTURE RESEARCH

Numerous investigations not discussed here have demonstrated potent pharmacologic effects of various PGs on the cutaneous vasculature. However, our knowledge of PGs' role(s) in the physiologic regulation of this vascular bed is incomplete. Studies by others and our own work amply demonstrate the potential for endogenous generation of PGs in or near skin vessels, but do not clarify which, if any, physiological interventions might activate the cutaneous PG synthetase system and whether this effects local changes in blood flow.

One area that certainly warrants further investigation concerns the possible involvement of PGs in local vascular responses to heat stimuli. It has already been demonstrated (2) that local production of PGs by skin increases in response to heat injury. Further experiments, perhaps utilizing PGSI and radioactive microspheres, could ascertain whether this response (e.g., increased PG synthesis) to traumatic heat stimuli contributes to local changes in blood flow. Prostaglandins might also modulate cutaneous vascular responses to less traumatic heat stimuli. Although it is felt that PGs might be involved in the central regulation of body temperature, it is not known whether an increase in the ambient temperature elicits elevated PG synthesis which could contribute to local vasodilatation. Again, this question could be approached utilizing PGSI and microspheres. It would also be important to determine whether any PG involvement uncovered is operative in the conscious animal.

The PGs might also be involved in cutaneous neurogenic vasodilator mechanisms. As discussed above, the present data suggest that vasodilator PGs are not responsible for sustained sympathetic vasodilatation in the dog's paw; however, this question should be reexamined using PGSIs in concentrations which are shown to, in fact, suppress PG synthesis in the dog's paw. As shown here and in other studies (unpublished) in our laboratories, it is difficult to reduce in situ paw vascular responses to AA by PGSI in concentrations that are effective in vitro. The specificity of any observed PGSI alteration of sympathetic vasodilatation could be assessed by simultaneous monitoring of the activity of other vasodilator systems (e.g., sympathetic cholinergic vasodilatation in skeletal muscle).

In view of the recent advances concerning PG and non-PG products of AA metabolism, the need for additional studies to clarify the pharmacologic effects of these compounds is clear. Insight into the potential endogenous generation and effects of these compounds (e.g., PG endoperoxide intermediates, thromboxanes, HETE, PGI) on cutaneous vessels could be gained from a combination of approaches, including study of pharmacologic effects of purified compounds, effects of AA in the presence of PGSI (indomethacin and ETA) and in the presence of inhibitors of PGI formation [15-hydroperoxy-AA (40)], and measurement of AA metabolites in the paw venous effluent.

ACKNOWLEDGMENT

This work was supported by National Institutes of Health Grants HL-08570, HL-15447, and HL-17871.

REFERENCES

1. Dunham, E. W., Rolewicz, T., and Zimmerman, B. G. Prostaglandin as the possible mediator of cutaneous sympathetic vasodilation. Fed. Proc. 27:536, 1968.
2. Ängaård, E., and Jonsson, C. E. Efflux of prostaglandins in lymph from scalded tissue. Acta physiol. scand. 81:440-447, 1971.
3. Jouvenaz, G. H., Nugteren, D. H., Beerthius, R. K., and van Dorp, D. A. A sensitive method for the determination of prostaglandins by gas chromatography with electron-capture detection. Biochim. Biophys. Acta 202:231-234, 1970.
4. Ziboh, V. A., and Hsia, S. L. Prostaglandin E_2: biosynthesis and effects on glucose and lipid metabolism in rat skin. Arch. Biochem. Biophys. 146:100-109, 1971.

5. Tan, W. C., and Privett, O. S. Studies on detection and synthesis of prostaglandins in tail skin of the rat. Lipids 8:166-169, 1973.
6. Söndergaard, J., and Greaves, M. W. Pharmacological studies in inflammation due to exposure to ultraviolet radiation. J. Pathol. 101: 93-97, 1970.
7. Greaves, M. W., Söndergaard, J., and McDonald-Gibson, W. Recovery of prostaglandins in human cutaneous inflammation. Br. Med. J. 2:258-260, 1971.
8. Jonsson, C. E. Biosynthesis and metabolism of prostaglandin E_2 in human skin. Scand. J. Clin. Lab. Invest. 29:289-296, 1972.
9. Ängaård, E., and Strandberg, K. J. Efflux of prostaglandin from cat paws perfused with compound 48/80. Acta physiol. scand. 82:333-344, 1971.
10. Celander, O., and Folkow, B. A comparison of the sympathetic vasomotor fibre control of the vessels within the skin and the muscles. Acta physiol. scand. 29:241-250, 1953.
11. Davis, D. L., and Hamilton, W. F. Small vessel responses of the dog paw. Am. J. Physiol. 196:1316-1321, 1959.
12. Zimmerman, B. G. Sympathetic vasodilatation in the dog's paw. J. Pharmacol. Exp. Ther. 152:81-87, 1966.
13. Folkow, B., and Sivertsson, R. Aspects of the difference in vascular "reactivity" between cutaneous resistance vessels and A-V anastomoses. Angiologica 1:338-345, 1964.
14. Zimmerman, B. G., and Whitmore, L. Transmitter release in skin and muscle blood vessels during sympathetic stimulation. Am. J. Physiol. 212:1043-1053, 1967.
15. Folkow, B. Autoregulation in muscle and skin. Circ. Res. 14/15(Suppl. I):19-29, 1964.
16. Henriksen, O., Nielsen, S. L., Paaske, W. P., and Sejrsen, P. Autoregulation of blood flow in human cutaneous tissue. Acta physiol. scand. 89:538-543, 1973.
17. Gomer, S. K., and Zimmerman, B. G. Effect of indomethacin and other agents on sustained sympathetic vasodilatation in the dog's paw. 5th Int. Congr. Pharmacol., p. 84, 1972.
18. Zimmerman, B. G., Ryan, M. J., Gomer, S., and Kraft, E. Effect of the prostaglandin synthesis inhibitors indomethacin and eicosa-5,8,11, 14-tetraynoic acid on adrenergic responses in dog cutaneous vasculature. J. Pharmacol. Exp. Ther. 187:315-323, 1973.
19. Hedqvist, P. Control by prostaglandin E_2 of sympathetic neurotransmission in the spleen. Life Sci. Part I Physiol. Pharmacol. 9:269-278, 1970.
20. Hedqvist, P., Stjärne, L., and Wennmalm, A. Inhibition by prostaglandin E_2 of sympathetic neurotransmission in the rabbit heart. Acta physiol. scand. 79:139-141, 1970.

21. Kadowitz, P. J., Sweet, C. S., and Brody, M. J. Differential effects of prostaglandins E_1, E_2, $F_{1\alpha}$ and $F_{2\alpha}$ in the dog hindpaw. J. Pharmacol. Exp. Ther. 177:641-649, 1971.
22. Kadowitz, P. J. Effect of prostaglandins E_1, E_2 and A_2 on vascular resistance and responses to noradrenaline, nerve stimulation and angiotensin in dog hindlimb. Br. J. Pharmacol. 46:395-400, 1972.
23. Piper, P. J., and Vane, J. R. Release of prostaglandins from lung and other tissues. Ann. N.Y. Acad. Sci. 180:363-385, 1971.
24. Satoh, S., and Zimmerman, B. G. Renal effect of meclofenamate in presence and absence of superfusion bioassay. Am. J. Physiol. 230: 711-714, 1976.
25. Ryan, M. J., and Zimmerman, B. G. Effect of prostaglandin precursors, dihomo-γ-linolenic acid and arachidonic acid on the vasoconstrictor response to norepinephrine in the dog paw. Prostaglandins 6:179-192, 1974.
26. Terragno, D. A., Crowshaw, K., Terragno, N. A., and McGiff, J. C. Prostaglandin synthesis by bovine mesenteric arteries and veins. Circ. Res. 36(Suppl. I):76-80, 1975.
27. Goldberg, M. R., Joiner, P. D., Greenberg, S., Hyman, A. L., and Kadowitz, P. J. Effects of indomethacin on venoconstrictor responses to bradykinin and norepinephrine. Prostaglandins 9:385-390, 1975.
28. Goldberg, M. R., Chapnick, B. M., Joiner, P. D., Hyman, A. L., and Kadowitz, P. J. Influence of inhibitors of prostaglandin synthesis on venoconstrictor responses to bradykinin. J. Pharmacol. Exp. Ther. 198:357-365, 1976.
29. Coimbra, A., Ribeiro-Silva, A., and Oswald, W. Fine structural and autoradiographic study of the adrenergic innervation of the dog lateral saphenous vein. Blood Vessels 11:128-144, 1974.
30. Dunham, E. W., Haddox, M. K., and Goldberg, N. D. Alteration of vein cyclic 3':5' nucleotide concentrations during changes in contractility. Proc. Natl. Acad. Sci. USA 71:815-819, 1974.
31. Müller-Schweinitzer, E., and Brundell, J. Enhanced prostaglandin synthesis contributes to the venoconstrictor activity of ergotamine. Blood Vessels 12:193-205, 1975.
32. Müller-Schweinitzer, E., and Brundell, J. Modification of canine vascular smooth muscle responses to dihydroergotamine by endogenous prostaglandin synthesis. Eur. J. Pharmacol. 34:197-206, 1975.
33. Paton, W. D. M. A pendulum auxotonic lever. J. Physiol. 137:35P-36P, 1957.
34. Dunham, E. W., and Zimmerman, B. G. Release of prostaglandin-like material from dog kidney during nerve stimulation. Am. J. Physiol. 219:1279-1285, 1970.
35. Dunham, E. W., and Anders, M. W. High-speed liquid chromatographic analysis of prostaglandins in rat kidney. Prostaglandins 4:85-92, 1973.

36. Kulkarni, P. S., Roberts, R., and Needleman, P. Paradoxical synthesis of a coronary dilating substance from arachidonate. Prostaglandins 12:337-353, 1976.
37. Danon, A., Chang, L., Sweetman, B., Nies, A., and Oates, J. Synthesis of prostaglandins by the rat renal papilla in vitro; mechanism of stimulation by angiotensin II. Biochim. Biophys. Acta 388:71-83, 1975.
38. Ryan, M. J., Sugawara, K., Kraft, E., and Zimmerman, B. G. J. Pharmacol. Exp. Ther. 200:606-613, 1977.
39. Bridenbaugh, G. A., Flynn, J. T., and Lefer, A. M. Arachidonic acid in splanchnic artery occlusion shock. Am. J. Physiol. 231:112-119, 1976.
40. Moncada, S., Gryglewski, R., Bunting, S., and Vane, J. A lipid peroxide inhibits the enzyme in blood vessel microsomes that generates from prostaglandin endoperoxides the substance (prostaglandin X) which prevents platelet aggregation. Prostaglandins 12:715-737, 1976.

5 Prostaglandins and Uterine Blood Flow

KENNETH E. CLARK* / MICHAEL J. BRODY / University of Iowa College of Medicine, Iowa City, Iowa

The uterus is a dynamic organ whose hemodynamics are changing constantly. Like other vascular beds the basic factors regulating uterine blood flow are arterial pressure and vascular resistance. While arterial pressure remains relatively constant, uterine vascular resistance is dramatically altered, for example, during the estrous cycle (1) and pregnancy (2).

The role of prostaglandins in uterine physiology has been extensively investigated and numerous reviews dealing with the function of these acidic lipids in reproduction are available (3,4). The present chapter is limited to the effect of prostaglandins on uterine hemodynamics in both the nonpregnant and pregnant state. At present, the majority of observations in this area of research have been in experimental animals. Based on these experimental observations, it appears that these agents may play a major role in regulating uterine blood flow. In addition, increasing amounts of experimental evidence indicate that, at least in some cases of toxemia in pregnancy, the underlying etiology may be a failure in the production of vasodilator prostaglandins by the uteroplacental unit.

METHOD FOR STUDYING UTERINE HEMODYNAMICS

Much of the research on the effects of prostaglandins on the nonpregnant uterine vasculature has been carried out in our laboratories using the pump-perfused canine uterus (5). In this model, nonpregnant mongrel dogs were anesthetized with pentobarbital sodium and placed in the supine position. The exact phase of the estrous cycle in each animal was not known, except that these animals were not in heat. Animals were intubated so that the positive pressure ventilation could be administered via a respirator when required. The brachial artery and vein were cannulated to allow continuous monitoring

*Present affiliation: University of Cincinnati College of Medicine, Cincinnati, Ohio

of systemic arterial pressure and administration of drugs, respectively. The uterus was exposed via a midline incision and the uterine vasculature was completely isolated by ligating the ovarian artery and collateral arteries in the mesometrium. Following heparinization, the uterine artery was cannulated and the uterus perfused with a pulsatile pump at a constant rate of flow with blood from the femoral artery. Uterine perfusion pressure was determined from a T fitting placed between the pump and point of cannulation of the uterine artery. Uterine blood flow was adjusted until uterine perfusion pressure was approximately equal to systemic arterial blood pressure. Since blood flow remained constant throughout all experiments using this model, changes in uterine perfusion pressure reflect changes in uterine vascular resistance; i.e., decreases in uterine perfusion pressure are due to decreases in uterine vascular resistance (vasodilation). Uterine perfusion pressure and systemic arterial blood pressure were recorded. Periarterial uterine nerve stimulation was accomplished by placing the uterine artery, vein, and surrounding tissue on a bipolar stainless steel electrode. A detailed description of these methods is printed elsewhere (5).

The pump-perfused canine uterus provides a stable preparation to investigate the direct and indirect effects of both exogenous and endogenous prostaglandins. This vascular bed is innervated by sympathetic vasoconstrictor fibers, and frequency-dependent vasoconstrictor responses to uterine nerve stimulation have been obtained (5). The preparation also provides for direct intraarterial injection of norepinephrine, which allows for assessment of the effects of prostaglandins and other agents on adrenergic neurotransmission at both pre- and postjunctional levels.

EFFECTS OF EXOGENOUS PROSTAGLANDINS ON UTERINE VASCULAR RESISTANCE

Prostaglandins have two major actions on uterine vascular smooth muscle: (1) Direct effects producing either relaxation or vasoconstriction and (2) indirect effects produced by modifying adrenergic vasoconstrictor activity. The direct effects of these compounds on uterine vascular resistance have been reported (6, 7). These studies were carried out in the nonpregnant pump-perfused canine uterus. In these studies, the effects of PGA_1, PGE_1, PGE_2, and $PGF_{2\alpha}$ on uterine vascular resistance were determined. PGA_1, PGE_1, and PGE_2 were all found to be potent uterine vasodilators. When the relative vasodilator potencies of these compounds was determined in the same five preparations, the following order of vasodilator potency was determined by using a parallel-line bioassay (8): $PGE_1 > (9X)\ PGE_2 > (3X)\ PGA_1$ (7). $PGF_{2\alpha}$, on the other hand, did not have any intrinsic activity in the nonpregnant canine uterus at concentrations as high as 20 μg/ml of uterine blood flow (6). In contrast to the potent uterine vasodilator nature of PGE_1 in the nonpregnant animal, infusion of PGE_1 in doses from 1 to 100 μg/min into the uterine arterial vasculature of one horn of the near-term pregnant canine uterus produced no significant alterations in uterine perfusion pressure. As in the nonpregnant animal, $PGF_{2\alpha}$ did not alter uterine vascular resistance in the pump-perfused pregnant canine uterus. Other vasodilators, such as nitroglycerin, were also inactive, suggesting that little vascular tone is present in this preparation in late pregnancy (6).

In contrast, Nakajima and coworkers (9) reported that PGE_1 increases, while $PGF_{2\alpha}$ decreases, uterine blood flow in the autoperfused near-term pregnant canine uterus. These investigators injected a bolus of either PGE_1 (10-20 μg) or $PGF_{2\alpha}$ (10-100 μg) into the vasculature of a single conceptal segment of the pregnant horn, doses that probably result in much higher local concentrations than those used by Clark and coworkers (6).

Rankin and Phernetton (10) have reported that PGE_2 can significantly increase uterine blood flow in the unanesthetized late-term pregnant sheep. In these experiments, PGE_2 was given to the fetus and the increase in uterine blood flow was observed following placental transfer. This method was chosen because bolus administration of PGE_2 into the maternal left ventricle led to increased intrauterine pressure, which they suggested masked the PGE_2 induced uterine vasodilation. One of the major problems with this observation is the fact that PGE_2 must cross the placenta (rich in the prostaglandin dehydrogenase enzyme), pass into the maternal venous circulation, through the maternal lungs (known to be effective in degradation of PGEs), and then act on the uterine and renal vasculature. Thus the vasodilation observed may be due to the formation of a metabolite rather than the parent compound. Since uterine blood flow was measured using microspheres, the investigators had to know the exact time course of the events described above in order to detect the maximum effect. Data on uterine vascular effects might have been more reliable if lower doses of PGE_2, which might be below the threshold of myometrial effects, were given by intraarterial infusion to the mother.

Overall, it seems reasonable to conclude that prostaglandins can exert direct effects on the uterine vessels in both the pregnant and nonpregnant state; however, the vasodilator actions probably depend in large part on the existence of adequate vascular tone.

EFFECT OF EXOGENOUS PROSTAGLANDINS ON ADRENERGIC NEUROTRANSMISSION

Numerous reports exist on the effect of prostaglandins on adrenergic neurotransmission in nonuterine vascular beds (see Ref. 11). Research on the effect of exogenous prostaglandins on uterine adrenergic vasoconstrictor responses has been limited to the pump-perfused canine uterus (6, 7). In these experiments uterine vasoconstrictor responses to periarterial uterine sympathetic nerve stimulation and intraarterial injections of norepinephrine were determined during the intraarterial infusion of various prostaglandins. Each prostaglandin tested had differential effects on sympathetic neurotransmission and these effects (see Figs. 1-3) appear to be dose dependent.

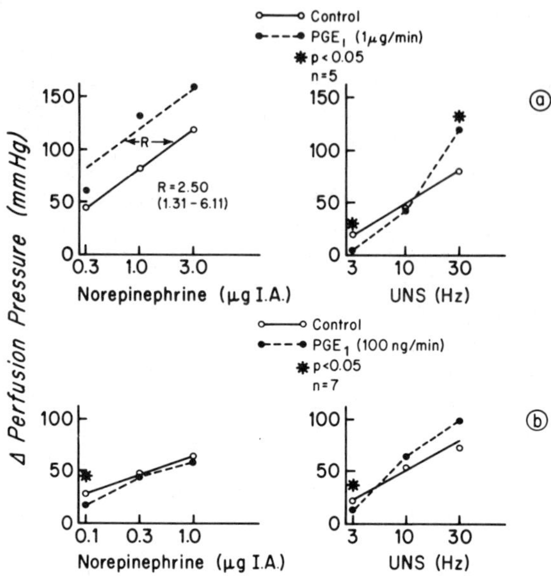

FIG. 1. (a) Effect of the intraarterial infusion of PGE_1 (1 μg/min) on uterine vasoconstrictor responses to uterine nerve stimulation and intraarterial norepinephrine in the nonpregnant dog. Each point is the mean of five animals. On the left, PGE_1 (1 μg/min) significantly shifted responses to intraarterial norepinephrine to the left in a parallel fashion and a relative potency ratio (R) of 2.50 with a 95% confidence interval of 1.31-6.11 was determined. On the right are shown vasoconstrictor responses to uterine nerve stimulations (UNS). PGE_1 (1 μg/min significantly depressed responses at 3 Hz, while it significantly potentiated responses at 30 Hz (paired t-test). (Adapted from Ref. 6 with permission from K. E. Clark, M. J. Ryan, and M. J. Brody, Effects of prostaglandins E_1 and $F_{2\alpha}$ on uterine hemodynamics and motility. In Advances in Biosciences, Vol. 9, S. Bergstrom (Ed.). Copyright 1973, Pergamon Press, Ltd.) (b) Effect of the intraarterial infusion of PGE_1 (100 ng/min) on uterine vasoconstrictor responses to intraarterial norepinephrine and uterine nerve stimulation. On the left, PGE_1 (100 ng/min) significantly depressed responses to the lowest dose of norepinephrine (0.1 μg I.A.), responses to higher doses of norepinephrine were not significantly altered. Right side: PGE_1 (100 ng/min) significantly depressed responses to uterine nerve stimulation at the lowest frequencies examined, 3 Hz (paired t test). Responses to uterine nerve stimulation were not significantly altered at higher frequencies (10 and 30 Hz). (Data from Ref. 7.)

PGE_1 1 μg/min (approximately 200 ng/ml of blood) produced a significant parallel shift in the dose-response curve to intraarterially injected norepinephrine. The potency ratio of 2.5 means that in the presence of PGE_1 the uterine vasculature responded to norepinephrine as if a 2.5 times greater dose had been administered. The effects on uterine nerve stimulation were biphasic, being significantly depressed at low frequency (3 Hz) and significantly potentiated at higher (30 Hz) frequency of stimulation (Fig. 1a). A tenfold reduction in PGE_1 concentration (approximately 20 ng/ml of blood) produced a completely different effect on norepinephrine-induced vasoconstrictor responses than was observed at the higher dose (Fig. 1b). At all the doses of norepinephrine tested responses were depressed. Responses to uterine nerve stimulation remained biphasic, like those seen at the higher dose of PGE_1 (Fig. 1b). Thus at this low dose of PGE_1 postjunctional responsiveness appears to be depressed since responses to both intraarterial nor-

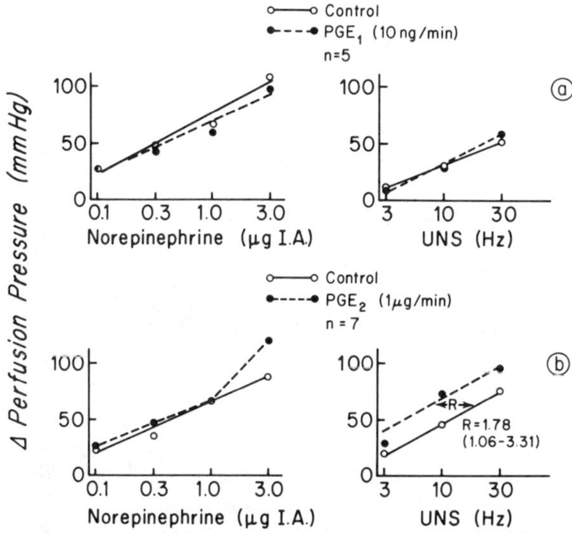

FIG. 2. (a) Effect of the intraarterial infusion of PGE_1 (10 ng/min) on uterine vasoconstrictor responses to intraarterial norepinephrine and uterine nerve stimulation (UNS). At this dose of PGE_1 (10 ng/min) neither responses to intraarterial norepinephrine nor uterine nerve stimulation were significantly altered, although uterine vascular resistance was significantly decreased. (Data from Ref. 7.) (b) Effect of the intraarterial infusion of PGE_2 (1 μg/min) on uterine vasoconstrictor responses to intraarterial norepinephrine and uterine nerve stimulation. Left-hand side: Responses to intraarterial norepinephrine were not significantly altered by PGE_2 (1 μg/min). Right-hand side: PGE_2 (1 μg/min) significantly shifted responses to uterine nerve stimulation to the left in a parallel fashion and a relative potency ratio of 2.50 and a 95% confidence interval of 1.06-3.31 was determined. (Data from Ref. 7.)

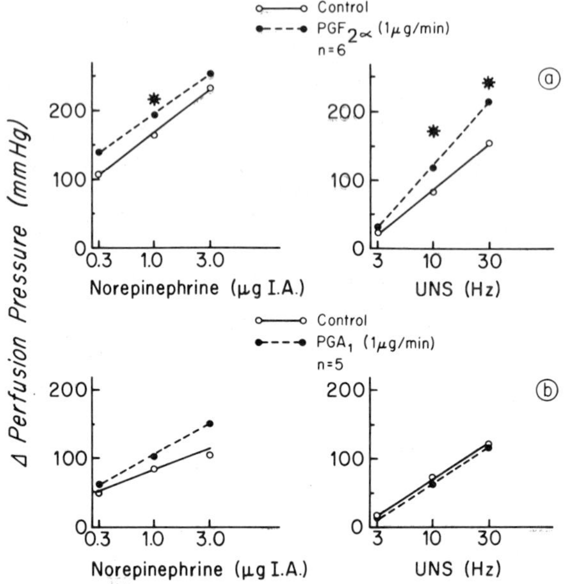

FIG. 3. (a) Effect of the intraarterial infusion of $PGF_{2\alpha}$ (1 μg/min) on uterine vasoconstrictor responses to intraarterial norepinephrine and uterine nerve stimulation (UNS). Left side: $PGF_{2\alpha}$ (1 μg/min) significantly increased (paired t test) vasoconstrictor responses to the intraarterial injection of 1 μg of norepinephrine. Responses at lower and higher doses were nonsignificantly increased. Right side: $PGF_{2\alpha}$ (1 μg/min) significantly increased ($^*p < 0.05$, paired t test) vasoconstrictor responses to uterine nerve stimulation at 10 and 30 Hz, but the lowest frequency tested (3 Hz) was not modified. (Adapted from Ref. 6 with permission from K. E. Clark, M. J. Ryan, and M. J. Brody, Effects of prostaglandins E_1 and $F_{2\alpha}$ on uterine hemodynamics and motility. In Advances in Biosciences, Vol. 9, S. Bergstrom (Ed.). Copyright 1973, Pergamon Press, Ltd.) (b) Effect of the intraarterial influsion of PGA_1 (1 μg/min) on uterine vasoconstrictor responses to intraarterial norepinephrine and uterine nerve stimulation. PGA_1 (1 μg/min) did not significantly alter vasoconstrictor respones to either norepinephrine or uterine nerve stimulation. (Data from Ref. 7.)

epinephrine and low-frequency uterine nerve stimulation were depressed. When the doe of PGE_1 was reduced further to 10 ng/min (approximately 2 ng/ml of blood), vasoconstrictor responses to norepinephrine and uterine nerve stimulation were no longer significantly modified (Fig. 2a) by PGE_1.

These results demonstrate that the effect of PGE_1 on adrenergic neurotransmission is dose dependent. Prostaglandins of the E series have generally been reported to depress vasoconstrictor responses to catecholamines in most vascular beds (11). Using high doses of PGE_1 (1 μg/min), responses to norepinephrine were potentiated (6). A similar observation has been made in another reproductive tissue, isolated seminal vesicles of guinea pigs (12). Lowering the concentration of PGE_1 leads to depression of postjunctional responsiveness to catecholamines, an action seen in most other vascular beds (11).

PGE_2 decreased uterine vascular resistance as did PGE_1, but unlike PGE_1 it acted prejunctionally (Fig. 2b) to produce a significant leftward shift in the dose-response curve to uterine nerve stimulation (7). The effect appears to be prejunctional in nature since responses to intraarterially injected norepinephrine were not significantly altered, while responses to nerve stimulation were potentiated. Kadowitz and coworkers (13, 14) observed similar effects in the perfused hindpaw preparation, whereas PGE_2 depressed responses to both intraarterial injections of norepinephrine and sympathetic nerve stimulation in the hindlimb (15). The effect of PGE_2 in the hindlimb appears to be due to postjunctional depression of the vascular smooth muscle to catecholamines (15). PGE_2 has also been shown to have different effects in other vascular beds (see Ref. 7 for discussion), suggesting that these effects on adrenergic vasoconstrictor responses appear to be organ, species, and concentration dependent.

$PGF_{2\alpha}$ (approximately 200 ng/ml of blood) potentiated responses to both intraarterial norepinephrine and uterine nerve stimulation. The effects of $PGF_{2\alpha}$ on responses to uterine nerve stimulation (Fig. 3a) were greater than those to norepinephrine, suggesting that $PGF_{2\alpha}$, like PGE_2, may act directly on the adrenergic nerve terminal to facilitate release of norepinephrine. The effects of $PGF_{2\alpha}$ on adrenergic neurotransmission in the uterus are similar to those seen in other vascular beds (14, 16).

The effect of PGA_1 on adrenergic neurotransmission is illustrated in Fig. 3b. Like PGE_1 and PGE_2, PGA_1 produced a significant reduction in uterine vascular resistance, but failed to significantly alter adrenergic vasoconstrictor responses. The failure to alter neurotransmission in the uterus is in contrast to the effects of PGA_1 in the perfused canine hindpaw, where vasoconstrictor responses to both intraarterial norepinephrine and sympathetic nerve stimulation were significantly depressed (13, 17).

In conclusion, prostaglandins of the A, E, and F series have differential effects on uterine adrenergic vasoconstrictor responses. These effects are dose dependent and appear to vary between species and organs. It is worth noting that the direct effect of these vasoactive agents can be separated from their effects on adrenergic neurotransmission. PGE_1 (lowest dose) and PGA_1 significantly reduced uterine vascular resistance without significantly modifying adrenergic vasoconstrictor responses. The results observed with $PGF_{2\alpha}$ provide additional evidence that the vasomotor effects of prostaglandins can be separated from their actions on adrenergic neurotransmission. $PGF_{2\alpha}$, unlike PGA_1 and PGE_1, does not alter uterine vascular resistance but potentiates responses to both intraarterial norepinephrine and uterine nerve stimulation.

ENDOGENOUS PROSTAGLANDINS

Prostaglandins of the E and F series are effectively cleared in a single pass through the lungs. If endogenous prostaglandins are to play an important role in regulating uterine hemodynamics, it is likely that they would be produced locally in the uterus. Prostaglandins have been shown to be synthesized in uterine tissue and uterine tissue levels are influenced by sex hormones (18, 19). The role of endogenous prostaglandins in regulating uterine vascular resistance has been extensively studied in the pump-perfused canine uterus (20). If endogenous prostaglandins play a role in regulating uterine hemodynamics, it would be expected: (1) that uterine venous prostaglandin levels would be elevated above arterial levels, and (2) that inhibition of endogenous prostaglandin production would lead to altered uterine vascular resistance.

Blood levels of immunoreactive PGEs and PGFs in arterial and uterine venous samples were determined by the radioimmunoassay of Van Orden and Farley (21). Prostaglandin F levels were 290 ± 105 pg/ml in arterial blood and significantly elevated to 1620 ± 119 pg/ml in uterine venous plasma. Prostaglandin E levels were relatively low in arterial plasma (280 ± 66 pg/ml) but extremely high in uterine venous plasma (4650 ± 750 pg/ml). These data suggested that prostaglandins of the E series appear to be present in concentrations consistent with a role in sustaining uterine blood flow. These elevated venous PGE and PGF levels were relatively specific for the uterus since venous prostaglandins from a second vascular bed, the gracilus muscle, were significantly lower (see Table 1).

The effect of endogenous prostaglandins on uterine vascular resistance and adrenergic neurotransmission is dependent on the summation of the effects of each prostaglandin present. In order to evaluate the effect of tonically released endogenous prostaglandins on uterine vascular resistance, the prostaglandin synthesis inhibitor meclofenamate (22) was infused intraarterially into the perfused uterus. In addition, a second vascular bed, the gracilis muscle, was used to determine the specificity of the inhibitor (20). The results of these experiments are shown in Table 1. During the mecofenamate infusion, uterine perfusion pressure was significantly elevated while immunoreactive PGEs were significantly reduced in uterine venous blood. These results are in contrast to the effect of meclofenamate on gracilis muscle vascular resistance. Gracilis muscle perfusion pressure was not significantly altered by meclofenamate and prostaglandin levels were not changed in gracilis muscle venous blood, suggesting that PGEs do not appear to play an important role in maintaining skeletal muscle blood flow. From these data it appears that prostaglandins of the E series may help sustain uterine blood flow in this nonpregnant animal preparation, since inhibition of their formation results in increased uterine vascular resistance.

Similar results have been reported in the pregnant dog (23), pregnant rabbits (24), and pregnant monkeys (25). In all three of these species administration of the prostaglandin synthesis inhibitor indomethacin led to reduced

TABLE 1 Effect of the Prostaglandin Synthesis Inhibitor Meclofenamate on Uterine and Gracilis Muscle Perfusion Pressure (mmHg, $\bar{x}$ diff. ± SE) and Uterine and Gracilis Muscle Venous Immunoreactive Prostaglandin Levels (ng/ml of plasma, $\bar{x}$ diff. ± SE)

	Uterine (n = 6)			Gracilis Muscle (n = 4)		
	Perfusion pressure			Perfusion pressure		
	Before meclofenamate	During meclofenamate	$\bar{x}$ ± SE	Before meclofenamate	During meclofenamate	$\bar{x}$ ± SE
	165	226	61 ± 7[a]	167	172	5 ± 5
	Uterine Venous Prostaglandin in level			Gracilus Muscle Venous PGE and PGF levels		
	Before meclofenamate	During meclofenamate	$\bar{x}$ ± SE	Before meclofenamate	During meclofenamate	$\bar{x}$ ± SE
PGE	4.65	2.28	2.37 ± 0.55[b]	0.96	0.52	0.44 ± 0.16
PGF	1.62	1.2	0.41 ± 0.40	0.32	0.26	0.06 ± 0.14

[a] $p < 0.001$.

[b] $p < 0.01$.

Source: Data from Ref. 20.

uterine blood flow, a decrease in uterine venous PGEs, and elevation of systemic arterial pressure. Thus vasodilator prostaglandins of the E series appear to play an important role in regulating uterine vascular resistance in both the nonpregnant and pregnant state. Since toxemia of pregnancy is know to be associated with reduced uterine blood flow (26,27), the observations described above have led to the postulation by numerous investigators that toxemia of pregnancy might be due in part to a lower than normal uterine production of vasodilator prostaglandins (20,23-25). Additional evidence in support of the postulate that toxemia is due to inadequate uterine production of vasodilator prostaglandin has recently been reported by Demers and Gabbe (28), who showed that prostaglandin E levels were significantly decreased in placental tissue from preeclamptic patients, while $PGF_{2\alpha}$ levels were significantly elevated above normal. A recent review of the role of prostaglandins in toxemia of pregnancy can be found elsewhere (29).

In addition to the direct effect on uterine vascular resistance, endogenous prostaglandins modify adrenergic vasoconstrictor responses in the uterine vasculature (20). Responses to intraarterially injected norepinephrine were significantly shifted to the left in the presence of meclofenamate, as were responses to uterine nerve stimulation (20). The magnitudes of the shifts were approximately the same, with potency ratios averaging 2.17 for norepinephrine and 1.71 for nerve stimulation. These data suggest that endogenous prostaglandins ordinarily act on uterine vascular smooth muscle to depress adrenergic responses to sympathetic nerve stimulation and to blood-borne catecholamines. This modulating effect is uncovered by removing the tonic formation of uterine prostaglandins.

In order to determine if the facilitation of vasoconstrictor responses in the uterine vascular smooth muscle was due to the lack of endogenous prostaglandins or a direct action by meclofenamate on the vascular smooth muscle, vasoconstrictor responses to norepinephrine were obtained prior to and during the infusion of meclofenamate in the gracilis muscle preparation. In contrast to the uterus, responses to intraarterial doses of norepinephrine in the gracilis muscle were not potentiated except at the highest dose of norepinephrine (20).

The effects of endogenous prostaglandins on adrenergic vasoconstrictor stimuli have not been evaluated in the pregnant uterus. However, it seems reasonable to expect that similar depression of vasoconstrictor responses would be observed. The ability of endogenous prostaglandins to relax vascular smooth muscle while simultaneously depressing vasoconstrictor responses is consistent with the proposed role of prostaglandins as humoral modulators of uterine hemodynamics. Since each prostaglandin has slightly different effects on vascular resistance and adrenergic neurotransmission, it seems possible that fluctuating levels of these humoral agents might be able to act like a fine tuning mechanism to meet the constantly changing hemodynamic needs of this organ.

EFFECT OF SYMPATHETIC NERVE STIMULATION ON RELEASE OF PROSTAGLANDINS

Both sympathetic nerve stimulation and norepinephrine have been shown to release prostaglandins from kidney, spleen, and other tissues (28,30-32). To determine if release of prostaglandins in the canine uterine vasculature was under neurogenic control, levels of immunoreactive prostaglandins of the E and F series were measured in uterine venous plasma during uterine nerve stimulation and intraarterial injections of norepinephrine (20). In these experiments neither PGE nor PGF uterine venous levels were significantly modified by these adrenergic vasoconstrictor stimuli. These results suggest that release of PGEs and PGFs may not be under neurogenic control, but rather may represent a tonic uterine synthesis of prostaglandins. An alternative interpretation of these data is that neurogenically released prostaglandins might be metabolized locally and thus would not be detected in uterine venous effluent. A third possibility is that prostaglandin-induced modification of adrenergic neurotransmission might be due to either an active prostaglandin intermediate such as an endoperoxide (33) or prostacyclin, substances that would not be detected by the assay method used in the present studies.

In the pump-perfused canine uterine preparation, uterine blood flow remains constant even during adrenergic vasoconstrictor responses which increase uterine vascular resistance. In vivo, vasoconstriction would lead to reduced uterine blood flow. The present data suggest that the tonic release of prostaglandins in the canine uterus would remain constant and thus the concentration of vasodilator prostaglandins per milliliter of blood would increase, leading to relaxation of the uterine vascular smooth muscle and a return of uterine blood flow toward control levels. Thus vasodilator prostaglandins may be important in maintaining uterine blood flow in the presence of both neurogenic and humoral vasoconstrictor influences. Greiss and Anderson (34) have recently presented evidence that uteri of both nonpregnant and pregnant sheep are able to autoregulate blood flow. The possibility that this uterine autoregulation is mediated by vasodilator prostaglandins seems reasonable but at present has not been investigated.

PROSTAGLANDIN RECEPTORS IN UTERINE VASCULAR SMOOTH MUSCLE

The concept that prostaglandin receptors exist in tissue is not new. Eliasson in 1966 (35) reported that minor alterations in prostaglandin structure produced differential effects in the smooth muscle of reproductive tissues. Pickles (36) examined the effects of six different prostaglandins on both human and guinea pig myometrium and on rabbit ileum. Based on the differential effects he observed, he hypothesized that two or more types of prostaglandin receptors must exist. Numerous reports have appeared in the literature dealing with specific binding studies (see 37,38). In these reports, binding sites for prostaglandins exhibited high affinity, saturability, and reversibility, suggesting that prostaglandin receptors do exist. These receptor sites are specific for one prostaglandin, but a second prostaglandin can compete for these binding sites.

As mentioned earlier, PGE_1, PGE_2, and PGA_1 are potent uterine vasodilators in the canine uterus (6, 7), whereas $PGF_{2\alpha}$ is without intrinsic activity on the uterine vasculature of this preparation (6). Thus if vasodilator prostaglandin receptors exist in uterine vascular smooth muscle, $PGF_{2\alpha}$ would be an excellent candidate for competitively antagonizing these vasoactive agents (37). Experiments were undertaken using the nonpregnant pump-perfused canine uterus model. Vasodilator responses to intraarterial infu-

TABLE 2 Mean Vasodilator Responses to PGA_1, PGE_1, or PGE_2 Infusion and Intraarterial Injections of Glyceryl Trinitrate (GTN) Before and During the Infusion of $PGF_{2\alpha}$ (10 μg/min)

Dose	Before $PGF_{2\alpha}$	During $PGF_{2\alpha}$	Mean difference ± SE	n
Antagonism of PGE_1-induced vasodilation by $PGF_{2\alpha}$ [a]				
PGE_1 10 ng/min	14	7	-7 ± 2*	6
PGE_1 100 ng/min	39	17	-22 ± 3*	6
PGE_1 1000 ng/min	75	57	-18 ± 4*	6
GTN 1.0 μg	21	23	+1 ± 4	4
Antagonism of PGE_2-induced vasodilation by $PGF_{2\alpha}$				
PGE_2 500 ng/min	29	20	-9 ± 6	5
PGE_2 1000 ng/min	33	23	-10 ± 1*	5
PGE_2 2000 ng/min	36	24	-12 ± 11	5
GTN 3 μg	21	25	+4 ± 3	5
10 μg	36	50	+14 ± 7	5
Antagonism of PGA_1-induced vasodilation by $PGF_{2\alpha}$				
PGA_1 500 ng/min	16	10	-6 ± 2*	4
PGA_1 1000 ng/min	18	8	-11 ± 5	4
PGA_1 2000 ng/min	30	17	-13 ± 5*	4
GTN 3 μg	32	31	-1 ± 1	3
10 μg	45	42	-3 ± 2	3

[a] Vasodilator responses (mmHg decrease).
Source: From Ref. 37.

sions of several doses of either PGE_1, PGE_2 or PGA_1 or intraarterial injection of the direct-acting vasodilator glyceryl trinitrate (GTN) were obtained (Table 2). Following control responses, a continuous intraarterial infusion of $PGF_{2\alpha}$ was started and vasodilator responses to the prostaglandins and GTN were repeated. Vasodilator responses to PGA_1, PGE_1, and PGE_2 were decreased during the infusion of $PGF_{2\alpha}$, suggesting that $PGF_{2\alpha}$ was able to compete with these vasodilator prostaglandins for receptor sites (Table 2). While dilator responses to PGE_1, PGE_2, and PGA_1 were reduced, responses to GTN were not significantly altered (Table 2). This suggests that the interaction between prostaglandins was specific and not merely the result of vasodilatation. Following cessation of the $PGF_{2\alpha}$ infusion, responses to the vasodilator prostaglandins returned toward control levels.

The importance of the observation that $PGF_{2\alpha}$ can antagonize PGA- and PGE-induced uterine vasodilation lies in the fact that vasodilator prostaglandins appear to play an important role in regulating uterine blood flow in both the nonpregnant (20) and pregnant uterus (23-25). The effect of endogenous prostaglandins on uterine blood flow may well depend upon the summation of PGA, PGE, and PGF effects. High uterine levels of $PGF_{2\alpha}$ might be able to reduce or modulate uterine blood flow by competitive antagonism of vasodilator prostaglandins. In addition, $PGF_{2\alpha}$ facilitates neurogenic vasoconstrictor responses in the canine uterus (6), while PGEs depress adrenergic neurotransmission (7). Thus in high concentrations, $PGF_{2\alpha}$ could produce reduction in uterine blood flow by two different mechanisms: (1) the competitive antagonism of vasodilator prostaglandins, and (2) the potentiation of adrenergic neurotransmission leading to increased vascular resistance.

Wakeling and coworkers (38) have reported that in uterine tissue of hamsters PGE_1 binding sites are affected by the stage of the estrous cycle, being maximal at proestrus. The possibility that cyclic changes occur in the number and structure of prostaglandin receptors in uterine vascular smooth muscle, although conceivable, has not been investigated. If the number of prostaglandin receptors in the vascular smooth muscle is under hormonal control, additional prostaglandin-mediated modulation of uterine hemodynamics might occur during pregnancy or the estrous or menstrual cycle. To add to the complexity of the role of prostaglandins in regulating uterine blood flow, estrogen has been shown to increase prostaglandin levels (18, 19, 39) and this increase in prostaglandin may be associated with estrogen-induced uterine vasodilation (19, 39).

EFFECTS OF PROSTAGLANDINS ON UTERINE BLOOD FLOW DISTRIBUTION

Since prostaglandins have been shown to be synthesized locally in the uterus (18, 19, 39), the possibility exists that these humoral agents may play an important role in the relative distribution of blood flow within the uterus. To determine if either exogenous or endogenous prostaglandins could alter blood flow distribution between the endometrium and myometrium, the following experiments were carried out (40).

Both horns of the canine uterus were pump perfused independently using separate perfusion pumps (5). Following stabilization of uterine perfusion pressure, radiolabeled microspheres (15 ± 5 μM, 3M Nuclear Products) were injected to evaluate the relative blood flow distribution between the endometrium and myometrium. Microspheres (^{141}Ce or ^{85}Sr) were suspended in a solution of saline and Tween 80 and were injected proximal to the perfusion pump of each horn to allow mixing with the arterial blood. Ten minutes later the experimental horn received an intraarterial infusion of either an exogenous prostaglandin (PGE_2, PGE_1, or $PGF_{2\alpha}$) or the prostaglandin synthesis inhibitor meclofenamate. The contralateral control horn received the corresponding vehicle. Except with the infusion of meclofenamate, uterine vascular resistance and the percent of blood flow to endometrium were not significantly modified in the control horn (Tables 3 and 4). Ten minutes after the initiation of this infusion, a second radiolabeled microsphere was injected. Each horn of the uterus was removed, divided into four or five pieces, and the endometrium and myometrium were separated.

Using this method the number of spheres or the amount of radioactivity is directly proportional to the blood flow to each tissue. In this preparation, uterine blood flow is held constant so that changes in the percent of blood flow to endometrium corresponds directly to modification of the amount of blood flow reaching each uterine tissue layer. In the canine uterus, the endometrium composes only a small percent (approximately 6%) of the uterine

TABLE 3 Effect of PGE_2, PGE_1, $PGF_{2\alpha}$, and the Prostaglandin Synthesis Inhibitor Meclofenamate on the Uterine Perfusion Pressure (mmHg)

Test agent (Dose/ml of uterine blood)	Control			Experimental		
	Before	Vehicle	$\bar{x} \pm SE$	Before	Test agent	$\bar{x} \pm SE$
PGE_2 (~170 ng/ml)	134	144	10 ± 4	141	110	-31 ± 4[a]
PGE_1 (~170 ng/ml)	128	148	20 ± 11	132	85	-47 ± 8[a]
PGE_1 (~1 ng/ml)	129	129	0 ± 2	147	115	-32 ± 8[a]
$PGF_{2\alpha}$ (~1 μg/ml)	164	174	10 ± 6	146	158	12 ± 6
Meclofenamate (5 μg/ml)	132	145	13 ± 3*	126	176	50 ± 8[a]

[a] $p < 0.05$.

TABLE 4 Effect of PGE_2, PGE_1, $PGF_{2\alpha}$, and the Prostaglandin Synthesis Inhibitor Meclofenamate on the Percent Endometrial Blood Flow on an Equal-Weight Basis

Agent (Dose/ml of uterine blood)	Control			n	Experimental		
	Before	Vehicle	$\bar{x} \pm$ SE		Before	Test agent	$\bar{x} \pm$ SE
PGE_2 (~170 ng/ml)	51	45	-6 ± 3	5	47	53	6 ± 6
PGE_1 (~170 ng/ml)	46	44	-2 ± 3	5	37	56	19 ± 4[a]
PGE_1 (~1 ng/ml)	38	37	-1 ± 4	5	35	51	16 ± 6[a]
$PGF_{2\alpha}$ (~1 μg/ml)	43	42	-1 ± 6	5	45	32	-13 ± 1[a]
Meclofenamate (5 μg/ml)	49	49	0 ± 1	5	45	53	8 ± 7

[a] $p < 0.05$.

tissue, and thus small changes in efficiency of separation of endometrium and myometrium would affect the calculated percent of uterine blood flow going to the endometrium. To avoid this error, the data were normalized on an equal-weight basis using the following equation:

$$\begin{matrix}\text{\% endometrium blood flow} \\ \text{(equal weight basis)}\end{matrix} = \frac{\text{cpm/100 mg endometrium} \times 100}{\begin{matrix}\text{cpm/100 mg endo + cpm/100 mg myo} \\ \text{(total cpm)}\end{matrix}}$$

The effect of exogenous prostaglandins and the prostaglandin synthesis inhibitor meclofenamate on uterine vascular resistance and blood flow distribution are shown in Tables 3 and 4. PGE_2 produced a significant reduction in uterine perfusion pressure but did not significantly alter the percent of blood flow going to the endometrium. This observation is in contrast to PGE_1, which produced a significant dose-related reduction in uterine vascular resistance (Table 3) and a significant increase in the percent of endometrial flow (Table 4). These data suggest that in the canine uterus PGE_1 has a greater effect on endometrial blood vessels than on myometrial blood vessels.

Although $PGF_{2\alpha}$ did not significantly alter uterine vascular resistance, it produced a significant reduction in the percent of endometrial blood flow (Table 4), indicating that $PGF_{2\alpha}$ produces selective constriction of endometrial vessels.

As in experiments described earlier, the prostaglandin synthesis inhibitor meclofenamate significantly increased uterine vascular resistance in the experimental horn (Table 3). Uterine perfusion pressure was also slightly increased in the control horn (Table 3), suggesting that either recirculating levels of meclofenamate or the meclofenamate vehicle produced slight vasoconstriction. However, meclofenamate did not significantly alter the percent of endometrial blood flow (Table 4), suggesting that under the conditions of the experiment endometrial and myometrial vessels are affected equally by endogenously produced prostaglandins.

These experiments demonstrate that prostaglandins have differential effects on uterine blood flow distribution. PGE_1 produces dose-related increases in endometrial blood flow, whereas PGE_2, although producing equivalent vasodilation, does not alter uterine blood flow distribution. In contrast, $PGF_{2\alpha}$ produces a significant reduction in the fraction of blood flow going to endometrium. This observation may be of special interest since Pickles and coworkers (41,42) suggested that $PGF_{2\alpha}$ levels are very high at menstruation, a time when endometrial vasoconstriction would be expected. The failure of meclofenamate to alter uterine blood flow distribution suggests that endogenous prostaglandins exert equal effects of myometrial and endometrial blood vessels, an action similar to the results observed with infusions of exogenous PGE_2.

Thus these endogenously occurring humoral agents may play an important role in determining the final distribution of blood flow within the uterus. Since prostaglandin levels in uterine tissues have been reported to be directly influenced by sex steroids (18,19,39), endogenously occurring prostaglandins may be responsible for modulating estrogen- and progesterone-related modifications in uterine hemodynamics. Thus the effect of these sex steroids on uterine blood flow distribution would be dependent on the final ratio of endogenous prostaglandins.

INTERRELATIONSHIP OF PROSTAGLANDINS AND ESTROGEN—POSSIBLE MEDIATION OF ESTROGEN-INDUCED INCREASES IN UTERINE BLOOD FLOW BY VASODILATOR PROSTAGLANDINS

The precise mechanism of estrogen-induced increases in uterine blood flow has eluded investigators for almost 50 years. This sex steroid is not considered to be a direct-acting vasodilating agent because a lag period of 30-60 min occurs before estrogen affects the uterine vasculature (43,44). The increase in uterine blood flow is not associated with a rise in systemic arterial blood pressure (44), indicating that uterine vascular resistance is decreased, i.e., vasodilation is occurring in the uterine vasculature. Estrogen and progesterone have been shown to increase both uterine venous and uterine tissue prostaglandins (3,18,19,39,45) and prostaglandins have been shown to fluctuate during the estrous cycle (3,45-48). In addition, Clark and coworkers (6,7) have shown that prostaglandins of the E series are extremely potent dilators of the uterine vasculature and that PGE_1 can redistribute uterine blood flow toward the endometrium (40). These observations appear to be consistent with a role for vasodilator prostaglandins in the estrogen response.

Studies by several investigators have added additional support to the concept that prostaglandins may be involved in the uterine responses to estrogen. Blatchley et al. (18) observed that during the estrous cycle of guinea pigs, PGE_2 levels in uteroovarian blood are less than 1 ng/ml until the day of proestrous, at which time PGEs increase to 55 ng/ml. This increase in uterine venous PGE_2 occurs at a time when endogenous estradiol levels would be rising. The level of PGE_2 measured by these investigators would be sufficient to produce a significant decrease in uterine vascular resistance in the dog (7).

Ryan and coworkers (19) reported that in the rat two structurally different inhibitors of prostaglandin synthesis, meclofenamate and indomethacin, can significantly attenuate estrogen-induced increases in uterine blood volume in a dose-related manner. In these experiments immunoreactive prostaglandins of the E and F series were also measured in rat uterine tissue. Following estrogen administration PGEs and PGFs were both significantly increased. When rats were pretreated with either indomethacin or meclofenamate, estrogen-induced increases in immunoreactive prostaglandins were significantly attenuated. The magnitude of reduction in uterine prostaglandin levels was greater than the reduction in the estrogen-induced increase in uterine blood volume. These data can be interpreted to mean that either prostaglandins are only partially responsible for the estrogen response in rats or that the reduction in immunoreactive prostaglandins reflects changes occurring in nonvascular tissue (endometrium and myometrium) rather than in uterine vascular smooth muscle.

Recent studies using this same rat model (49) have investigated the role of adrenergic mechanisms and their possible relationship to prostaglandins in estrogen-induced increases in uterine blood volume. When rats were pretreated with one of two structurally dissimilar α-adrenergic receptor blocking agents, either phentolamine or HEAT [BE-2254, 2-(β-(4-hydroxyphenyl)ethylaminomethyl)tetralonehydrochloride], the uterine blood volume response to estrogen was totally abolished, as was the normal estrogen-induced increase in uterine PGE and PGF levels. This blockade of the estrogen effect was not due to lowering of systemic arterial blood pressure since the ganglionic blocking agent hexamethonium, which had similar effects on arterial pressue, did not modify the normal uterine response to estrogen. In these experiments, attempts were also made to determine if the α-adrenergic receptor stimulant was released from uterine neuronal stores. Pretreatment of rats with reserpine, guanethidine, or 6-hydroxydopamine, although depleting adrenergic nerves, failed to modify the estrogen response. Thus at least in the rat, α-adrenergic receptor stimulant of humoral rather than local neuronal origin, appears to be necessary for a normal uterine vascular response to estrogen. In addition, since α-adrenergic receptor blockade significantly attenuated the normal estrogen induced increase in uterine PGEs and PGSs, it appears that a relationship exists between the α-adrenergic receptor and the increased production of prostaglandins which occurs following estrogen. The possibility that α-adrenergic receptors mediate estrogen-induced uterine vascular prostaglandin production has been investigated only in the rat; in the future these studies should be extended to other species.

If prostaglandins are responsible for estrogen-induced uterine vasodilation, these agents are probably produced locally in the blood vessel rather than in nonvascular uterine tissue. Blood vessels have the capacity to synthesize prostaglandins and the rate of synthesis can be increased by humoral agents such as bradykinin (50). Thus the possibility that estrogen gives rise to an increase in the enzymes of the prostaglandin synthetase system or phospholipase system (increased release of arachidonic acid), which eventually causes an increased production of vasodilator prostaglandins, and finally uterine vasodilation seems conceivable. Killam and coworkers (44) found that local intraarterial (uterine artery) administration of the protein synthesis inhibitor cyclohexamide could prevent the increase in uterine blood flow seen following administration of exogenous estrogen. When the infusion of cyclohexamide was stopped, a typical response to estrogen occurred following the hormonal time lag of 45 min. These results suggest that new protein synthesis (i.e., prostaglandin-related enzymes) is needed before the estrogen response can occur.

Barcikowski et al. (39) have reported that estradiol-17β increases PGFs (PGE levels were not measured) in uteroovarian venous blood of the autotransplanted uterine horn of the sheep. These investigators also noted that estrogen-induced increases in uterine blood flow as well as the increases in uterine venous PGF levels could be attenuated by the local infusion of the prostaglandin synthesis inhibitor indomethacin. In an extension of these experiments, Clark and coworkers (51) have reported that estrogen-induced increases in uterine blood flow in the nonpregnant unanesthetized sheep can be significantly attenuated by the intraarterial (uterine artery) infusion of a second prostaglandin synthesis inhibitor, meclofenamate. In these experiments intraarterial infusions of meclofenamate at a concentration of 5-10 μg/ml of uterine blood flow attenuated or in some cases ablated the response to estrogen without altering responses to the direct-acting vasodilator, nitroglycerin (K. E. Clark, unpublished observation, 1977). The problem with these studies is reproducibility; blockade has been obtained in all five of the sheep that have been studied, but following the initial blockade, second attempts to block the normal estrogen response have failed. A possible explanation for these conflicting results may be the local intraarterial infusion of meclofenamate alters the intimal lining of the uterine artery and prevents future access of the inhibitor to the site of prostaglandin synthesis or that estrogen receptor sites may be altered by the intraarterial infusion of this pharmacological agent. These possibilities as well as others are currently under investigation in our laboratories. Although vasodilator prostaglandins appear to be excellent candidates for the mediator of estrogen-induced increases in uterine blood flow, their role has not been demonstrated unequivocally.

CONCLUSION

Uterine blood flow is regulated by both arterial blood pressure and uterine vascular resistance. Prostaglandins produced in the uterus act on vascular smooth muscle to alter vascular resistance. This alteration is accomplished at two levels: (1) direct action on the vascular smooth muscle to produce constriction or relaxation, and (2) indirect action on adrenergic neurotransmission, leading to either facilitation or depression of vasoconstrictor influences mediated through uterine sympathetic innervation.

Prostaglandins of the E and A series are potent uterine vasodilators in the nonpregnant canine uterus, whereas $PGF_{2\alpha}$ lacks intrinsic vasomotor activity. Direct effects of prostaglandins on uterine vascular resistance are independent of their actions on adrenergic neurotransmission. Inhibition of endogenous prostaglandin synthesis leads to increased uterine vascular resistance and increased responsiveness to norepinephrine. Thus, like exogenous prostaglandins, endogenous prostaglandins act directly to relax uterine vascular smooth muscle and indirectly to depress postjunctional responsiveness of the vascular smooth muscle to both circulating and neurogenically released norepinephrine. During uterine sympathetic nerve stimulation, prostaglandins of the E and F series are not released in detectable amounts in uterine venous effluent. This observation is in contrast to several other vascular beds where prostaglandin release appears to be under neurogenic control. It seems possible that neurogenically released prostaglandins could be metabolized locally at the site of action (vascular smooth muscle) and thus not be reflected in venous effluent.

The observations that prostaglandins of the E and F series have differential effects on uterine blood flow distribution and that $PGF_{2\alpha}$ is able to antagonize competitively PGA- and PGE-induced uterine vasodilation suggest that these locally synthesized uterine prostaglandins may be important in modulating uterine hemodynamics at the local level. In addition, the prostaglandins appear to be important in maintaining adequate blood flow during periods of fluctuating metabolic requirements imposed upon the uterus by hormones such as estrogen or progesterone.

In the rat, estrogen-induced alterations in uterine blood flow appear to be at least partially mediated by vasodilator prostaglandins. The mechanism of prostaglandin formation and/or release during estrogen stimulation appears to involve activation of α-adrenergic receptors; however, the source of the adrenergic stimulant appears to be humoral rather than from uterine adrenergic nerves. Interactions between adrenergic systems and uterine prostaglandins require further identification. In contrast, the role of prostaglandins in mediating estrogen-induced increases in uterine blood flow in the sheep is questionable.

The physiological role of uterine vasodilator prostaglandins during pregnancy may have important clinical implications. Evidence that uterine blood flow is decreased in patients with toxemia and that placental levels of prostaglandins of the E series are depressed suggests a potential pathophysiological role. One of the underlying causes of toxemia might be a failure of the uterus to synthesize adequate amounts of vasodilator prostaglandins leading to reduced uterine blood flow. Further studies on functions of uterine prostaglandins may not only be important for uncovering mechanisms of normal blood flow regulation but may also help uncover the etiology of toxemia of pregnancy.

Finally, it is important to note the recent work of Terragno et al. (52), which showed that renal prostaglandin levels are significantly elevated in anesthetized acutely stressed dogs when compared to unanesthetized animals. This observation suggests that these humoral agents may play an important role in maintaining blood flow during acute stress. The possibility that some of the results on prostaglandins and uterine blood flow described in the present chapter are modified due to the effects of acute stress is currently being investigated.

ACKNOWLEDGMENT

Portions of the work reported here were supported by U.S. Public Health Service Grants HLP-14388 and HL-07121.

REFERENCES

1. Greiss, F. C., and Anderson, S. G. Uterine vascular changes during the ovarian cycle. Am. J. Obstet. Gynecol. 103(5):629-640, 1969.
2. Ladner, C., Brinkman, C. R., III, Weston, P., and Assali, N. S. Dynamics of uterine circulation in pregnant and nonpregnant sheep. Am. J. Physiol. 218(1):257-263, 1970.
3. Sabhsetwar, A. P. Prostaglandins and the reproductive cycle. Fed. Proc. 33:61-77, 1974.
4. Goldberg, V. J., and Ramwell, P. W. Role of prostaglandins in reproduction. Physiol. Rev. 55:325-351, 1975.
5. Ryan, M. J., Clark, K. E., and Brody, M. J. Neurogenic and mechanical control of canine uterine vascular resistance. Am. J. Physiol. 227(3):547-555, 1974.
6. Clark, K. E., Ryan, M. J., and Brody, M. J. Effects of prostaglandins E_1 and $F_{2\alpha}$ on uterine hemodynamics and motility. Adv. Biosci. 9: 779-782, 1973.
7. Clark, K. E., Ryan, M. J., and Brody, M. J. Effect of prostaglandins on vascular resistance and adrenergic vasoconstrictor responses in the canine uterus. Prostaglandins 12(1):71-82, 1976.
8. Finney, D. J. Statistical Methods in Biological Assay. Charles Griffin, London, 1952.

9. Nakajima, A., Manahe, Y., Tauchi, K., and Sagaguchi, M. Effect of prostaglandins on uterine blood flow in the pregnant dog. Acta Obstet. Gynaecol. Jap. 20(1):26-33, 1973.
10. Rankin, J. H. G., and Phernetton, T. M. Effect of prostaglandin E_2 on ovine maternal placental blood flow. Am. J. Physiol. 231(3):754-759, 1976.
11. Brody, M. J., and Kadowitz, P. J. Prostaglandins as modulators of the autonomic nervous system. Fed. Proc. 33(1):48-60, 1974.
12. Eliasson, R., and Risley, P. L. Potentiated response of isolated seminal vesicles to catecholamines and acetylcholine in the presence of PGE_1. Acta Physiol. Scand. 67:253-254, 1966.
13. Kadowitz, P. J., Sweet, C. S., and Brody, M. J. Effects of prostaglandins on adrenergic neurotransmission to vascular smooth muscle In Prostaglandins in Cellular Biology, P. W. Ramwell and B. B. Pharriss (Eds.). Plenum Press, New York, pp. 479-511, 1972.
14. Kadowitz, P. J., Sweet, C. S., and Brody, M. J. Differential effects of prostaglandin E_1, E_2, $F_{1\alpha}$ and $F_{2\alpha}$ on adrenergic vasoconstriction in the dog hindpaw. J. Pharmacol. Exp. Ther. 177:641-649, 1971.
15. Kadowitz, P. J. Effect of prostaglandin E_1, E_2 and A_2 on vascular resistance and responses to noradrenaline, nerve stimulation and antiotensin in the dog hindlimb. Br. J. Pharmacol. 46:395-400, 1972.
16. Kadowitz, P. J., Sweet, C. S., and Brody, M. J. Potentiation of adrenergic venomotor responses by angiotensin, prostaglandin $F_{2\alpha}$ and cocaine. J. Pharmacol. Exp. Ther. 176:167-173, 1971.
17. Kadowitz, P. J., Sweet, C. S., and Brody, M. J. Blockade of adrenergic vasoconstrictor responses in the dog by prostaglandins E_1 and A_1. J. Pharmacol. Exp. Ther. 179:563-572, 1971.
18. Blatchley, F. R., Donovan, B. T., Horton, E. W., and Poyser, N. L. The release of prostaglandins and progestins into the utero-ovarian venous blood of guinea pigs during the oestrous cycle and following oestrogen treatment. J. Physiol. (Lond.) 223:69, 1972.
19. Ryan, M. J., Clark, K. E., Van Orden, D. E., Farley, D., Edvinsson, L., Sjoberg, N. O., Van Orden, L. S., III, and Brody, M. J. Role of prostaglandins in estrogen-induced uterine hyperemia. Prostaglandins 5:257-268, 1974.
20. Clark, K. E., Farley, D. B., Van Orden, D. E., and Brody, M. J. Role of endogenous prostaglandins in regulation of uterine blood flow and adrenergic neurotransmission. Am. J. Obstet. Gynecol. 127:455-461, 1977.
21. Van Orden, D. E., and Farley, D. B. Prostaglandin $F_{2\alpha}$ radioimmunoassay utilizing polyethylene glycol separation technique. Prostaglandins 4:215-231, 1973.
22. Gryglewski, R., and Vane, J. R. The release of prostaglandins and rabbit aorta contractile substance (RCS) from the rabbit spleen and its antagonism by anti-inflammatory agents. Br. J. Pharmacol. 45:37-47, 1972.

23. Terragno, N. A., Terragno, D. A., Pacholegzh, D., and McGiff, J. C. Prostaglandins and the regulation of the uterine blood flow in pregnancy. Nature (Lond.) 249:57-58, 1974.
24. Venuto, R. C., O'Dorisio, T., Stein, J. H., and Ferris, T. R. Uterine prostaglandin E (PGE) secretion and uterine blood flow in the rabbit. J. Clin. Invest. 55:193-197, 1975.
25. Franklin, G. O., Dowd, A. J., Caldwell, B. V., and Speroff, L. The effect of angiotensin-II intravenous infusion on plasma renin activity and prostaglandins A, E and F levels in the uterine vein of the pregnant monkey. Prostaglandins 6(4):271-280, 1974.
26. Browne, J. C. M., and Veal, N. The maternal placental blood flow in normotensive women. J. Obstet. Gynaecol. Br. Commonw. 60:141-150, 1953.
27. Landerman, R., and Knapp, R. Na^{24} uterine muscle clearance in late pregnancy. Am. J. Obstet. Gynecol. 80:92-103, 1960.
28. Demers, L. M., and Gabbe, S. G. Placental prostaglandin levels in preeclampsia. Am. J. Obstet. Gynecol. 126(1):137-139, 1976.
29. Speroff, L. An autoregulatory role for prostaglandins in placental hemodynamics: their possible influence on blood pressure in pregnancy. J. Reprod. Med. 15(5):181-188, 1975.
30. Davies, B. N., and Withrington, P. G. The effects of PGE_1 and E_2 on the smooth muscle of the dog spleen and on its responses to catecholamines, angiotensin and nerve stimulation. Br. J. Pharmacol. Chemther. 321:136-144, 1967.
31. Ramwell, P. W., and Shaw, J. E. Biological significance of the prostaglandins. Recent Prog. Horm. Res. 26:139-187, 1970.
32. McGiff, J. C., Crowshaw, K., Terragno, N. A., Malik, K. U., and Lonigro, A. J. Differential effect of noradrenaline and renal nerve stimulation on vascular resistance in the dog kidney and the release of prostaglandin E-like substance. Clin. Sci. 42:223-233, 1972.
33. Kolata, G. B. Thromboxanes: the power behind the prostaglandins? Science 190:770-771, 1975.
34. Greiss, F. C., and Anderson, S. G. Pressure-flow relationship in the nonpregnant uterine vascular bed. Am. J. Obstet. Gynecol. 118:763-772, 1974.
35. Eliasson, R. Mode of action of prostaglandins on the human nonpregnant myometrium. Biochem. Pharmacol. 15:755, 1966.
36. Pickles, V. R. The myometrial actions of six prostaglandins: consideration of a receptor hypothesis. In Prostaglandins (Proc. 2nd Nobel Symp.), S. Bergstrom and B. Samuelsson (Eds.). Interscience, New York, pp. 79-83, 1967.
37. Clark, K. E., and Brody, M. J. Competitive antagonism of prostaglandin (PG) E_1, E_2 and A_1 induced vasodilation by $PGF_{2\alpha}$ in the canine uterus. Blood Vessels, 14:204-211, 1977.
38. Wakeling, A. E., Kirton, K. T., and Wyngarden, L. J. Prostaglandin receptors in the hamster uterus during the estrous cycle. Prostaglandins 4:1-8, 1973.

39. Barcikowski, B., Carlson, J. C., Wilson, L., and McCracken, J. A. The effect of endogenous and exogenous estradiol-17-β on the release of prostaglandin $F_{2\alpha}$ from the ovine uterus. Endocrinology 95:1340-1349, 1974.
40. Clark, K. E., and Van Orden, D. E. Effect of prostaglandins (PG's) and meclofenamic acid (MA) on blood flow distribution in the canine uterus. Fed. Proc. 35(3):447 (abstr.), 1976.
41. Pickles, V. R., Hall, W. J., Best, F. A., and Smith, G. N. Prostaglandins in endometrium and menstrual fluid from normal and dysmenorrhoeic subjects. J. Obstet. Gynaecol. Br. Commonw. 72:185-192, 1965.
42. Pickles, V. R. Prostaglandins in the human endometrium. Int. J. Fertil. 12:335-338, 1967.
43. Brody, M. J., Clark, K. E., Edvinsson, L., Owman, Ch., and Sjoberg, N. O. Determination of uterine blood volume and correlation with ovarian function. Proc. Soc. Exp. Biol. Med. 147:91-96, 1974.
44. Killam, A. P., Rosenfeld, C. R., Battaglia, F. C., Makowski, E. L., and Meschia, G. Effect of estrogens on the uterine flow of oophorectomized ewes. Am. J. Obstet. Gynecol. 115:1045-1052, 1973.
45. Ham, E. A., Cirillo, V. J., Zanetli, M. E., and Kuehl, F. A., Jr. Estrogen-directed synthesis of specific prostaglandins in uterus. Proc. Natl. Acad. Sci. USA 72(4):1420-1424, 1975.
46. Bland, K. P., Horton, E. W., and Poyser, N. L. Levels of prostaglandin F_2 in the uterine venous blood of sheep during the oestrous cycle. Life Sci. 10(I):509-517, 1971.
47. Kuehl, F. A., Jr., Cirillo, V. J., Zanetli, M. E., Beveridge, G. C., and Ham, E. A. The effect of estrogen upon cyclic nucleotide and prostaglandin levels in the rat uterus. Adv. Prostaglandin Thromboxane Res. 1:313-323, 1976.
48. Shemesh, M., and Hansel, W. Levels of prostaglandin F (PGF) in bovine endometrium, uterine venous, ovarian arterial and jugular plasma during the estrous cycle. Proc. Soc. Exp. Biol. Med. 148:123-126, 1975.
49. Clark, K. E., Farley, D. B., Van Orden, D. E., and Brody, M. J. Estrogen-induced uterine hyperemia and edema persist during histamine receptor blockade. Proc. Soc. Exp. Biol. Med. 156:411-416, 1977.
50. Terragno, D. A., Crowshaw, K., Terragno, N. A., and McGiff, J. C. Prostaglandin synthesis by bovine mesenteric arteries and veins. Circ. Res. 36(6) (Suppl. I):76-80, 1975.
51. Clark, K. E., Van Orden, D. E., Meldrum, D. R., Brody, M. J., and Brinkman, C. R., III. Effect of the prostaglandin synthetase inhibitor meclofenamate on estrogen-induced increases in uterine blood flow in sheep. Gynecol. Invest. 7:25 (abstr.), 1976.
52. Terragno, N. A., Terragno, D. A., and McGiff, J. C. Contribution to the renal circulation in conscious, anesthetized, and laparotomized dogs. Circ. Res. 40(6):590-595, 1977.

6 Prostaglandins and Renal Function

ROCCO C. VENUTO / State University of New York at Buffalo, Buffalo, New York

THOMAS F. FERRIS / University of Minnesota Hospitals, Minneapolis, Minnesota

In the mid-1930s the postulation of an antihypertensive role for the kidney and the discovering of prostaglandins were concomitantly made (1-3), but their possible interrelationship was not appreciated. A number of investigators had demonstrated that the renal parenchyma, in the absence of excretory function, protected against the development of hypertension in experimental animals (4-6). Extensive experimentation by Muirhead pointed to the renal medulla (7-9), specifically the medullary interstitial cells, as the source of this antihypertensive effect (10-12). In 1965, Lee and colleagues identified prostaglandins in an acid lipid extract of rabbit renal medulla and demonstrated their potent vasodepressor activity (13). Further studies identified the prostaglandins in the renal medulla to possess a double bond at the 5,6-position, namely PGA_2, PGE_2, and $PGF_{2\alpha}$ (14,15). The presence of these vasoactive lipids in the kidney, primarily in the medulla, has stimulated extensive investigation into their potential role in control of blood pressure, renal blood flow, and salt and water excretion.

INTRARENAL SYNTHESIS AND DEGRADATION OF PROSTAGLANDINS

Renal prostaglandins are synthesized from the essential fatty acid arachidonic acid by a group of enzymes, designated prostaglandin synthetases (16). The substrate is first converted to a cyclic endoperoxide intermediate (17) and then to PGE_2 and $PGF_{2\alpha}$. Synthetase activity is greatest in the renal medulla, with the highest concentration localized in the microsomal fraction of cells from the inner medulla (18-20). Although earlier work by Crowshaw and

Szlyk (21) failed to detect prostaglandin synthesis in renal cortex, more recent studies by Anggard and others have shown that the renal cortex can synthesize prostaglandins. The renal cortex is rich in prostaglandin dehydrogenase (22,23) and the earlier report of a lack of prostaglandin synthesis in cortex was probably due to rapid degradation of prostaglandins.

Biochemical studies have demonstrated little storage of prostaglandins in the medulla, suggesting immediate synthesis and release (20,24,25). The major source of both precursor and synthetase is the medullary interstitial cells with their characteristic lipid granules (8,9,26,27). Collecting duct cells also possess synthetase activity.

In addition to a potential vasodepressor effect, the position and morphology of interstitial cells with large pseudopodlike projections (Fig. 1), which contact both ascending and descending vasa recti as well as collecting ducts, suggest that prostaglandins may play a role in controlling urinary concentration, sodium excretion, oxygen tension, or medullary blood flow (26). Evidence by Muirhead suggests that autotransplants of these cells increase in size and number in response to experimental hypertension with depletion of lipid content (9), suggesting increased synthesis (27,28). Nonencapsulated tumorlike collections of interstitial cells have been found in human kidneys (29).

In contrast to prostaglandin synthetase activity, the enzymes responsible for prostaglandin degradation, prostaglandin dehydrogenase, and Δ^{13}-reductase, are most abundant in the renal cortex (22,23). Epithelial cells in the chick ascending limb of the loop of Henle, distal convoluted tubule, renal pelvis, and tunica media of renal arteries and arterioles contain the highly specific 15-hydroxydehydrogenase enzyme (30). The concentration of these enzymes progressively falls as deeper portions of the kidney are sampled. The concentration of degrading enzymes in the renal cortex could reflect a systemic metabolic function of the kidney in addition to metabolizing locally formed prostaglandins.

In spite of these enzymes, a significant portion of PGE_2 and $PGF_{2\alpha}$ escapes intrarenal degradation. Increased synthesis of PGE_2 and $PGF_{2\alpha}$ is reflected in their elevation in both urine and renal venous blood (31-36). The exact mechanism of transport of renal prostaglandins into the urine and blood is unknown, but these routes of elimination give medullary prostaglandins exposure to both the distal nephron, where they may have an effect on sodium or water absorption and to the systemic circulation. In addition, inactive PGE metabolites of nonrenal origin are excreted in the urine (31,32,37).

Recent work employing gas-liquid chromatography-mass spectrophotometry have failed to confirm the original observation by Lee et al. that the prostaglandin A_2 is produced in significant quantities in vivo by the kidney (18,19). PGA_2 is readily formed by nonenzymatic dehydration of PGE_2 and probably represents dehydration of the abundant renal PGE_2 (38,39). This observation is of significance since PGA, a potent vasodilator, largely escapes

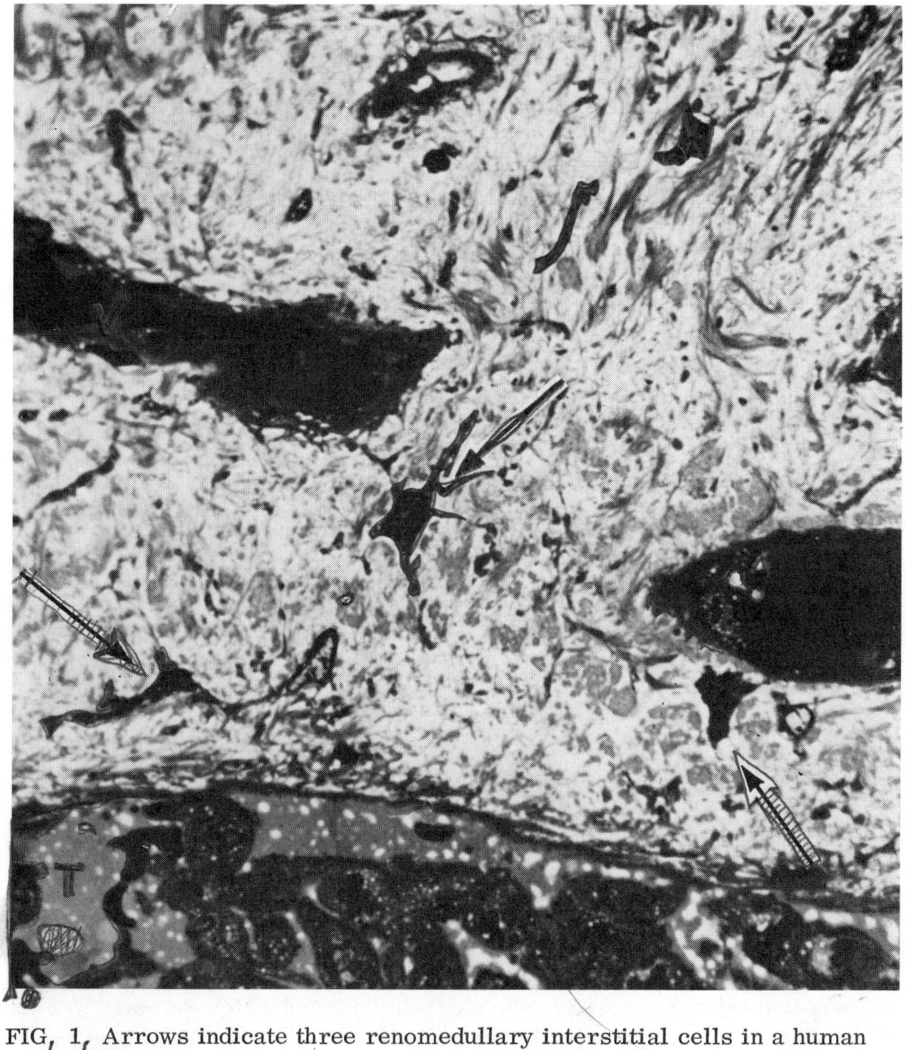

FIG. 1. Arrows indicate three renomedullary interstitial cells in a human kidney. V, small blood vessel; T, a collecting duct. X800. (Courtesy of Dr. A. Prezyna, State University of New York, School of Medicine, Buffalo, New York.)

metabolism in the pulmonary circulation (40,41), and has been postulated to play a significant role in the control of systemic blood pressure (42,43). A role for renal prostaglandins in blood pressure control is not totally dependent on the presence of PGA since PGE_2 is also a potent vasodilator. Originally

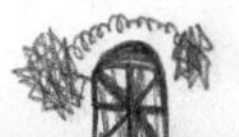

thought to be almost completely metabolized by a single passage through the pulmonary circulation (41), studies in humans have demonstrated that approximately 66% of PGE_2 injected into the right ventricle is metabolized during transit through the pulmonary capillary network (38). Thus under certain circumstances sufficient PGE may escape pulmonary metabolism to contribute to arterial PGE concentration. A role for renal PGE_2 has recently been suggested in Bartter's syndrome, where insensitivity to angiotensin is present (32), in pregnancy (44), and with certain kidney tumors (45).

PROSTAGLANDINS AND RENAL BLOOD FLOW

In humans approximately 20% of the cardiac output is delivered to the kidneys, which together weigh only 300 g. The constancy of renal blood flow over a wide range of perfusion pressure demonstrates that renal vascular resistance is quite variable (46). It is tempting to postulate that the renal prostaglandins play a role in maintenance of basal renal blood flow or in the change in renal vascular resistance which occurs in response to physiologic stimuli (39). Administration of prostaglandins of the E or A series to anesthetized dogs or hypertensive humans results in increased renal blood flow (47-50), but the significance of a prostaglandin infusion may be questioned. Pharmacologic doses are usually administered and infusions deliver prostaglandins primarily to renal cortex, in contrast to their primary medullary site of synthesis. To approximate the "in vivo" situation, two approaches have been employed. Tannenbaum et al. (51), Larsson and Anggard (52), and Chang et al. (53) have studied the effect of increasing prostaglandin synthesis by infusing specific substrate for prostaglandin synthesis, arachidonic acid. Sodium arachidonate infusions increase renal blood flow with a simultaneous increase in renal venous prostaglandin E as measured by bioassay. Since arachidonate solutions are unstable and capable of autooxidation to either a prostaglandin-like substance or conversion to a vasoactive hydroxy acid when administered intraarterially (54, 55), the effect of arachidonate may not indicate synthesis in medullary interstitial cells. However, inhibitors of prostaglandin synthesis administered during the arachidonate infusion block the increase in renal blood flow and increase in renal vein PGE. Tannenbaum et al. (51) demonstrated that injected prostaglandin E_2 resulted in a greater increase in renal blood flow than arachidonate, further supporting differences in the effect between infused and locally synthesized prostaglandins.

Juxtamedullary blood flow preferentially increases in both rabbits and dogs (52, 53) during the arachidonate infusion, which correlates with an effect primarily in the renal medulla. Medullary-generated prostaglandins may be transported to the renal cortex via the loop of Henle to the distal convoluted tubule. Since only deep cortical nephrons have long loops of Henle that penetrate into the medulla, the effect of medullary prostaglandin synthesis should be primarily on deep cortical nephrons.

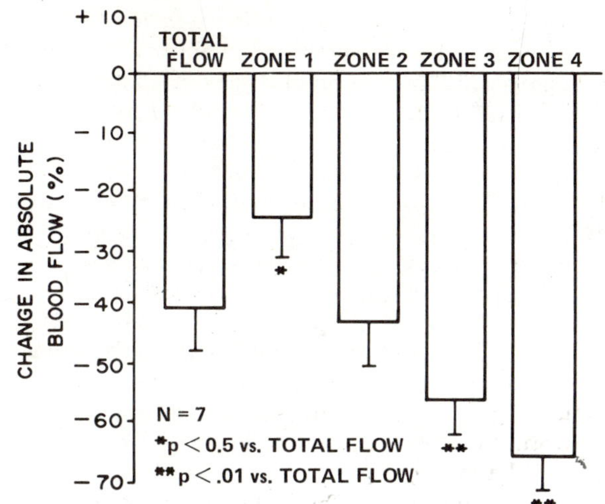

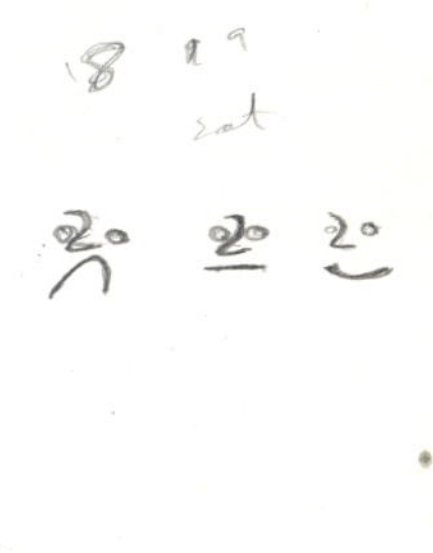

FIG. 2. Effect of indomethacin on absolute zonal blood flow. Data are presented as percent change in absolute blood flow in comparison to control observations. (From Ref. 58.)

A widely used technique to avoid difficulties with infusions of prostaglandins or arachidonate employs inhibitors of prostaglandin synthesis (56). Lonigro and associates demonstrated that the administration of meclofenamate or indomethacin, two structurally dissimilar antiinflammatory agents, reduced renal blood flow in isolated kidneys and in the anesthetized dog (57). The decrease in renal blood flow was associated with a fall in renal venous prostaglandin E by bioassay. Kirschenbaum and colleagues (58), using radiolabeled microspheres, confirmed the reduction in total renal blood flow and demonstrated that the reduction in cortical perfusion was most severe in the juxtamedullary cortex (Fig. 2). These findings were confirmed in the isolated perfused kidney by Itskovitz et al. (59), and Solez et al., using the radiolabeled albumin technique, found substantial reduction in rat medullary plasma flow following indomethacin (60). As with the arachidonic acid infusion, these studies suggest that basal renal blood flow, especially to the inner cortical and medullary regions, is dependent on prostaglandin synthesis. However, these studies were in anesthetized animals, and subsequent studies in conscious animals have demonstrated that little or no change in renal blood flow occurs following administration of synthesis inhibitors (61-63). Both the noncompetitive inhibitors, indomethacin and meclofenamate, or the competitive inhibitor, RO-20-5720, had similar effects. Although Swain et al. (62) demonstrated substantial reduction of renal blood flow with high doses of meclofenamate in the conscious animal, more recent studies have confirmed the observation that conscious dogs do not have a reduction in renal blood flow following administration of prostaglandin synthesis inhibitors (63-65). It seems to be the surgical preparation, more than anesthesia, that is responsible for the difference (64). The effect of prostaglandin inhibition correlates with renal prostaglandin synthesis. In the conscious animal renal venous blood contains low levels of PGE, as measured by bioassay, whereas following laparotomy a threefold increase in PGE secretion occurs (64). Basal renal PGE secretion is unaffected by up to 10 mg/kg indomethacin, whereas the increased secretion induced by laparotomy is reduced with indomethacin. These observations suggest that little PGE is produced under basal conditions but if the animal is stressed, a variety of hormonal and nervous stimuli increase prostaglandin synthesis. Angiotensin, norepinephrine, and stimulation of the renal nerve increase PGE synthesis and the different response to indomethacin following barbiturate anesthesia may be a reflection of this. Barbiturate induces an increase in renin secretion, which is countered by increased prostaglandin synthesis, so that renal blood flow remains stable. Flow at this point, however, is dependent on prostaglandin synthesis and will fall with prostaglandin synthesis inhibitors (66). Renin is one of the major factors influencing renal prostaglandin synthesis. Angiotensin increases renal venous PGE concentration (34,35,67,68), and the increased release of PGE is associated with tachyphylaxis to the renal vasoconstrictive effect of angiotensin. Indomethacin administration heightens the vasoconstrictive effect of angiotensin and abolishes tachyphylaxis (68,69). Studies in anesthetized dogs (70) and rats (71) have demonstrated that vasoconstriction induced by indomethacin is diminished or reversed by angiotensin blockade with Saralasin (72), whereas the effect of epinephine or stimulation of the renal nerve on PGE synthesis is not blocked by Saralasin (73). The modulating effect of prostaglandin E on the vasoconstrictive action of angiotensin is seen in other vascular beds (73,74).

Indomethacin and other inhibitors of prostaglandin synthesis suppress renin release (75,76), an effect independent of change in renal blood flow since Anggard has demonstrated that indomethacin suppresses renin release from renal cortical slices. Kotchen and Miller demonstrated in vitro inhibition of angiotensin generation with extremely large quantities of prostaglandin A but not E (77).

Prostaglandins play a role in the renal hemodynamic response to various stimuli. Indomethacin and salicylate block the redistribution of blood flow to deep cortex normally seen after hemorrhage (78,79), and renal blood flow, usually relatively constant following modest hemorrhagic hypotension, falls dramatically after pretreatment with salicylate (80). Although these studies were performed in anesthetized animals, Swain et al. (62) demonstrated that renal ischemia induced by angiotensin or methoxamine was increased in indomethacin-treated, chronically instrumented conscious dogs and reactive hyperemia was almost completely abolished.

Increased synthesis of prostaglandin E is not restricted to circumstances in which renal blood flow is reduced. Bradykinin, a potent renal vasodilator, also increases the concentration of PGE in the venous effluent of the canine kidney (81). However, the increased flow is not dependent on elevated synthesis of PGE, and Chapnick et al. (82) have found in indomethacin-treated anesthetized rats that bradykinin stimulates release of catecholamines (83), which may increase prostaglandin synthesis rather than being a direct effect of bradykinin. An interrelationship between prostaglandin synthesis and the autonomic nervous system is well documented in both extrarenal (72, 84, 85) and the renal vascular bed (36, 78, 79). Since renal renin release is dependent, in part, on sympathetic stimulation (86-88) and renal prostaglandin synthesis is increased by both angiotensin and sympathetic nervous activity, the role of PGE synthesis may modulate the response of the renal vasculature to autonomic nervous activity.

Bartter's syndrome (32) and, in both rabbit and humans (90), pregnancy (89) are characterized by increased urinary PGE excretion. In pregnancy there is a striking decrease in renal vascular resistance as renal blood flow and glomerular filtration increase approximately 50%. Bartter's syndrome, a disease associated with insensitivity to the pressor effect of angiotensin, has certain similarities to pregnancy. In both, angiotensin insensitivity is present, which necessitates increased renin secretion for maintenance of blood pressure. Treatment of Bartter's syndrome with indomethacin reduces renin and aldosterone secretion and partially restores angiotensin sensitivity to normal. Renal biopsy specimens in patients with Bartter's syndrome have demonstrated hyperplasia of the interstitial cells of the renal medulla (91). The cause of the increased renal PGE synthesis is not known, but recent studies by Galvez et al. have demonstrated that potassium depletion increases urinary PGE in the dog (92) (Fig. 3). Thus some patients with Bartter's syndrome may have a potassium-losing nephropathy which increases medullary PGE synthesis with the development of angiotensin resistance. Although treatment with indomethacin in Bartter's syndrome causes a rise in serum potassium, potassium wasting persists. The partial correction of the hypokalemia may represent correction of that part of the K wasting caused by the hyperaldosteronism. Potassium wasting has persisted in at least two children with Bartter's syndrome following bilateral total adrenalectomy (93).

The increase in renal blood flow following administration of furosemide and ethyacrynic acid is blunted by prostaglandin inhibition (94, 95). Since both drugs increase renin secretion, the increase in renal blood flow may be dependent on angiotensin increasing prostaglandin synthesis.

In the isolated kidney, pretreated with indomethacin, Herbaczynska-Cedro and Vane originally reported failure of autoregulation during decreased perfusion pressure (96). Subsequent studies in the intact animal (97, 98) and in isolated perfused kidney (99) have failed to verify this observation. Although a rise in renal resistance occurs in anesthetized indomethacin-treated animals, blood flow remains constant over a wide range of perfusing pressure (Fig. 4). Thus the autoregulatory capacity of the kidney appears to be due to intrinsic qualities of smooth muscle independent of prostaglandin synthesis.

In summary, the renal vasodilating prostaglandins, notably PGE_2, do not appear to have a major role in the maintenance of basal renal blood flow or in the autoregulatory capacity of the kidney. This also appears to be true of the more recently discovered vasodilatory product of, primarily, renal

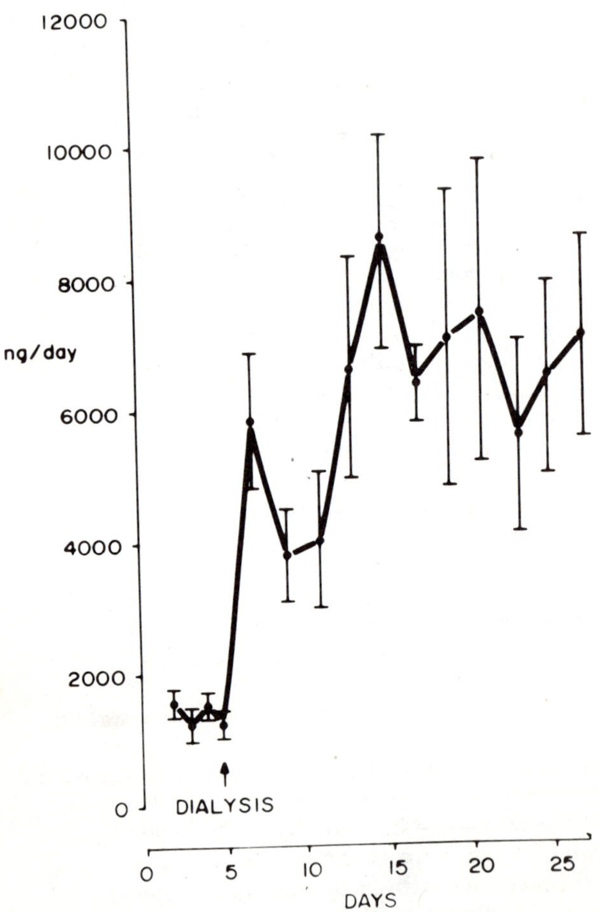

FIG. 3. Urinary PGE excretion in 12 dogs after potassium deficiency by dialysis on day 5 followed by a low-potassium diet. (From Ref. 92, by permission of the American Heart Association, Inc.)

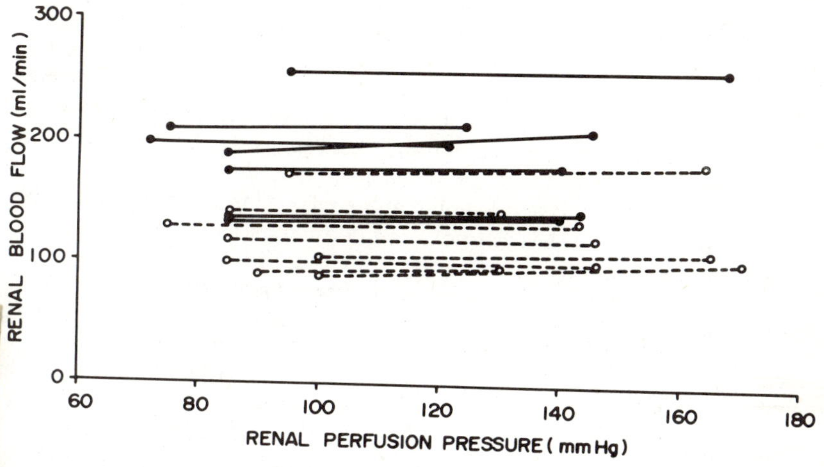

FIG. 4. Effect of inhibition of prostaglandin synthesis on renal autoregulation. The lines connect the initial perfusion pressure and the lowest pressure at which renal resistance continued to decrease during aortic constriction. Control, solid line; prostaglandin inhibition, dashed line. (From Ref. 97.)

cortical metabolism of arachidonic acid, PGI_2 (prostacyclin) (100, 101). The major function of these vasoactive lipids appears to be the modulation of the increase in renal resistance which occurs in response to vasoconstrictive stimuli such as activation of the autonomic nervous system or the renin-angiotensin system. The role of the potential vasoconstrictor renal prostaglandin $PGF_{2\alpha}$ in the control of renal blood flow is not completely defined but appears to be limited. Similarly, thromboxane A_2, another vasoconstrictor product of arachidonic acid metabolism, is produced in such small quantities under physiologic conditions that its role under these conditions also appears to be minor (102).

PROSTAGLANDINS AND NATRIURESIS

Administration of prostaglandin E and A causes increased excretion of sodium in animals (48, 49) and humans (103, 104). Free water clearance, a measure of sodium chloride reabsorption in the ascending limb of the loop of Henle, increases during the natriuresis, so the inhibitory effect of prostaglandin E and A on sodium absorption is probably in the proximal tubule. PGA and PGE, like all vasodilators, increase renal blood flow without change in glomerular filtration; the fall in filtration fraction reduces oncotic pressure and increases hydrostatic pressure in the peritubular capillary, both of which reduce proximal tubular sodium absorption (104, 105). Infusion of the more recently discovered PGI_2 infusion in dogs causes an increase in sodium excretion and renal blood flow without an increase in either glomerular filtration rate or free water clearance (106). This suggests that the increase in free water clearance seen with PGE and PGA may be the result of alternative mechanisms. PGE, for example, antagonizes the effect of antidiuretic hormore (ADH) (107); PGI_2 has not yet been defined as having this effect.

Tannenbaum et al. (51) contrasted intraarterial infusion of PGE_2 and arachidonate in dogs and found low doses of arachidonate increased sodium excretion without significant change in renal blood flow or glomerular filtration rate, implying a direct natriuretic role of endogenous prostaglandins. However, renal blood flow, even at the lowest dose of arachidonate, 1 μg/kg per min, was higher in the infused than the contralateral kidney. Renal vein PGE_2 rose with arachidonate infusion and the natriuretic effect could be blocked by administering an inhibitor of prostaglandin synthesis. An infusion of PGE_2 also caused natriuresis but increased renal blood flow. These studies suggested a natriuretic role for prostaglandins independent of change in renal blood flow, but Bay et al. (108) found that infusions of arachidonate during aortic constriction so that renal perfusion pressure was maintained constant at approximately 80 mmHg (MAP) caused no change in urinary sodium excretion. Since the renal vasculature was maximally vasodilated prior to the infusion, no further change was possible during the arachidonate infusion.

Several other investigators have evaluated the effect of intrarenal prostaglandins on renal sodium excretion. Tobian and O'Donnell (109) studied sodium-loaded and sodium-depleted rats and found that medullary PGE was decreased in sodium-loaded but increased in sodium-deprived rats. The authors postulated that heightened synthesis after sodium deprivation and the lowered levels after sodium loading pointed to PGE being antinatriuretic. However, Dunn has demonstrated that here is no correlation in the spontaneously hypertensive rat between medullary PGE concentration and the rate of prostaglandin synthesis in microsomes of medullary cells (110). Thus medullary PGE content may not reflect the rate of prostaglandin synthesis. Lower medullary PGE may reflect increased utilization with higher tissue levels present during reduced prostaglandin activity. In support of this view, Tan et al. have demonstrated in rats that increasing sodium intake is associated with increased urinary PGE_2 excretion (111).

Conflicting data have been reported in studies utilizing prostaglandin inhibitors to assess the role of renal prostaglandins in sodium excretion. Since prostaglandin synthesis inhibition in anesthetized animals usually reduces renal blood flow, their effect on sodium excretion, independent of renal hemodynamics, is difficult to determine. Kirschenbaum and Stein reported that intrarenal prostaglandins may be antinatriuretic since in conscious dogs meclofenamate or RO-20-5720, a competitive inhibitor of prostaglandin synthesis, caused a slight increase in sodium excretion during a water diuresis without a change in renal blood flow or glomerular filtration rate (63).

Sreenivasan et al. (112) demonstrated that although meclofenamate and RO-20-5720 reduced urinary prostaglandin E_2 excretion in conscious chronically instrumented dogs following a modest sodium load (2% of body weight of 0.45 NaCl), the decrease in sodium excretion observed was not statistically significant. Furthermore, Altsheler et al. (65) and Dusing et al. (113) reported a substantial decrease in sodium excretion when conscious dogs and rats, respectively, received inhibitors of prostaglandin synthesis following even larger sodium loads. Glomerular filtration rate and renal blood flow were nearly constant in all these studies. This suggests that the status of the plasma volume may have a major effect on renal prostaglandin synthesis. Sodium excretion following sodium loading in intact animals may be renal prostaglandin dependent.

Donker and associates demonstrated modest sodium retention and a slight decrease in glomerular filtration rate in humans given indomethacin (114). Prior treatment with a low-sodium diet heightened this effect. Sodium-restricted patients with nephrotic syndrome (115) and a patient with congestive heart failure (116) also have been demonstrated to drop both glomerular filtration rate and sodium excretion when treated with indomethacin. These studies suggest that when the plasma volume is truly depleted or perceived as depleted, as in congestive heart failure, reduced sodium excretion as a consequence of treatment with inhibitor of prostaglandin synthesis may be related primarily to changes in renal hemodynamics. This would be similar to the situation in anesthetized animals. Since inhibitors of prostaglandin synthesis can interfere with a number of enzymes in addition to PG synthetase (117), all the aforementioned studies must be accepted with caution.

In vitro studies also have variable results, depending on the model. Prostaglandin E_1 increases sodium transport across the toad bladder (118) and frog skin (119, 120), suggesting a sodium-retaining effect. In contrast, studies on the isolated perfused rabbit tubules indicate that PGE_2 can cause direct tubular inhibition of sodium reabsorption (121, 122).

On the basis of present evidence, the effect of prostaglandin synthesis on sodium excretion is at least in part explained by the concomitant changes in renal hemodynamics which occur. The status of the plasma volume also appears to be a major determinant of the role of prostaglandin in sodium excretion. Evidence suggests that in both volume-expanded and volume-contracted states, prostaglandins may have a role in sodium handling, but perhaps by different mechanisms. A species-specific direct tubular effect of prostaglandins on renal sodium handling is also possible. Further studies are obviously needed to clarify the physiological role of renal prostaglandin synthesis in control of blood pressure, renal blood flow, and sodium and water excretion.

REFERENCES

1. von Euler, U. S. Über die spezifische blutdrucksenkende Substanz des menschlichen Prostata—und Samenblasensekretes. Klin. Wochenschr. 14:1182, 1935.
2. Goldblatt, M. W. Properties of human seminal plasma. J. Physiol. (Lond.) 84:208, 1935.
3. Fasciolo, J. D., Houssay, B. A., and Taquini, A. C. The blood pressure raising secretion of the ischemic kidney. J. Physiol. (Lond.) 94:281, 1938.
4. Grollman, A., Muirhead, E. E., and Vanatta, J. Role of the kidney in pathogenesis of hypertension as determined by a study of the effects of bilateral nephrectomy and other experimental procedures on the blood pressure of the dog. Am. J. Physiol. 157:21, 1949.
5. Floyer, M. A. Further studies on the mechanism of experimental hypertension in the rat. Clin. Sci. 14:163, 1955.
6. Green, J. A., Lucas, J., and Floyer, M. A. The effect of the kidney in altering the response to the circulation to fluid loading. Clin. Sci. 48:41, 1970.
7. Muirhead, E. E., Stirman, J. A., and Jones, F. Renal autoexplantation and protection against renoprival hypertensive cardiovascular disease and hemolysis. J. Clin. Invest. 39:266, 1960.
8. Muirhead, E. E., Brooks, B., Pitcock, J. A., and Stephenson, P. The renomedullary antihypertensive function in accelerated (malignant) hypertension: with observations on the renomedullary interstitial cells. J. Clin. Invest. 51:181, 1972.
9. Muirhead, E. E., Germain, G., Leach, B. E., Pitcock, J. A., Stephenson, P., Brooks, B., Brosius, W. L., Daniels, E. G., and Hinman, J. W. Production of renomedullary prostaglandins by renomedullary interstitial cells grown in tissue cultures. Circ. Res. 31 (Suppl. II):161, 1972.
10. Lee, J. B., Hickler, R. B., Saravis, C. A., and Thorn, G. W. Sustained depressor effects of renomedullary extracts. Circulation 26:747, 1962.
11. Lee, J. B., Hickler, R. B., Saravis, C. A., and Thorn, G. W. Sustained depressor effects of renal medullary extract in the normotensive rat. Circ. Res. 13:359, 1963.
12. Muirhead, E. E., Brown, G. B., Germain, G. S., and Leach, B. E. The renal medulla as an antihypertensive organ. J. Lab. Clin. Med. 76:641, 1970.
13. Lee, J. B., Covino, B. G., Takman, B. H., and Smith, E. R. Renomedullary vasodepressor substance, medullin. Isolation. Chemical characterization and physiological properties. Circ. Res. 17:57, 1965.
14. Lee, J. B., Crowshaw, K., Takman, B. H., and Attrep, K. A. The identification of prostaglandins $F_{2\alpha}$ and A_2 from rabbit kidney medulla. Biochem. J. 105:1251, 1967.

15. Daniels, E. G., Hinman, J. W., Leach, B. E., and Muirhead, E. E. Identification of prostaglandin E_2 as the principal vasopressor lipid of rabbit renal medulla. Nature (Lond.) 215:1298, 1967.
16. Hamberg, M. Biosynthesis of prostaglandins in the renal medulla of rabbit. Fed. Eur. Biochem. Soc. Lett. 5:127, 1969.
17. Hamberg, M., Svenson, J., Wakabayashi, T., and Samuelsson, B. Isolation and structure of two prostaglandin endoperoxides which cause platelet aggregation. Proc. Natl. Acad. Sci. USA 71:345, 1974.
18. Crowshaw, K. The incorporation of (1-^{14}C) arachidonic acid into the lipids of rabbit renal slices and conversion to prostaglandins E_2 and F_2. Prostaglandins 3:607, 1973.
19. Davis, H. A., and Horton, E. W. Output of prostaglandins from the rabbit kidney, its increase on renal nerve stimulation and its inhibition by indomethacin. Br. J. Pharmacol. 46:658, 1972.
20. Anggard, E., Bohman, S. O., Griffin, J. E., Larsson, C., and Maunsbach, A. B. Subcellular localization of the prostaglandin system in the rabbit renal papilla. Acta Physiol. Scand. 84:231, 1972.
21. Crowshaw, K., and Szlyk, J. Z. Distribution of prostaglandins in the rabbit kidney. Biochem. J. 116:421, 1970.
22. Larsson, C., and Anggard, E. Regional differences in the formation and metabolism of prostaglandins in the rabbit kidney. Eur. J. Pharmacol. 21:30, 1973.
23. Anggard, E., Larsson, C., and Samuelsson, B. The distribution of 15-hydroxyprostaglandin dehydrogenase and prostaglandin A^{13} reductase in tissues of the swine. Acta Physiol. Scand. 81:396, 1971.
24. Crowshaw, K. The incorporation of (1-^{14}C) arachidonic acid into the lipids of rabbit renal slices and conversion to prostaglandins E_2 and $F_{2\alpha}$. Prostaglandins 3:607, 1973.
25. Jouvenza, G. H. Sensitive method of the determination of prostaglandins by gas chromatography with electron capture detection. Biochim. Biophys. Acta 202:231, 1970.
26. Osvaldo, D., and Latta, H. Interstitial cells of the renal medulla. J. Ultrastruct. Res. 15:589, 1966.
27. Muehrcke, R. C., Mandal, A. K., and Volini, F. I. A pathophysiological review of the renal medullary interstitial cells and their relationship to hypertension. Circ. Res. 27(Suppl. I):109, 1970.
28. Tobian, L., Ishii, M., and Duke, M. Relationship of cytoplasmic granules in renal papillary interstitial cells to post salt hypertension. J. Lab. Clin. Med. 73:309, 1969.
29. Prezyna, A., Attalah, A., Vance, K., Schoolman, M., and Lee, J. A newly recognized structure of renomedullary interstitial cell origin associated with high prostaglandin content. Prostaglandins 3:669, 1973.
30. Nissen, H. M., and Anderson, H. On the localization of a prostaglandin-dehydrogenase activity in the kidney. Histochemie 14:189, 1963.
31. Frolich, J. C., Wilson, T. W., Sweetman, B. J., Smigel, M., Nies, A. S.,

Carr, K., Watson, T. J., and Oates, J. A. Urinary prostaglandin identification and origin. J. Clin. Invest. 55:763, 1975.

32. Gill, J. R., Frolich, J. C., Bowden, R. E., Taylor, A. A., Keiser, H. R., Seyberth, H. W., Oates, J. A., and Bartter, J. C. Bartter's syndrome: a disorder characterized by high urinary prostaglandins and a dependence of hyperreninemia on prostaglandin synthesis. Am. J. Med. 61:43, 1976.
33. Davis, H. A. Output of prostaglandins from the rabbit kidney on renal nerve stimulation. J. Physiol. (Lond.) 201:76, 1969.
34. McGiff, J. C., Crowshaw, K., Terragno, N. A., Lonigro, A. J., Strand, J. C., Williamson, M. A., Lee, J. B., and Ng, K. K. F. Prostaglandin-like substances appearing in canine renal venous blood during renal ischemia. Circ. Res. 27:765, 1970.
35. McGiff, J. C., Crowshaw, K., Terragno, N. A., and Lonigro, A. J. Release of a prostaglandin-like substance into renal venous blood in response to angiotensin II. Circ. Res. 27(Suppl. I):121, 1970.
36. McGiff, J. C., Crowshaw, K., Terragno, N. A., Malik, K. U., and Lonigro, A. J. Differential effect of noradrenaline and renal nerve stimulation on vascular resistance in the dog kidney and the release of a prostaglandin E-like substance. Clin. Sci. 42:223, 1972.
37. Seyberth, H. W., Segre, G. V., Morgan, J. L., Sweetman, B. J., Potts, J. T., Jr., and Oates, J. A. Prostaglandins as mediators of hypercalcemia associated with certain types of cancer. N. Engl. J. Med. 293:1278, 1975.
38. Golub, M., Zia, P., Matsuno, M., and Horton, R. Metabolism of prostaglandins A and E in man. J. Clin. Invest. 56:1404, 1975.
39. McGiff, J. C., Crowshaw, K., and Itskovitz, H. D. Prostaglandins and renal function. Fed. Proc. 33:39, 1974.
40. Horton, E. W., and Jones, R. L. Prostaglandins A_1, A_2, and 19-hydroxy A_1: their actions on smooth muscle and their inactivation on passage through the pulmonary and hepatic portal vascular beds. Br. J. Pharmacol. 37:705, 1969.
41. McGiff, J. C., Terragno, N. A., Strand, J. C., Lee, J. B., and Lonigro, A. J. Selective passage of prostaglandins across the lung. Nature (Lond.) 223:742, 1969.
42. Lee, J. B. Chemical and physiological properties of renal prostaglandins, the antihypertensive effects of medullin in essential hypertension. In Prostaglandins. Almqvist & Wiksell, Stockholm, p. 197, 1966.
43. Carr, A. A. Hemodynamic and renal effects of a prostaglandin PGA_1, in subjects with essential hypertension. Am. J. Med. Sci. 259:21, 1970.
44. Venuto, R. C., O'Dorisio, T., Stein, J. H., and Ferris, T. F. Uterine prostaglandin E secretion and uterine blood flow in the pregnant rabbit. J. Clin. Invest. 55:193, 1975.

45. Zusman, R. M., Snider, J. J., Cline, A., Caldwell, B. B., and Speroff, L. Antihypertensive function of a renal-cell carcinoma. N. Engl. J. Med. 290:843, 1974.
46. Stein, J. H. The renal circulation. In The Kidney, D. Brenner and F. Rector (Edits.). Saunders, Philadelphia, p. 215, 1976.
47. Vander, A. J. Direct effects of prostaglandin on renal function and renin release in anesthetized dog. Am. J. Physiol. 214:218, 1968.
48. Johnston, H. H., Herzon, J. P., and Lauier, D. P. Effect of prostaglandin E_1 on renal hemodynamics, sodium and water excretion. Am. J. Physiol. 213:939, 1967.
49. Martinez-Maldonado, M., Tsaparas, N., Eknoyan, G., and Suki, W. W. Renal actions of prostaglandins. Comparison with acetylcholine and volume expansion. Am. J. Physiol. 222:1147, 1972.
50. Gross, J. B., and Bartter, J. C. Effects of prostaglandins E_1, A_1 and F_2 on renal handling of salt and water. Am. J. Physiol. 225:218, 1973.
51. Tannenbaum, J., Splawinski, J. A., Oates, J. A., and Nies, A. S. Enhanced renal prostaglandin production in the dog: effects on renal function. Circ. Res. 36:197, 1975.
52. Larsson, C., and Anggard, E. Increased juxtamedullary blood flow on stimulation of intrarenal prostaglandin biosynthesis. Eur. J. Pharmacol. 25:326, 1974.
53. Chang, L. C. T., Splawinski, J. A., Oates, J. A., and Nies, A. S. Enhanced renal prostaglandin production in the dog: II. Effects on intrarenal hemodynamics. Circ. Res. 36:204, 1975.
54. Nutgeren, D. H. Arachidonate lipoxygenase in blood platelets. Biochim. Biophys. Acta 380:299, 1975.
55. Splawinski, J. A., Nies, A. S., Sweetman, B., and Oates, J. A. The effects of arachidonic acid, prostaglandin E_2 and prostaglandin F_2 on the longitudinal stomach strip of the rat. J. Pharmacol. Exp. Ther. 197:501, 1973.
56. Flower, R. J. Drugs which inhibit prostaglandin biosynthesis. Pharmacol. Rev. 26:33, 1974.
57. Lonigro, A. J., Itskovitz, H. D., Crowshaw, K., and McGiff, J. C. Dependency of renal blood flow on prostaglandin synthesis in the dog. Circ. Res. 32:712, 1973.
58. Kirschenbaum, M. A., White, N., Stein, J. H., and Ferris, T. F. Redistribution of renal cortical blood flow during inhibition of prostaglandin synthesis. Am. J. Physiol. 227:801, 1974.
59. Itskovitz, H. D., Terrango, N. A., and McGiff, J. C. Effect of a renal prostaglandin on distribution of blood flow in the isolated canine kidney. Circ. Res. 34:770, 1974.
60. Solez, K., Fox, J. A., Miller, M., and Heptinstall, R. H. Effects of indomethacin on renal inner medullary plasma flow. Prostaglandins 7:91, 1974.
61. Zins, G. R. Renal prostaglandins. Am. J. Med. 58:14, 1975.

62. Swain, J. A., Heyndrckx, G. R., Boetcher, D. A., and Vatner, S. F. Prostaglandin control of renal circulation in the unanesthetized dog and baboon. Am. J. Physiol. 229:826, 1975.
63. Kirschenbaum, M. A., and Stein, J. H. The effect of inhibition of prostaglandin synthesis on urinary sodium excretion in the conscious dog. J. Clin. Invest. 57:517, 1976.
64. Terragno, N., Terragno, D., McGiff, J. Contribution of prostaglandins to the renal circulation in the conscious, anesthetized and laparotomized dogs. Circ. Res. 40:590, 1977.
65. Altsheler, P., Klahr., S., Rosenbaum, R., Slatopolsky, E. Effects of inhibitors of prostaglandin synthesis on renal sodium excretion in normal dogs and dogs with decreased renal mass. Am. J. Physiol. 4:F338, 1978.
66. Burger, B. M., Hopkins, T., Tulloch, A., and Hollenberg, N. K. The role of angiotensin in the canine renal vascular response to barbiturate anesthesia. Circ. Res. 38:196, 1976.
67. Needleman, P., Kauffman, A. H., Douglas, J. R., Johnson, E. M., and Marshall, G. R. Specific stimulation and inhibition of renal prostaglandin release by angiotensin analogs. Am. J. Physiol. 224:1415, 1973.
68. Aiken, J. W., and Vane, J. R. Intrarenal prostaglandin release attenuates the renal vasoconstrictor activity of angiotensin. J. Pharmacol. Exp. Ther. 184:678, 1973.
69. Itskovitz, H. D., and McGiff, J. C. Hormonal regulation of the renal circulation. Circ. Res. 35(Suppl. I):65, 1974.
70. Satoh, S., and Zimmerman, B. G. Influence of the renin-angiotensin system on the effect of prostaglandin synthesis inhibitor in the renal vasculature. Circ. Res. 36(Suppl. I):89, 1975.
71. Mimran, A., Casellas, D., Dupont, M., and Barjon, P. Effects of a competitive angiotensin antagonist on the renal haemodynamic changes induced by inhibition of prostaglandin synthesis in rats. Clin. Sci. Mol. Med. 48:299, 1975.
72. Davis, J. O., Freeman, R. H., Johnson, J. A., and Spielman, M. Agents which block the action of the renin-angiotensin system. Circ. Res. 34:279, 1974.
73. Kadowitz, P. J. Effects of prostaglandin E_1, E_2 and A_2 on vascular resistance and responses to noradrenaline, nerve stimulation and angiotensin in the dog hindlimb. Br. J. Pharmacol. 46:395, 1972.
74. Aiken, J. W. Effects of prostaglandin synthesis inhibitors on angiotensin tachyphylaxis in the isolated coeliac and mesenteric arteries of the rabbit. Pol. J. Pharmacol. Pharm. 26:217, 1974.
75. Romero, J. C., Strong, C. G., and Ott, C. E. The effect of indomethacin on the renin angiotensin system. J. Clin. Invest. 58:282, 1976.
76. Patak, R. V., Mookerjee, B. K., Bentzel, C. J., Hysert, P. E., Babej, M., and Lee, J. B. Antagonism of the effects of furosemide by indomethacin in normal and hypertensive man. Prostaglandins 10:649, 1976.

77. Kotchen, I. A., and Miller, M. C. Effect of prostaglandins on renin reactivity. Am. J. Physiol. 226:314, 1974.
78. Needleman, P., Douglas, J. R., Jakschuk, B., Stoecklein, P. B., and Johnson, E. M. Release of renal prostaglandins by catecholamines: relationship to renal endocrine function. J. Pharmacol. Exp. Ther. 188:453, 1974.
79. Needleman, P., Marshall, G. R., and Johnson, E. M. Determinants and modification of adrenergic and vascular resistance in the kidney. Am. J. Physiol. 227:665, 1974.
80. Data, J., Chang, L. C., and Nies, A. S. Alterations of canine vascular response to hemorrhage by inhibitors of prostaglandin synthesis. Am. J. Physiol. 230
81. McGiff, J. C., Terragno, N. A., Malik, K. U., and Lonigro, A. J. Release of prostaglandin E-like substance from canine kidney by bradykinin. Circ. Res. 31:36, 1972.
82. Chapnick, B. M., Paustian, P. W., Joiner, P. D., Human, A. L., and Kadowitz, P. J. Influence of prostaglandin synthesis on renal vascular resistance and on renal vascular responses to vasopressor and vasodilator agents in the cat. Circ. Res. 40:348, 1977.
83. Feldberg, W., and Lewis, G. P. Action of peptides on the adrenal medulla release of adrenaline by bradykinin and angiotensin. J. Physiol. (Lond.), 171:98, 1964.
84. Kadowitz, P. J., Sweet, C. S., and Brody, M. J. Differential effects of prostaglandins E_1, E_2, F_2 and $F_{2\alpha}$ on adrenergic vasoconstriction in the dog hindpaw. J. Pharmacol. Exp. Ther. 76:167, 1971.
85. Hedqvist, P. Control by prostaglandin E_2 of sympathetic neurotransmission in the spleen. Life Sci. 9:269, 1970.
86. Vander, J. F. Effect of catecholamine and the renal nerves on renin secretion in anesthetized dogs. Am. J. Physiol. 209:659, 1965.
87. Winer, N., Chiksi, D. S., and Walkenhorst, W. G. Effects of cyclic AMP sympathomimetic amine and adrenergic receptor antagonists on renin secretion. Circ. Res. 29:239, 1971.
88. Vandongen, R., Peart, W. S., and Boyd, G. W. Adrenergic stimulation of renin secretion in the isolated perfused rat kidney. Circ. Res. 32: 290, 1973.
89. Venuto, R. C. The role of prostaglandin E in the renal function of pregnant rabbits. Clin. Res. 27:432a (abstr.), 1979.
90. Ferris, T. F. Unpublished observation.
91. Verberchkmoes, R., VanDamme, B., Clement, J., Amery, A., and Michielsen, P. Bartter's syndrome with hyperplasia of renomedullary cells: successful treatment with indomethacin. Kidney Int. 9:302, 1976.
92. Galvez, O. G., Bay, W. H., Roberts, B. W., and Ferris, T. F. The hemodynamic effects of potassium deficiency. Circ. Res. 40(Suppl. I): 11-16, 1977.
93. Trygstad, C. W., Mangos, J. A., Bloodworth, J. M. B., Jr. A sib-

ship with Bartter's syndrome: failure of total adrenalectomy to correct the potassium wasting. Pediatrics 44:235, 1969.

94. Williamson, H. E., Bowland, W. A., and Marchand, G. R. Inhibition of ethacrynic acid induced increase in renal blood flow in indomethacin. Prostaglandins 8:297, 1974.
95. Bailie, M. D., Barbour, J. A., and Hook, J. B. Effects of indomethacin on furosemide-induced changes in renal blood flow. Proc. Soc. Exp. Med. Biol. 148:1173, 1975.
96. Herbaczynska-Cedro, K., and Vane, J. R. Contribution of intrarenal generation of prostaglandin to autoregulation of renal blood flow in the dog. Circ. Res. 33:428, 1973.
97. Venuto, R. C., O'Dorisio, T., Ferris, T. F., and Stein, J. H. Prostaglandins and renal function: II. The Effect of prostaglandin inhibition on autoregulation of blood flow in the intact kidney of the dog. Prostaglandins 9:817, 1975.
98. Anderson, R. J., Taker, M. S., Cronin, R. E., McDonald, K. M., and Schrier, R. W. Effect of B-adrenergic blockade and inhibitors of angiotensin II and prostaglandins on renal autoregulation. Am. J. Physiol. 229:731, 1975.
99. Kaloyanides, G. J., Ahrens, R. E., Shepherd, J. A., and DiBona, G. F. Inhibition of prostaglandin E_2 secretion: failure to abolish autoregulation in the isolated dog kidney. Circ. Res. 38:67, 1976.
100. Moncado, S., Guyglewski, R., Bunting, S., and Vane, J. R. An enzyme isolated from arteries transforms prostaglandin endoperoxides to an unstable substance that inhibits platelet aggregation. Nature (Lond.) 263:663, 1976.
101. Pace-Asciak, C. R., and Rangaraj, G. Distribution of prostaglandin biosynthetic pathways in several rat tissue formation of 6-ketoprostaglandin F_1. Biochim. Biophys. Acta 486:579, 1977.
102. Morrison, A. R., Nishikawa, K., and Needleman, P. Unmasking of thromboxane A_2 synthesis by ureteral obstruction in the rabbit kidney. Nature (Lond.) 267:259, 1977.
103. Lee, J. B., McGiff, J. C., Kannegiessir, H., Ayken, Y. Y., Mudd, J. G., and Frawley, T. F. Antihypertensive renal effects of prostaglandin A_1 in patients with essential hypertension. Ann. Intern. Med. 74:703, 1971.
104. Fichman, M. P., Littenburg, G., Brooker, G., and Horton, R. Effect of prostaglandin A_1 on renal and adrenal function in man. Circ. Res. 30/31(Suppl. II):19, 1972.
105. Strandhoy, J. W., Ott, C. E., Schneider, E. G., Willis, L. R., Beck, N. P., Davis, B. B., and Knox, F. G. Effects of prostaglandins E_1 and E_2 on renal sodium reabsorption and Starling forces. Am. J. Physiol. 226:1015, 1974.
106. Gerber, J. C., Nies, A. S., Friesinger, G. C., Gerkens, J. E., Branch, R. A., and Oates, J. A. The effect of PGI_2 on canine renal

function and hemodynamics. Prostaglandins 16:519, 1978.

107. Grantham, J. J., and Orloff, J. Effect of prostaglandin E, on the permeability response of the isolated collected tubule to vasopressin, adenosine 3',5'-monophosphate and theophylline. J. Clin. Invest. 47: 1154, 1968.

108. Bay, W. H., Mishkind, M. H., Lane, G. E., and Ferris, T. F. Studies of the mechanism of natriuresis with prostaglandin E. J. Lab. Clin. Med. 93:78-84, 1979.

109. Tobian, L., and O'Donnell, M. Renal prostaglandins in relation to sodium regulation and hypertension. Fed. Proc. 35:2388, 1976.

110. Dunn, M. J. Renal prostaglandin synthesis in the spontaneously hypertensive rat. J. Clin. Invest. 58:862, 1976.

111. Tan, S., Sandwisch, D., and Mulrow, P. Salt intake as a determinant of renal prostaglandin E_2 production. Clin. Res. 26:693A (abstr.), 1978.

112. Sreenivasan, V., Walker, B., Mookerjee, B., Krasney, J., and Venuto, R. The effect of inhibition of prostaglandin synthesis on the natriuresis of furosemide in conscious dogs. Hypertension 3:59, 1981.

113. Dusing, R., Melder, B., and Kramer, J. H. Prostaglandins and renal function in acute extracellular volume expansion. Prostaglandins 12:3, 1976.

114. Donker, A., Arisz, L., Brentjens, J., Van Der Hem, S., and Hollemans, H. The effect of indomethacin on kidney function and plasma renin activity in man. Nephron 17:288, 1976.

115. Arisz, L., Brentjens, J., Donker, A., and Van Der Hem, G. The effect of indomethacin on proteinuria and the kidney function in the nephrotic syndrome. Acta Med. Scand. 199:121, 1976.

116. Walshe, J., and Venuto, R. Acute oliguric renal failure induced by indomethacin: possible mechanism. Ann. Intern. Med. 91:47, 1979.

117. Dunn, M., and Hood, V. Prostaglandins and the kidney. Am. J. Physiol. 233(3): F169, 1977.

118. Lipson, L. C., and Sharp, G. W. Effect of prostaglandin E_1 on sodium transport and osmotic water flow in toad bladder. Am. J. Physiol. 220:1046, 1971.

119. Fassina, G., Carpenedo, F., and Santi, R. Effect of prostaglandin E_1 on isolated short-circuited frog skin. Life Sci. 8:181, 1969.

120. Barr, E., and Hall, W. J. Stimulation of sodium movement across frog skin by prostaglandin E_1. J. Physiol. (Lond.) 200:83, 1969.

121. Kauker, M. Prostaglandin E_2 effect from the luminal side on renal tubular ^{22}Na efflux: tracer microinjection studies. Proc. Soc. Exp. Biol. Med. 154:274, 1977.

122. Stokes, J., and Kokko, J. Inhibition of sodium transport by prostaglandin E_2 across the isolated, perfused rabbit collecting tubule. J. Clin. Invest. 59:1099, 1977.

7 Prostaglandins and the Renin-Angiotensin-Aldosterone System

MERRILL L. OVERTURF / ROBERT E. DRUILHET* / and WALTER M. KIRKENDALL / The University of Texas Medical School, Houston, Texas

The series of biochemical transformations and the attending physiological sequelae, known collectively as the renin-angiotensin-aldosterone system (RAAS), have achieved scientific and clinical prominence. Besides the enormous number of research papers that have been published during the past several years concerning various aspects of the RAAS, it has also been the subject of recent monographs (Oparil, 1976; Oparil and Katholi, 1977), book chapters (Soffer, 1976; Genest et al., 1977), journal reviews (Skeggs et al., 1976; Erdös, 1976; Peart, 1978), and symposia (Buckley and Ferrario, 1977; Davis, 1977; Ganten et al., 1978).

One reason it has commanded so much attention is that it has been linked, to various degrees, to the etiology and pathology of various types of hypertension and other disturbances of cardiovascular function. The RAAS has profound pharmacological effects which relate to the well-known pressor activity of angiotensin II (AII) and its steroidogenic effects on aldosterone. Angiotensin causes strong vasoconstriction of the cardiovascular system, particularly in the precapillary vessels of skin, splanchnic mesentery, and the kidney. Subtle effects are observed in the vessels of skeletal muscle, adrenals, heart, and brain; the pulmonary and heart vasculature appear to be unaffected by AII. Systemic pressure elevation and stimulation of the sympathetic system due to AII mask apparent effects on either the heart or coronary vessels, as in vitro experiments show that AII increases the strength and rate of cardiac contraction. Correspondingly, the elevated systemic blood pressure presumably provides adequate coronary flow so that despite inotropic and chronotropic effects and increased work load, coronary insufficiency seldom ensues. Stimulation of the central and peripheral nervous system by AII also contributes to the overall cardiovascular response through increased sympathetic outflow, potentiation of adrenergic transmission, and stimulatory action of sympathetic ganglia.

*Present affiliation: OBI Hughes

Angiotensin II has a stimulatory effect on the adrenal gland, where it causes release of catecholamines from the medulla and aldosterone from the cortex. These effects lead to increased sympathomimetic activity and alterations of sodium-potassium balance. Additionally, AII has direct effects on the kidney and the renal vascular bed which can lead to either diuresis or sodium retention. These variable effects depend on dose, species, posture, sodium balance, and other factors.

Until quite recently, renin was thought to be a physiologically passive protein in that its only known action was to form angiotensin I (AI). However, clinical observations of malignant hypertension where renin activity is very high, as well as experimental data, have led to speculation regarding its vasculotoxicity. It has even been suggested recently that renin may play an important role in atherogenesis.

There are numerous clinical conditions ascribed to derangements of the RAAS. The most significant disease which embraces the RAAS is hypertension. There is little doubt that the high blood pressure which accompanies functional stenosis of the renal artery is due to increased activity of the RAAS. In the case of hypertension and nephrosclerosis, the conclusions are more tenuous, for it is argued by some that hypertension secondarily involves the arterioles of the kidney, thereby producing nephrosclerosis, while others believe that nephrosclerosis is the primary event leading to hypertension. It is not clear as to which occurs first, the lesions or the increased pressure. The possible role of the RAAS in hypertensive disease where renin activity is normal or below normal, such as primary aldosteronism and essential hypertension, has also caused much speculation. There are

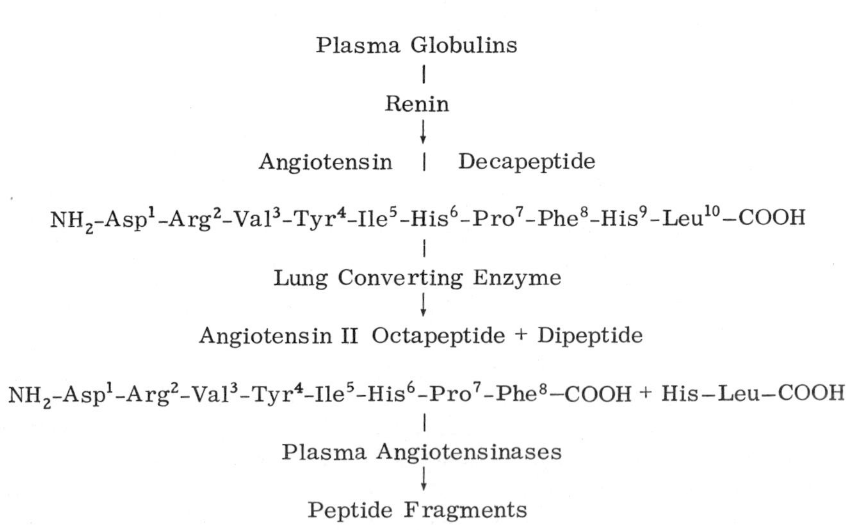

FIG. 1. Essentials of the renin-angiotensin sequence (human forms shown).

some diseases where hypertension is absent, even though high levels of renin and circulating AII are in evidence. Examples of these include adrenal cortical insufficiency, low-output congestive heart failure with hyperaldosteronism, and Bartter's syndrome. These seemingly paradoxical situations indicate that the complete story of the RAAS is not known.

The purpose of this chapter is to review selected literature published largely since 1975 concerning the RAAS and attempt to differentiate clearly that which is known from that which is suspected, and identify those areas where additional studies are needed.

Until recently, the components and transformations of the renin-angiotensin sequence could be simply described (Fig. 1). Renin, a proteolytic enzyme, is released from the kidney into the circulatory system. Here, it comes into contact with renin substrate, angiotensinogen, which is derived from the liver. The hydrolytic action of renin on renin substrate at the Leu-Leu bond yields angiotensin I, a decapeptide intermediate that is without significant physiological activity. The majority of the AI formed is subsequently hydrolyzed at the Phe-His bond by lung angiotensin-converting enzyme (ACE) to yield the active octapeptide, angiotensin II. Various peptidases of plasma inactivate AII by hydrolysis to peptide fragments. It is now recognized that the biochemical formation and degradation of AI and AII is much more complex than this catechistic description.

RENIN SUBSTRATES

The formation, purification, assay, and properties of renin substrates (angiotensinogens) have been reviewed (Skeggs, 1974). Proteins which can serve as renin substrates (RS) were first isolated from the α_2-globulins of hog plasma and since then RS have been demonstrated in lymph, liver, and most recently, kidney (Morris and Johnston, 1976a) and brain (Printz et al., 1978; Morris and Reid, 1978).

Skeggs et al. (1957) demonstrated that a tryptic digest of horse plasma protein produced a tetradecapeptide (TDP) that could serve as a renin substrate. Sequential analysis showed that the N-terminus was composed of aspartic acid and the preceding nine amino acids were in the same sequence as those in AI; the tetrapeptide (Leu-Val-Tyr-Ser) was attached to the C-terminal leucine of the AI sequence. The structure of TDP renin substrate was subsequently confirmed by synthesis (Skeggs et al., 1958) and the kinetics of the TDP-renin reaction was determined (Montague et al., 1966; Skeggs et al., 1968). Several studies have since made use of this substrate (Ganten et al., 1971; Boucher et al., 1974) and the labeled 3-[^{14}C]valine-TDP substrate (Mendelsohn and Johnston, 1971; Overturf et al., 1974). It has the obvious advantages of having a chemically defined structure and it permits the direct measurement of AI.

Much information regarding the metabolism of AI and its metabolites could be obtained from the availability of a series of TDP compounds containing various radiolabeled amino acids; however, they are not available. The development of dual-labeled TDP would also provide a potent tool for the study of renin renin-substrate reactions. Bath and Gregerman (1972) synthesized a labeled polymeric renin substrate (N-acetyl-poly-L-glutamyl-[125]-tridecapeptide) and a [^{14}C]cyanate-labeled protein substrate for renin has recently been developed (Lentz et al., 1976). However, the low sensitivity of the methods involved in the use of these substrates severely limits their usefulness.

Skeggs et al. (1963) demonstrated that hog plasma RS existed in multiple forms, with three of the major forms having a molecular weight of about 58,000. With further purification of three of the five major forms (A, B, and C), subfractions of B and C were obtained (B_1-B_2, C_1-C_2). Three forms (A, C_1, and C_2) were found to be glycoproteins with nearly identical amino acid sequences. However, there were substantial differences in their glucosamine, sialic acid, and hexose content. The Michaelis constants were also different (Skeggs et al., 1967). A comparative study of renin substrates of eight mammalian species indicated considerable differences in their electrophoretic mobility and on this basis they were divided into two main groups: those moving with α_2-globulins (cow, sheep, pig, and rabbit) and those moving as α_1-globulins (human, dog, rat, and mouse) (Gordon and Sachin, 1975).

Purified renin substrates have recently been obtained from plasma of various sources (human, hog, rabbit, and rat). It has been found that they have different molecular weights and all of them exhibit microheterogeneity (Tewksbury et al., 1977; Printz et al., 1977; Faiers et al., 1977; Dorer et al., 1978).

Early evidence from observations of hepatotectomized animals strongly suggested that the liver is the major source of plasma RS. The clear demonstration that liver synthesizes and releases RS was accomplished by the perfusion of radiolabeled amino acids into isolated rat livers (Nasjletti and Masson, 1972). Nasjletti and Masson (1973) extended their studies by investigating whether AII might alter RS formation. They found that renin, AI, and AII administration stimulated RS formation by the liver and thus proposed a positive feedback mechanism. A recent study has shown that isolated hepatocytes can synthesize and secrete angiotensinogen (Weigand et al., 1977).

Little is known about the specific mechanisms that regulate RS formation. However, several physiological states are associated with variations in RS levels. Plasma renin substrate levels are found to be elevated during pregnancy, postnephrectomy, and upon the administration of various substances such as ACTH, cortisone, diethylstilbestrol, and oral contraceptives. It has been reported that the average K_m value for homologous substrate and human renin was 0.782 nmol/ml in a normal population (Gould and Green, 1971). The K_m for the reaction of human renin on human substrate of women who were either receiving oral contraceptives or were essential hypertensives was 0.931 nmol/ml; the K_m values were much higher in malignant hypertensives with an average of 3.160 nmol/ml. Although these data are interesting and may have important clinical significance, the validity of enzyme kinetic data obtained from such crude enzyme and substrate preparations can be questioned.

Intrinsic plasma RS concentrations are of practical importance in terms of the clinical assay of renin activity, where renin activity is equated with the generation of AI in plasma during an incubation period (Kirkendall et al., 1975). It is held by some investigators (Skinner, 1967; Weinberger et al., 1969), although not by all (Haas and Goldblatt, 1967; Rieger et al., 1972), that plasma substrate concentration is seldom great enough to provide zero-order kinetics. If substrate concentration is rate limiting, the velocity at which a certain plasma sample forms angiotensin I (PRA) would be a variable determined not only by the concentration of renin, but also by the substrate concentration. Indeed, the control of substrate concentration is of prime importance in the kinetics of all enzyme reactions. Considering the commonly used clinical radioimmunoassay procedures for determining PRA, the use of endogenous substrate precludes this important requisite. The existence of naturally occurring plasma renin activators and inhibitors further complicates kinetic studies of renin-substrate reactions in plasma and will be discussed later in the text.

RENAL RENIN SYNTHESIS AND STORAGE

There is little doubt that the renal juxtaglomerular apparatus, which is comprised of the juxtaglomerular (JG) cells and the macula densa, is the center of renal renin synthesis and secretion (reviews by Thurau and Mason, 1974; Davis and Freeman, 1976). However, there is no information regarding the biochemical synthesis of renal renin; thus it has not been possible to dissociate renin synthesis from renin release.

Renin is found in a concentration gradient, with the highest concentration being in the JG cells of the renal afferent arteriole and the lowest amount present in the efferent arteriolar wall and the mesangial cells. Similarly, a renin concentration gradient is present in the renal cortex, with the greatest amount being in the outer cortex with decreasing concentrations inward. Most of the renin is released into the renal circulation via the lumen of the afferent arteriole, although some is secreted into the renal lymph.

Catheterization of the renal vein, aorta, and inferior vena cava is used experimentally and clinically to obtain blood samples for the determination of plasma renin activity and renin secretion rates. This renal catheterization technique is used clinically for determining possible kidney and renal vasculature involvement in hypertensive patients. Plasma renin activity (PRA) is also frequently measured in peripheral venous blood of hypertensives as a screening procedure. However, it has limited diagnostic usefulness, for at best it is an indirect measurement which represents a net estimation of the renin activity released by the kidney and the rate of renin catabolism.

RENAL RENIN-RELEASE MECHANISMS

During the past several years there has been great emphasis placed on the elucidation of the mechanisms that control renin release (reviews by Chonko et al., 1975; Davis and Freeman, 1976; Zanchetti et al., 1976; Peart, 1978). There are many events which are known to provoke renin release. Some of these stimuli include postural changes, acute and chronic salt depletion, hemorrhage, and renal artery stenosis. Although it is recognized that there is a plethora of experimental, physiological, and pathological conditions that affect renin secretion, the proposed mechanisms are still contested. Indeed, there is still controversy regarding the role of renin per se in cardiovascular homeostasis and the participation of renin in various pathological conditions, such as renovascular hypertension. However, in our opinion the development of compounds, such as analogs of AII, that block specific components of the RAAS has adequately shown that the RAAS is actively involved in several pathological states.

There are three major conditions that are known to induce renin release: (1) decreased sodium reaching the macula densa, (2) decreased blood pressure at the juxtaglomerular cells, and (3) increased sympathetic nervous system activity and increased levels of circulating catecholamines. Davis and Freeman (1976) broadly classified the various mechanisms controlling kidney renin release accordingly: (1) intrarenal sensors comprising the renal vascular receptors of the afferent arterioles which sense changes in perfusion pressure (baroreceptor theory) and sodium sensors located in the macula densa of the distal tubules (macula densa theory); (2) sympathetic activity of the renal nerves; and (3) humoral agents, some of which increase PRA, such as sodium ions, chloride ions, potassium ions, epinephrine, arachidonic acid, prostaglandin E_2, and norepinephrine, whereas others, such as angiotensin II and antidiuretic hormone, decrease PRA. Recent studies indicate that dopamine (Imbs et al., 1975) and calcium (Yamamoto et al., 1974) should be added to the "humoral" category.

An excellent study using the specific AII analog P-113 (Saralasin) has substantiated the view that circulating AII inhibits renin release by direct intrarenal action involving negative feedback control of renin release via end-product inhibition (Keeton et al., 1976). From the observations that propranolol reduced saralasin-induced renin release under all experimental conditions, it was concluded that the "short-loop" feedback mechanism is closely associated with intrarenal β-adrenergic receptors.

There is presently much interest in determining the precise role of the renal sympathetic nerves and catecholamines in renin release. It is generally held that it is the intrarenal β-adrenergic receptors and not the α-receptors which mediate the increased renin response to renal nerve stimulation and circulating catecholamines (Zanchetti et al., 1976; Johnson et al., 1976). Numerous studies have shown that many stimuli that increase renin release are inhibited by a β-adrenergic blocker (propranolol), but not by

α-blockers (phentolamine or phenoxybenzamine) (Ganong, 1972; Michelakis and McAllister, 1972; Johnson et al., 1976).

It has been postulated that the β-adrenergic stimulus to the kidney increases renin release via the cyclic adenosine monophosphate (AMP) system in the kidney (Winer et al., 1972; Beck et al., 1972). Allison et al. (1972) found that dibutyryl cyclic AMP, but not 5'-AMP or cyclic AMP, was associated with an increase in PRA in dogs. Unfortunately, the results were confounded, since the increase in PRA was accompanied by a decrease in plasma potassium concentration, a well-known stimulus of renin secretion. Another study of the role of the β-adrenergic stimulus-dependent cyclic AMP system in the dog kidney on renin release has been performed (Beck et al., 1975). Lithium was used to inhibit the effect of β-adrenergic stimulation of cyclic AMP generation, since lithium, unlike propranolol, inhibits the catecholamine-dependent cyclic AMP generation in the kidney without altering the hemodynamic effects of β-adrenergic stimulation. Additionally, the natriuretic effect of lithium was controlled by the administration of sodium chloride. They concluded that the increase in PRA observed after an injection of isoproterenol, a sympathomimetic amine, in lithium-treated dogs was probably not mediated through the β-adrenergic stimulus-dependent cyclic AMP in the kidney.

A study by Mancia et al. (1975) has shown that blocking vagal traffic (section of the cervical nerves and denervation or vascular isolation of the carotid sinuses) from the cardiopulmonary region caused a significant increase in renin release that was abolished after renal denervation. They concluded that the vagally innervated receptors in the cardiopulmonary region exert a tonic reflex inhibition of renin release by decreasing the sympathetic nerve activity to the kidney.

A recent study was conducted to determine whether renal hypertension of either the one-kidney (one kidney clipped and contralateral nephrectomy—low renin) or the two-kidney type (one kidney clipped and contralateral kidney left untouched—high renin) could be maintained for an extended period of time in guanethidine-sympathectomized rats (Douglas et al., 1975). They found that the absence of the peripheral sympathetic nervous system had no effect on the development and maintenance of hypertension in either hypertensive model.

Bravo and associates (1975) studied 69 essential hypertensive patients by examining the relationship between changes in PRA and arterial pressure in response to a β-adrenergic blocking agent, propranolol. PRA did not correlate well with blood pressure in either the patients receiving propranolol alone or in those patients who received a combination of diuretics and propranolol. Long-term β-adrenergic blockage did not inhibit the increases of PRA induced by either diuretics or rapid sodium depletion. They concluded, therefore, that β-adrenergic blockage can reduce blood pressure by mechanisms other than suppression of PRA and that although the β-adrenergic nervous system is important, it is not essential for renin release.

In vivo experiments aimed at defining the precise role that the sympathetic system has in regulating renin release have all been hampered by the complex nature of the RAAS. That is, the RAAS is very sensitive to many stimuli, particularly those that affect renal function and volume and electrolyte homeostasis. Similarly, it has been difficult to separate the effects of the sympathetic nervous system from other mechanisms that are known to effect renin release: sodium load at the macula densa, humoral agents, and stimulation of the vascular receptors in the renal afferent arterioles. Finally, the β-adrenergic drugs, which have been used as pharmacological probes, have various nonspecific effects which make cause-and-effect conclusions suspect. For example, the effect on renin release ascribed to the blocking of β-receptors with propranolol might also be due to other effects which propranolol has, such as its effects on the central nervous system, its ability to decrease glomerular filtration rate, and its blood pressure-lowering effect. Indeed, there is spirited controversy concerning whether renin suppression is an important mechanism for the hypotensive action of propranolol, as claimed by Buhler et al. (1973). However, as suggested by Stokes et al. (1974), differences in sodium balance between the patient populations may have contributed to the apparent discrepancies in many of the results obtained.

A study by Zanchetti and Stella (1975) used a combined experimental approach to separate the renin-releasing and vasomotor effects of sympathetic stimulation. Their techniques entailed stimulation of the vasomotor center in the brain stem known to give equal renin-releasing and vasoconstrictor responses on the two sides, and leaving one kidney innervated with the contralateral kidney being either denervated or treated with phenoxybenzamine or propanolol. They obtained evidence that sympathetic stimulation can induce renin release from the kidney independently of local vasomotor changes.

Despite the number of difficulties inherent in in vivo studies of the RAAS, it appears that the vast majority of recent studies credit a profound effect on renin release by intrarenal β-adrenergic receptors. Certainly, there is dwindling support for a role for α-adrenergic receptors in the control of renin release.

To avoid the "nonspecific" effects of drugs such as β-blockers, confounding effects of feedback loops, and other stimuli which operate in vivo, attention has been directed toward developing in vitro systems. Predictably, even the results obtained by the "simplified" in vitro approach have been controversial. For example, in vitro rat kidney slice incubations have led Braverman et al. (1971) and Corsini et al. (1974) to conclude that renin secretion from kidney slices may be taking place at a maximal rate and thus the system is not responsive to the usual in vivo stimuli (e.g., epinephrine, norepinephrine, and furosemide). A rat kidney slice technique developed by Weinberger and Rosner (1972) and its subsequent extensive use (Aoi et al., 1974; Weinberger et al., 1975; Aoi et al. 1976) has proven to be sensitive to direct stimulatory effects of epinephrine and norepinephrine on renin release (Aoi et al., 1974). A later study using the Weinberger perfusion technique gave in vitro evidence that the sympathetic nerve fibers of the JG apparatus are able to release epinephrine and stimulate renin release by a theophylline-amplified β-adenergic mechanism (Aoi et al., 1976). Significantly, tyramine-induced stimulation of renin release was blocked by propranolol and cocaine, but not by the α-antagonist phentolamine. The development of this model represents a significant advance toward the better understanding of the kidney and the RAAS. Specifically, it allows for the study of renin release which is devoid of complicating humoral, neurogenic, and hemodynamic factors. It should find wide application in the study of drugs affecting renin release, renin accelerators, renin inhibitors, and general intrarenal metabolism.

A somewhat different in vitro technique was developed by Hofbauer et al. (1974). This model entails perfusion of isolated rat kidneys with a defined medium at a constant pressure. It shares many of the desirable attributes of the kidney slice technique; however, it is more difficult to use. It does offer the added advantage of allowing the study of pressure-flow relationships in the intact kidney.

RENAL AND PLASMA RENINS

Kidney renin (EC 3.4.99.19), being the apparent initiator of the reaction leading to the formation of AII, with its attendant physiological and pathological sequelae, is becoming a more difficult subject. It can no longer be held that renin is a specific enzyme; rather, "renin" is most accurately conceived of as a family of enzymes, which hydrolyze leucyl-leucyl bonds at positions 10 and 11 of renin substrates.

It has been observed that PRA in some normal subjects and patients increase with storage, even at -20°C (Osmond et al., 1973a; Sealey and Laragh, 1975; Sealey et al., 1976). It appeared that the increase in PRA was not due to changes in renin substrate or to changes brought about by plasma activators or inhibitors. Rather, it was speculated that the increase was due to the activation of an inactive form of renin called "prorenin." The possibility that the increase in PRA was due to pseudorenin was ruled untenable on the basis of pH optima. Sealey and Laragh (1975) also observed that prorenin changed according to changes in sodium balance in some low-renin patients and was absent in others. These observations have stimulated additional studies aimed at determining possible diagnostic, physiological, and clinical relevance of prorenin.

There are several studies which report the existence of inactive forms of renin in humans (Morris and Lumbers, 1972; Skinner et al., 1975; Day et al., 1976; deLeiva et al., 1976; Derkx et al., 1976), rabbits (Leckie and McConnell, 1975), hogs (Boyd, 1974; Lauritzen et al., 1976), and rats (Morris and Johnston, 1976b). These renins appear to be activated by exposure to acid. However, the physiological importance of these observations is not as apparent as the observations that some enzymes have been shown to activate certain renins.

Numerous studies regarding the occurrence of multiple molecular weight forms of plasma and kidney renin, renin proenzymes, and the activation of renin by chemical and physical means have been reviewed (Overturf et al., 1979a). Many, but not all, of the studies have been able to demonstrate multiple molecular weight forms of renin, and most studies indicate that renin activity is enhanced by acid treatment (Rubin, 1972; Skinner et al., 1975) and by subjecting renin to low temperatures (Osmond et al., 1973a; Sealey et al., 1976).

Investigations have also shown that various proteases, including trypsin (Morris and Lumbers, 1972; Day and Luetscher, 1974; Cooper et al., 1977), pepsin (Morris and Lumbers, 1972; Day and Luetscher, 1975; Morris, 1978), cathepsin D (Morris, 1978), and urinary kallikrein (Sealey et al., 1978), when added to plasma or crude renin-substrate preparations, resulted in an apparent increase of renin activity, as measured by increased angiotensin I generation. A recent study using purified hog kidney renin and purified homologous substrate has shown that thrombin, as well as urinary kallikrein, can increase high molecular weight renin activity without a demonstrable change in molecular weight; plasmin was without effect (Overturf et al., 1979b).

A review of the literature concerning multiple molecular weight forms and activatable forms of renin leads to several conclusions:

1. Inactive plasma and kidney proteins exist which are referred to as "inactive renins" and "cryoactivatable renins." Some can be "activated" to generate angiotensin I by treatment with acid, enzymes, or low temperature.
2. The biochemical nature of inactive renins and cryoactivatable renins is largely unknown. In some species, the activation process is accompanied by a change in the molecular weight of the proteins, whereas in other species no change is noted. Nothing is known regarding the Mw of cryoactivatable renins.
3. There is no biochemical evidence that acid activatable renins are the same substances as cryoactivatable renins. There are some observations that indicate that they sometimes respond to stimuli known to affect renal renin release.
4. No physiological function has been positively ascribed to these "inactive" proteins. Indeed, the in vivo transformation to the active form has only been inferred.
5. No specific enzyme(s) has been clearly identified with the physiological transformation of either inactive or cryoactivatable renins, however, pepsin, trypsin, kallikrein, thrombin, and cathepsin D have been associated with it.

Interest has recently been shown in obtaining pure renal renins (review by Haber and Slater, 1977). The techniques of affinity chromotography have been applied to hog kidney renin using pepstatin renin inhibitor (Murakami and Inagami, 1975; Devaux et al., 1975), short peptide analogs of renin substrate (Majstoravich et al., 1974) and the synthetic competitive inhibitor of D-Leu^6-octapeptide (Poulsen et al., 1975). A study of the purification of human renin using a pepstatin-aminohexylagarose column demonstrated three discrete renin activity peaks; the first peak had a specific activity of 206 GU/mg protein, which represented a 137,000-fold purification (Inagami et al., 1976). In addition, the glycoprotein nature of renin from rabbit and human kidney has been demonstrated by affinity chromatography on concanavalin A-Sepharose (Printz and Dworschack, 1977). The recent discovery that Affi-Gel Blue (Cibacron Blue F3GA-agarose matrix) affinity chromatography allows for the convenient separation of active and inactive renin adds an important dimension to the study of renins (Inagami et al., 1978; Johnson et al., 1979).

EXTRARENAL RENIN SYNTHESIS, STORAGE, AND RELEASE

Within the past several years, it has become established that enzymes which are similar, but perhaps not identical, to renal renin are ubiquitous in the extrarenal tissues of many mammals (review by Ganten et al., 1976). Tissues particularly rich in so-called extrarenal renins (ERRs) include mouse submaxillary glands, rabbit uterus, and human lung tumors. They have also been reported to occur in tissues such as blood vessels, brain, adrenal gland, heart, spleen, skeletal muscle, and various tissue culture cells. Ganten et al. (1976) concluded that ERRs or "angiotensinogenases" probably exist in most tissues, although the specific tissue subcellular localization has not been well studied.

Very little is known about the synthesis and release of ERRs. However, it has been observed from cell culture studies that ERR synthesis in chorion and myometrical cells proceeds at a high rate and releases large amounts of ERR into the culture medium (Symonds et al., 1968). The majority of the ERR activity in other systems appears to be cellularly bound (Ganten et al., 1975a;b; Fischer et al., 1975).

A recent study by Poulsen and colleagues, using a classical cell-free translation system, reported that mouse submaxillary gland renin was synthesized as a 50,000-dalton single-chain polypeptide (Poulsen et al., 1979). This is an interesting report in view of another study that determined that the only form of renin in the submaxillary gland of mice was the fully active 40,000-dalton form (Nielsen et al., 1979).

There is also a dearth of information regarding stimuli that cause the release of ERR. It has been reported that renin release in the submaxillary salivary glands of the mouse is dependent on activation of α-receptors

(Menzie et al., 1974), which is the reverse of the situation in renal renin stimulation. There is clearly much more work to be done in order to define the synthesis, storage, and release of ERR. Examples of its role in the production of physiologically significant amounts of AI (AII) is increasing and recent data indicate that ERR may even participate, via the formation of AII, in the regulation of protein synthesis and cell proliferation (Khairallah et al., 1972; Ganten et al., 1976).

EXTRARENAL RENINS

A review of extrarenal tissue renins has recently been written (Ganten et al., 1976). It was suggested that the trivial term "iso-renin" be used to designate extrarenal renin in recognition that it is not established whether or not the extrarenal enzymes are isoenzymes to kidney renins in strict biochemical accord. Furthermore, it was suggested that the systemic nomenclature be applied to renin where it becomes "angiotensinogen hydrolase" or "angiotensinogenase." These terms circumvent the controversy regarding whether extrarenal tissue renins are biochemically identical to, or different from, the kidney enzymes. Because these terms are not universally accepted, extrarenal renins will be abbreviated in this section as "ERRs" and renal renins as "RRs." Other parts of this review deal exclusively with renins that have a renal origin and are referred to simply as renins.

Since few ERRs have been studied in pure form, it cannot be stated that they share physiochemical characteristics. They are termed "renins" because they, like renal renins: (1) specifically hydrolyze the leucyl-leucyl bond in positions 10 and 11 of synthetic renin substrate, (2) form AI from naturally occurring renin substrates, and (3) do not degrade AII. Similarly, studies using various inhibitors do show that some RRs and ERRs are closely related, if not identical. However, the lack of pure enzymes and substrates make kinetic data difficult to evaluate.

Renins from submaxillary glands of mice have been obtained in crystalline form (Cohen et al., 1972). Four enzyme fractions (A, B, C, D) with molecular weights ranging from 36,000 to 43,000 were obtained, and a positive periodic acid-Schiff reaction indicated that submaxillary renins, like renal renins, are glycoproteins. Whether there are four different renins which exist naturally, or whether they are purification artifacts, is conjecture. Membrane-bound (microsomal) renin has recently been isolated from submaxillary gland and kidney of both the mouse and the rat (Wilson et al., 1976). It was suggested that this renin may represent the less active higher molecular weight renin precursor of soluble renin. The study also demonstrated that this submaxillary renin fraction was elevated by the treatment of young female mice with androgenic or anabolic steroids.

There are several major impediments to the study of ERR. For example, the natural substrate is unknown. It is not certain whether plasma substrate or tissue-renin substrate is used to generate AI in vivo. The lack of purified "natural" ERR substrate severely complicates studies regarding inhibitors and kinetics of ERR. Research regarding naturally occurring ERR precursors, activators, and inactivators thus awaits substrate identification, as well as enzyme purification. There is, however, evidence that such substances occur (Morris and Lumbers, 1972; Leckie, 1973). Finally, ERR per se has only recently been measured directly (Michelakis et al., 1974). Most studies have estimated renin activity indirectly by measuring the amount of AI formed upon incubation by the radioimmunoassay (RIA) procedure of Haber et al. (1969). The many pitfalls regarding the RIA measurement of renin activity have been considered (Oparil et al., 1974; Kirkendall et al., 1975). Undoubtedly, much of the contestable data regarding the RAAS stems from difficulties involving this assay.

Although the amount of ERR activity in some organs, such as the submaxillary gland and the uterus of pregnant rats, exceeds the renin activity of renal tissue, evidence for a biological role is lacking. Since PRA after bilateral nephrectomy is often, but not always, found to be low or nonexistent (Berman et al., 1972; Oparil et al., 1974; McKenzie and Montgomerie, 1969; Yu et al., 1972) it has been inferred that ERR sources do not contribute significant quantities of renin to the plasma pool. Some observations have also led to the notion that the ERR system is a tissue enzyme system having mainly local actions. Other studies, however, have indicated that plasma renin activity could be stimulated in the absence of kidney tissue (Menzie et al., 1974). Also, Genest et al. (1975) have reported a case of malignant hypertension with high PRA in a patient with renin-producing pulmonary carcinoma. Significantly, the patient's kidney renin was suppressed below normal levels. While their study demonstrated that ERR can contribute to the plasma renin pool in certain instances, there is much work to be done to show whether ERR has any physiologic importance under normal circumstances.

Evidence has recently accumulated regarding the existence of novel renal (see "Renal and Plasma Renins") and extrarenal renins in humans. This renin form has been termed "big renin" since it has a molecular weight of 63,000 versus approximately 40,000 for "normal RR" (review by Day et al., 1976). A big renin (MW = 46,000) and a "big big renin" (MW = 140,000) have recently been reported from normal hog kidney (Murakami et al., 1976). Initial observations regarding big renin from plasma and tumors were made during the study of a hypertensive child with a Wilm's tumor (Day and Leutscher, 1974) and subsequently extended to amniotic fluids and kidney extracts (Day et al., 1975). Other significant considerations regarding human big renins are: (1) big renin is activated tenfold at pH 3.3; (2) it is not thought to be converted to normal kidney renin (MW = 40,000); (3) hypertension can result from the secretion of large quantities of big renin from a renal tumor; and (4) big renin does not appear to respond to physiologic changes that stimulate or suppress normal PRA. A review of other work regarding activatable renins has led to the following conclusions:

(1) human big renin is not normal renin bound to a protein, for its molecular weight does not change after acidification; (2) there is good evidence that there are extrarenal origins of big renin; and (3) evidence is needed to reliably conclude that big renin is either a zymogen or prohormone of renin (Day et al., 1976).

An ubiquitous enzyme termed "pseudorenin" by Skeggs et al. (1969, 1972) must also be dealt with when considering renins. It may be considered a renin form, since it hydrolyzes both synthetic renin substrate and purified natural renin substrate to form AI, and, like common kidney renin (MW = 40,000), it does not hydrolyze AI or synthetic substrates that do not contain tyrosine in position 13. Unlike common renin, it does not react with natural substrate in the presence of plasma, presumably due to the occurrence of unidentified plasma inhibitor(s). Also, renin and pseudorenin have distinctly different ion exchange elution patterns and different pH optima. Pseudorenin and cathepsin D, a major proteinase of animal tissues, share many biochemical properties (Barrett, 1973; Knight and Barrett, 1976).

The major current controversy regards the existence of brain renin. Some studies have resulted in the conclusion that there is a brain renin that acts on brain angiotensinogen to form angiotensin I (Rettig et al., 1978; Ganten and Speck, 1978). On the other hand, other studies have led to the conclusion that brain renin is closely related to, or identical with, cathepsin D (Day and Reid, 1976; Hackenthal et al., 1978a; Hackenthal et al., 1978b). Two recent critical reviews concerning the existence of a brain renin-angiotensin system have concluded that its existence is doubtful (Ramsay, 1979; Reid, 1979).

MEDIATORS OF RENIN ACTIVITY

Many studies have attempted to isolate activators and inhibitors of renin activity from kidney tissue and plasma. Indications that such substances exist come from such diverse observations as: (1) there is a hyperresponsiveness to renin after bilateral nephrectomy (Montague, 1968); (2) variable amounts of AI are formed after the addition of a constant amount of renin to various plasma samples (Pickens et al., 1965); (3) some clinical PRA samples cause unexpected decreases in rat blood pressure during bioassay determinations (personal observations); and (4) the maximum velocity of in vitro AII generation increases after removal of the normal contralateral kidney in rat experimental renovascular hypertension (Lazar et al., 1971).

Phospholipids isolated from acetone extracts of dog kidney were shown to inhibit the action of dog renin on dog renin substrate in vitro and to reduce the blood pressure of chronic and renal hypertensive rats and dogs in vivo (Sen et al., 1967; Smeby et al., 1967). The lysophosphatide derivative of the phospholipid was more potent than the parent phospholipid in terms of its ability to decrease blood pressure (Smeby et al., 1967). The parent phospholipid was termed preinhibitor because the "active" inhibitor was derived from the phospholipid by in vitro phospholipase hydrolysis (Sen et al., 1968). Lipid preinhibitors were subsequently found in dog (Tinker et al., 1973) and human plasma (Baggio et al., 1973); human erythrocytes (Ostrovsky et al., 1967); anephric human blood (Osmond et al., 1969b); rat, liver, heart, and erythrocytes (Osmond et al., 1969a; Osmond, 1972); and shark kidney (Turcotte et al., 1973).

Initially, preinhibitor was thought to be structurally similar to bovine phosphatidylserine, but later studies indicated that the preinhibitor was a phosphatidylethanolamine and the "active" inhibitor was therefore its lysophosphatidyl derivative (Osmond et al., 1969a; Tinker et al., 1973). The active inhibitor from shark kidney was also identified as a polyunsaturated lysophosphatidylethanolamine (Turcotte et al., 1973). Synthetic lysophosphatidylethanolamines (Pfeiffer et al., 1971), dilinolenyl phosphatidylethanolamines (Rahkit et al., 1969), and ethanolamine derivatives esterified with 1-adamantyl moieties (Pfeiffer et al., 1972) have also been found to inhibit renin in vitro.

Tinker et al. (1973) reexamined dog kidney phospholipids and the question of renin inhibition. They were unable to confirm the earlier studies which indicated in vivo renin inhibition; neither were they able to confirm renin inhibition by dog kidney lysophosphatidylethanolamines in vitro. Other studies which failed to find a decrease in the circulating levels of preinhibitor from blood of anephric rats (Osmond et al., 1969a), dogs (Ostrovsky et al., 1967), and humans (Osmond et al., 1969b) led to the conclusion that the kidney may not be the only source of preinhibitor.

Osmond et al. (1973b, c) investigated the possible renal influence on plasma phospholipase activity with the idea that if phospholipase is secreted by the kidney, nephrectomy would reduce or abolish the formation of the lysophospholipid inhibitor and produce a deficiency of renin-inhibiting capacity. Nephrectomy did not decrease the degradation of phosphatidylethanolamines to lysophosphatidylethanolamines; hence additional questions were raised regarding phospholipid renin inhibitors. Similar studies involving phospholipase A_2 in nephrectomized rats provided evidence that phospholipase A_2 could be regulating renin inhibitor and thus the level of renin activity (Zachariah et al., 1975). The in vitro effects of various purified human kidney lipids on human renin activity have been determined (Overturf et al., 1976). Triglycerides, 1-monoacyl and 2-monacyl phosphatidylethanolamines, and phosphatidylcholines significantly inhibited human kidney renin activity. Intact phospholipids slightly increased renin activity even at low concentrations, but renin activity was not affected by cholesterol, phosphatidylserines, or synthetic glyceryl ethers. From structural studies it was concluded that lipid-induced renin inhibition does not require either an ethanolamine moiety, acyl group unsaturation, or the presence of a hydroxyl group at the glycerol 2-position. No structural-activity relationships were adduced which could describe the lipid-renin interactions.

Early studies provided evidence for a naturally occurring acetone soluble (lipid?) renin-inhibiting factor in normal and uremic plasma (Kotchen et al., 1975). It was suggested that the increased reactivity of renin in uremic plasma was due to a deficiency of the inhibiting factor. More recent investigations concluded that neutral lipid from the acetone extracts of plasma are responsible for renin inhibition (Kotchen et al., 1976; Kotchen et al., 1977). Subsequent studies showed that acetone extraction of plasma actually decreased plasma renin reactivity in relation to control values (Druilhet et al., 1979). In addition, it was found that acetone extraction of plasma denatured renin substrate and that this was at least partially responsible for the observed apparent decrease in renin activity of acetone-extracted plasma. These results are in direct opposition to the circulating lipid-renin inhibitor hypothesis. Kinetic studies have also failed to provide evidence for the presence of activators or inhibitors in human serum (Gould et al., 1979). A recent study demonstrated that under physiological conditions, native plasma lipids of normal human subjects, when bound to their respective apoproteins, did not appear to inhibit the renin reaction at physiological concentrations (Eggena et al., 1979).

Renin has also been shown to be variably inhibited by such diverse substances as heparin (Sealey et al., 1967), bile (Hiwada et al., 1969), sodium deoxycholate (Hiwada et al., 1971), esters of synthetic tetrapeptides (Kokubu et al., 1973; Majstoravich et al., 1974), analogs of an octapeptide segment of renin substrate (Poulsen et al., 1973), C-terminal carbinol analogs related to renin substrate (Shigezane and Mizoguchi, 1973), and hemoglobins, fibrinogen, albumin, and β-lactoglobulin B (Workman et al., 1974). Scharpe et al. (1976) have recently shown that human plasma alpha$_1$-antitrypsin is a competitive inhibitor of pig kidney renin. Other common proteinase inhibitors, such as alpha$_2$-macroglobulin and C1 inactivator, had no inhibitory effect on the renin-angiotensinogen reaction.

Evidence has recently been obtained that inactive rabbit kidney renin (MW = 55,000) contains a renin-inhibiting protein component (MW = 13,000) that can be dissociated by exposure to pH 2.5 at 4°C to yield active renin (MW = 37,000) and a renin inhibitor (Leckie and McConnell, 1975). It was concluded that the activation of renin is the result of destruction of the inhibitor by acid; thus the inactive form (big renin) may be a renin proenzyme or a storage form of active renin-inhibitor complex.

Pepstatin A, an n-acylated low molecular weight pentapeptide obtained from culture filtrates of actinomycetes (Umezawa et al., 1970) is a potent inhibitor of hog renin in vitro and in vivo (Aoyagi et al., 1972; Miller et al. 1972; Scholkens and Jung, 1974) and human plasma and kidney renins in vitro (Overturf et al., 1974). Pepstatin A also reduces blood pressure in unilaterally nephrectomized rats and cats and in rats with acute and chronic renal hypertension (Miller et al., 1972). The dipsogenic response due to the injection of renin and renin substrate intracranially is also reduced by pepstatin (Epstein et al., 1974).

An isomeric pepstatin, pepstatin G, is the n-capryl substitution of the pentapeptide backbone of pepstatin A and is nearly four times more active against hog kidney renin than pepstatin A (Aoyagi et al., 1972). No information regarding its efficacy against human renins is available. A pepstatin (S-PI) with an acetyl group at the R_1 position was isolated from the culture filtrate of Streptomyces naniwaensis (Murao and Satoi, 1970; Satoi and Murao, 1973). It was found to be more active than pepstatin A (pepstatin with an isovaleryl group at the R_1 position) against human kidney renins at low concentrations (Overturf et al., 1977). Two other low molecular weight streptomyces products, leupeptin and antipain, were much less potent inhibitors. A review of the chemistry and pharmacology of these inhibitors is available (Aoyagi and Umezawa, 1975).

Considering the low toxicity of pepstatins and their high degree of effectiveness in inhibiting renins, their possible diagnostic and therapeutic values suggest important additional studies. Since it has been found that the activity of the pepstatins against renin increases with increasing numbers of carbon atoms in the acyl group (Aoyagi et al., 1972), even more potent renin inhibitors might result from long-chain hydrophobic substitutions on the pentapeptide backbone.

Prostaglandin A in high concentrations, but not prostaglandin E, has been reported to competitively inhibit renin (Kotchen et al., 1974). However, contrary results have indicated that the inhibitory action of renal PGE_2 is greater than that of PGA_2 (Eggena et al., 1975) (see "Renin-Angiotensin-System Prostaglandins and Kallikrein-Kinin System").

The existence of plasma "renin activators" has been suggested from studies of patients with renal hypertension, hypertensive cardiovascular renal disease (Sambhi and Wiedeman, 1972), and benign essential hypertension (Sambhi et al., 1974). Since this activator was nonlipid, nondialyzable, and heat labile, it was considered to be a protein (Sambhi et al., 1974). Cooper et al. (1974) demonstrated trypsin-induced increases in PRA. Later studies seem to indicate that the modifier in plasma from essential hypertensive patients increases the V_{max} and K_m of the system and that it acts like an uncompetitive activator (Sambhi et al., 1975). Studies aimed at isolating and identifying the activator, as well as its origin, should receive high research priority.

ANGIOTENSIN I

The decapeptide product of the reaction of renin on renin substrate, angiotensin I, is generally considered to be biologically inactive. Despite numerous attempts to show that AI is an effector hormone, it has usually been found that the effects ascribed to the action of AI were actually due to AII which was rapidly produced by the local action of AI converting enzymes. Probable exceptions are the experimental observations of direct stimulatory effects of AI on the adrenal medulla which induce catecholamine secretion

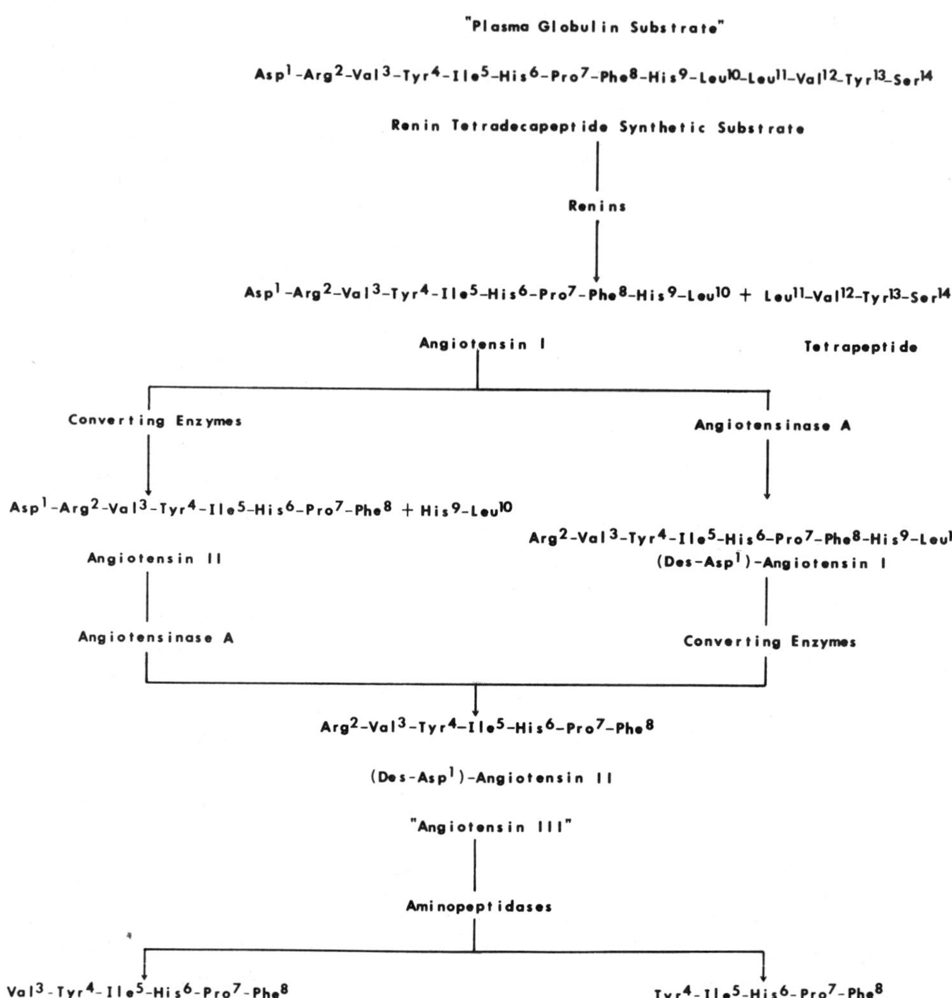

FIG. 2. Pathways for the formation of [Des-Asp^1]angiotensin II. (Modified with permission from B. S. Tsai, M. J. Peach, M. C. Khosla, and F. M. Bumpus, Synthesis and evaluation of [Des-Asp^1]angiotensin I as a precursor for [Des-Asp^2]angiotensin II ("angiotensin III"), J. Med. Chem. 18:1180-1183, Copyright 1975 American Chemical Society.)

(Peach, 1971) and stimulation by AI of the central nervous system (Solomon et al., 1974). However, even in these cases, the physiological importance of AI is questioned on the basis of the very rapid conversion of AI to AII in vivo.

Renewed interest in AI has been stimulated by observations regarding the biological activities of the Des-aspartic acid heptapeptide derivative of AII (AIII). Although the possible metabolic sequence was first suggested by Blair-West et al. (1971), it has only recently been shown that AIII can be formed directly from AI by the sequential action of aminopeptidases and converting enzymes (Fig. 2). Thus it is predictable that interest in AI as a precursor of AIII will receive future research interest.

ANGIOTENSIN I CONVERTING ENZYMES

Since comprehensive reviews have recently dealt with angiotensin I converting enzyme (ACE) (Soffer, 1976; Erdös, 1977), this section is limited to a brief overview of the subject and a discussion of some of the latest research involving a typical ACE (kininase II, EC 3.4.15.1), nontypical converting enzymes, and recently developed ACE inhibitors. Methods for the measurement of ACE in vitro and a discussion of the biological properties of ACE have been well reviewed (Bakhle, 1974).

Like renin, ACE is defined fundamentally in terms of its action, i.e., the conversion of AI to AII. Additional criteria were established by Skeggs and his colleagues in several publications from 1954-1956 (see listing in Bakhle, 1974). Together, these form a basis for distinguishing between the first AI converting enzyme described (a typical ACE) and those described subsequently.

Since the discovery of converting enzyme from horse plasma (Skeggs et al., 1954; Lentz et al., 1956), the subject has become increasingly complex. For many years, ACE was simply described as a plasma enzyme that converted AI to AII by cleaving the histidyl-leucine dipeptide from the C-terminus of AI. In vivo experiments later demonstrated that plasma conversion of AI to AII was inadequate to account for the unusually rapid formation of AII and that the most significant site of conversion was the pulmonary circulation (Ng and Vane, 1967; Biron and Huggins, 1968; Bakhle et al., 1969).

A significant hypothesis, which was later confirmed in part, was advanced; ACE from lung was identical to kininase I or carboxypeptidase-N, which inactivates bradykinin (Ng and Vane, 1968). One year previously, it was found that plasma contains (1) a carboxypeptidase (kininase I or carboxypeptidase arginine carboxypeptidase, EC 3.4.12.7) that inactivates bradykinin by the removal of the carboxy terminal arginine, and (2) a kininase II that releases Phe^{8}-Arg^{9} from bradykinin (Erdös and Yang, 1967). In accord with the Ng and Vane (1968) hypothesis, it was shown that the same enzyme that forms AII also inactivates bradykinin (Yang et al., 1970). However, it was found to be kininase II rather than kininase I.

Electrophoretically pure ACE was obtained from hog (Igic et al., 1972) and rabbit lung (Cushman and Cheung, 1972). While it is generally stated that it is bound to membranes, it should be remembered that it was first described in plasma and that various studies have demonstrated ACE in soluble fractions, as well as particulate fractions. Converting enzyme activity has now been found in many different tissues from every common laboratory mammal and man (review by Bakhle, 1974). Among the many surveys, it has been shown that only testicular tissue contains more ACE than lung tissue; however, the physiological significance of either testicular or seminal plasma ACE is unknown. Similarly, there is no ready explanation regarding the importance of the observation that mouse, rat, and rabbit lung contain eight times more activity than human lung (Depierre and Roth, 1972). The concentration of ACE in plasma also varies among different species. For example, dog serum has been reported to contain only 0.3 milliunit ACE/mg protein, while guinea pig plasma contains 15.5 milliunits/mg protein (Cushman and Cheung, 1972).

There is a considerable amount of information available regarding the biochemical properties of typical ACE. Most of the work has been done using rabbit, hog, and dog lung. The properties of typical ACE that have been most extensively investigated include: (1) molecular weight determinations, (2) pH and temperature effects, (3) substrate specificities, (4) effects of cations and anions, and (5) the effects of inhibitors. Recent studies have been made regarding the kinetics of typical converting enzymes, including measurements of the K_m (Dorer et al., 1975) and the effects of the ionic environment and pH on hog lung ACE in vitro (Dorer et al., 1976). Measurements have shown that the K_m for ACE with bradykinin as substrate is about 10 times lower than the K_m with AI as substrate (Dorer et al., 1975). Generally, there is no in vitro conversion of AI in the absence of chloride ions, whereas the inactivation of bradykinin by ACE is unaffected.

A wide molecular weight range (129,000-480,000) has been reported for ACE. These various results may be due to several factors, including (1) species differences, (2) differences in extraction procedures, (3) differences in ACE carbohydrate components, and/or (4) differences in methodologies. Another possibility includes the notion that ACE exists as polymeric species and that the lower molecular weight estimates represent monomeric forms. A good discussion regarding discrepancies of molecular weight determinations has been published (Soffer, 1976).

Recent studies of rabbit lung ACE have demonstrated that it is a glycoprotein (Soffer et al., 1974). Subsequent work indicated that the glycoprotein has a molecular weight of 129,000, that it is composed of a single polypeptide chain, and that it is associated with one molar equivalent of bound zinc (Das and Soffer, 1975). From these studies it would appear that at least some of the discrepancies regarding the molecular weight determinations have been due to the large oligosaccharide content of the protein, which can result in a high estimate of molecular weight as determined by gel-filtration chromatography.

Typical ACE can cleave many different substrates by the hydrolysis of dipeptides from the C-terminus. Protected C-terminal substrates such as Z-Phe-His-Leu (Piquilloud et al., 1970) and tripeptides such as His-His-Leu (Cushman and Cheung, 1971) can also serve as substrates. ACE can also cleave peptide bonds from substrates that do not contain the C-terminal sequence of AI, such as tripeptides of glycine (dansyl-Gly-Gly-Gly) (Igic et al., 1972) and chromophore substrates Z-Phe(NO_2)-Gly-Gly (Stevens et al., 1972). Dorer et al. (1975) have shown that hog lung ACE can form AI and AII from TDP renin substrate by the successive removal of three dipeptide units from the C-terminal end of TDP, and the velocity was found to be chloride dependent.

A recent study by Chiu et al. (1976) demonstrated that hog lung ACE can also form AIII, [Des-Asp^1]angiotensin II, from [Des-Asp^1]angiotensin I. Indeed, in vitro studies showed that the K_m of the reaction was one-third of that for the conversion of AI to AII. Since there is some evidence that [Des-Asp^1]AI is formed in vivo (Ryan et al., 1970), the conversion to AIII has great potential significance (see "Angiotensin II, Angiotensin III, and Aldosterone"). However, before any physiological importance can be ascribed, additional evidence is needed to establish that quantities of [Des-Asp^1]AI exist in vivo.

It has long been established that typical ACE has a requirement for chloride ions when AI is the substrate (Skeggs et al., 1954). Yet there is a great variation in the quantitative aspects of the chloride dependence, both in the amount of activation obtained and in the chloride concentration needed. Since the anion activator studies have been performed on relatively crude ACE preparations, future studies with homogenous enzyme preparations will allow better interpretation of the data. However, from a physiological viewpoint, it would not seem likely that in vivo levels of chloride would be insufficient to maintain ACE activity.

None of 13 common cations studied had any stimulatory effects on ACE with AI as the substrate (see the listing by Bakhle, 1974). The hydrolysis of different blocked substrates was variously inhibited and stimulated by different cations. There have been conflicting results regarding the effects of cations on EDTA-inhibited ACE, particularly in regard to zinc. When data from different studies were reviewed (Bakhle, 1974), it was concluded that either cobalt or manganese was the closest substitute for the cation in the native enzyme; zinc was only occasionally reported to be effective. Several years ago it was shown that ACE from rabbit lung (Cushman and Cheung, 1971) and human plasma (Fitz et al., 1971) which were inhibited by EDTA could be reactivated after removal of EDTA by dialysis. After prolonged dialysis against 1 mM EDTA, reactivation would only take place by the addition of $MnCl_2$ (40%), $Co(NO\ )_2$ (160%), and $ZnCl_2$ (100%) (Cushman and Cheung, 1971). Recently, it has been shown that typical ACE contains zinc (Das and Soffer, 1975).

Several studies have dealt with converting enzymes which are considered "atypical" because they do not fulfill the five criteria outlined for typical

ACE. An atypical ACE named "β-converting enzyme" (β-ACE) found in a crude extract of rat submaxillary gland was about 20 times more active than the so-called α-ACE (typical lung ACE) on a per gram of tissue basis (Boucher et al., 1972). In addition, the velocity of AI conversion by β-ACE was much greater than that of typical lung ACE.

Boucher et al. (1972) described the atypical ACE (β-ACE) from rat submaxillary gland which, unlike typical ACE, did not require Cl^-, was not inhibited by EDTA, did not significantly hydrolyze Z-Phe-His-Leu substrate, and had a slightly lower pH optimum (pH 6.5-7.2). Although they found that the presence of an unidentified β-ACE inhibitor in plasma rendered it inactive, they suggested that this enzyme may be physiologically active through the intracellular generation of AII. Accordingly, it may have an important role in AII generation at the tissue level, for there is a large amount of extrarenal renin activity in the rat submaxillary gland.

Subsequent studies of purified β-ACE by Boucher et al. (1974) led to its being renamed "tonin." These later studies revealed that tonin has several properties which, in addition to forming AII from AI, include: (1) cleaving the Phe-His bond from the synthetic tetradecapeptide (TDP) renin substrate to form AII directly; (2) being unaffected by the presence of Cl^-, EDTA, DFP, pepstatin, or Pyro-Glu-Lys-Tyr-Ala-Pro; and (3) having a molecular weight of about 31,400. Bradykinin had no inhibitory effect on tonin activity, whereas copper sulfate inhibited the conversion of AI to AII, but not the direct formation of AII from TDP. Plasma inhibited the reaction with AI, TDP, and natural substrate.

Boucher et al. (1974) found tonin in various tissues of the rat. These can be ranked in decreasing amounts as follows: adrenal gland; kidney medulla and inner cortex; kidney outer cortex; testes; spleen; and liver. Much additional work remains to resolve questions of the physiological importance of tonin.

Human lung ACE activity which produced histidyl-leucine from AI was demonstrated from an acetone-powder extraction (Fitz and Overturf, 1970). This enzyme preparation eluted from Sephadex G-150 at about the same volume as human plasma ACE. Both were inhibited by 0.03 M Na_2EDTA. Because of the low yield from the acetone powder, later studies dealt with the mild extraction of fresh tissue, and the enzyme fractions were obtained from Sephadex G-200. These studies resulted in the isolation of a native large molecular weight fraction (480,000) which hydrolyzed AI to AII. It was unaffected by 0.1 M EDTA and was free of angiotensinase and dipeptidase activity (Fitz and Overturf, 1972a,b). About 75% of the enzyme activity corresponded to a molecular weight of 480,000 and 25% of the activity was found in a fraction corresponding to about 175,000 daltons. A series of studies by Lee et al. (1971a-c) determined the molecular weight of hog and human plasma ACE, and hog and guinea pig lung ACE. They found that the molecular weight of all four samples was approximately 150,000 and that each was inhibited by EDTA. Their molecular weight studies were performed on both soluble and solubilized pellet fractions.

Another study of human lung ACE activity revealed atypical ACE fractions with molecular weights of 300,000, 450,000, and 600,000 (Fitz et al., 1974). None of the fractions was inhibited by EDTA, and Cl^- was not required for activity. Studies to determine whether human lung ACE inactivated bradykinin showed that ACE fractions from two different lungs did possess bradykininase activity, while a third lung preparation had only minimal activity (Overturf et al., 1975). Unlike ACE activity, bradykininase activity was inhibited by EDTA. Additional studies of the 450,000 and 600,000 molecular weight human lung ACE fractions demonstrated that both fractions converted TDP renin substrate to AII directly (Boaz et al., 1975). Grandino and Paiva (1974) found a high molecular weight (400,000) ACE from hog and guinea pig plasma which did not possess kininase activity, did not require Cl^-, and could not be dissociated with 4 M urea. Urinary ACE has been partially purified and found to have molecular weight of 40,000, 290,000 and 140,000 by Sephadex G-200 gel filtration (Kokubu et al., 1978).

Some of the important studies concerning atypical human lung ACE which remain to be done include: (1) obtaining highly purified enzymes, (2) determining if the various ACE activities represent polymeric species, and (3) determining if variations of human lung ACE are due to physiological or pathological changes. The great impediment to studying human lung ACE is primarily due to the difficulty of obtaining quantities of "normal" fresh tissue.

There is a lack of information regarding either physiological or pathological correlates of plasma or lung ACE activity (Erdös, 1976). Since the major sites of ACE activity are located in the vascular endothelium of various organs (Caldwell et al., 1976) and on the luminal surface of pulmonary endothelial cells (Ryan et al., 1975), it is not unexpected that most investigators who have measured plasma ACE have failed to find significant variations in ACE activity. For example, clinical studies (Osborn et al., 1970; Zakheim et al., 1976) and animals studies (Bell and Bakhle, 1975) have failed to demonstrate altered ACE levels in various pathological states. Unexpectedly, variations in serum ACE levels were reported in clinical idiopathic respiratory distress (Mattioli et al., 1975), sarcoidosis (Lieberman, 1975; Silverstein et al., 1975), and experimental chronic alveolar hypoxia (Molteni et al., 1974).

The subject of kininase II inhibitors is complex. Many studies present discordant results which may be explained on the basis of (1) the use of ACE preparations of varying purities, (2) the lack of characterization of the ACE used, and (3) the lack of standardized preparations to quantitate the activity of the preparations. The ability to compare results is further diminished by the great variety of substrates and incubation conditions employed. It has been clearly demonstrated that the rate of hydrolysis depends on the structure of the substrate, the concentration of the ions, and the pH of the media (Dorer et al., 1976).

In order to provide a structured discussion of ACE inhibitors, Bakhle (1974) divided them into two major categories: "peptide" and "nonpeptide" inhibitors. The various types of peptide ACE inhibitors include (1) competitive alternate substrates, e.g., bradykinin, Met-Lys-bradykinin (Sander et al., 1971); (2) product inhibition, e.g., AII and His-Leu (Lee et al., 1971b), Phe-Arg (Sander et al., 1971); and (3) snake venom competitive and noncompetitive inhibitors (Bakhle, 1972; Cushman and Cheung, 1972). The nonapeptide (BPF_{9a} or SQ 20,881) isolated from the venon of Bothrops jararaca, and synthesized by Ondetti et al. (1971) has been used in clinical trials (Gavras et al., 1974).

Nonpeptide ACE inhibitors include chelating agents, sulfhydryl blocking agents, and the new drug captopril. The results of many studies using various inhibitors have been tabulated by Bakhle (1974). In general, it was found that EDTA and other chelating agents inhibit typical ACE; however, there are discrepancies regarding the efficacy of sulfhydryl blocking agents.

In vivo studies using ACE inhibitors, principally SQ 20,881 and captopril, have provided indirect evidence for the actions of ACE in various experimental and clinical conditions. Some of the experimental effects of SQ 20,881-ACE inhibition are: (1) negation of vasoconstrictor effects of infused or perfused AI (Collier et al., 1973; Zschiedrich et al., 1975), (2) decreased blood pressure in experimental hypertension (Romero et al., 1974; Miller et al., 1975), (3) attenuation of blood pressure of dogs in endotoxic and hemorrhagic shock (Erdős et al., 1974, (4) negation of the dipsogenic effects of AI after centrally administered SQ 20,881 (Summy-Long and Severs, 1974), and (5) prevention of pulmonary vascular changes of experimental chronic alveolar hypoxia in the rat (Zakheim et al., 1975). Recently, another synthetic peptide, SQ 20,858 (Ondetti et al., 1971), has been shown to be effective in lowering blood pressure in chronic renal hypertensive rats, presumably by the inhibition of ACE (Loyke, 1975).

Clinical studies using SQ 20,881 have indicated that it can reduce blood pressure in humans (Collier et al., 1973; Gavras et al., 1974; Pettinger et al., 1975) and it has been suggested that it may be used diagnostically to identify "renin-dependent" hypertension (Gavras et al., 1974). While it is well known that SQ 20,881 has a prolonged action and lacks toxicity and agonistic properties (Pettinger et al., 1975), it should be noted that it is not orally effective and that it does inhibit bradykininase activity, thereby prolonging the vasodepressor effects of bradykinin (Nasjletti et al., 1975). These dual actions of SQ 20,881 make in vivo interpretations of cause and effect quite difficult.

Recently, a novel compound has been systematically developed that is a potent, orally active antihypertensive agent (Cushman et al., 1977; Ondetti et al., 1977). Captopril, also known as SQ 14,225 (D-3-mercapto-2-methylpropanoyl-L-proline), is a highly active competitive inhibitor of ACE, having a K_i of 0.0017 μM (Cushman et al., 1977). It is a relatively nontoxic compound; e.g., the acute oral LD_{50} in rats is about 6000 mg/kg (Sibley et al., 1978). A comprehensive review of the literature regarding the effects of captopril on normal blood pressure, renal hypertension (one-kidney and two-kidney), and genetic (spontaneous) hypertension cannot be given here, but a summary is provided and a recent review is available (Rubin et al., 1978).

1. Inhibition of pressor responses to AI without inhibition of the pressor responses to AII indicate that captopril is a potent inhibitor of ACE in conscious animals. It is probable that the antihypertensive response to captopril results from the decrease in AII and the accumulation of endogenous bradykinin, which in turn may lead to increased release of prostaglandins.
2. Captopril has a large margin of safety in acute studies.
3. Captopril augments the vasodepressor effects of exogenously administered bradykinin in experimental animals.
4. Two-kidney renal hypertensive (high-renin) rats respond with reduced blood pressure and increased PRA to daily doses of captopril for periods of up to 1 year. The addition of a daily dosage of a thiazide diuretic augments both the antihypertensive and life prolongation effects of captopril in two-kidney renal hypertensive rats.
5. Spontaneously (normal or low-renin?) hypertensive rats show only a moderate blood pressure lowering response to captopril.
6. As a result of captopril administration, PRA sharply increases in normotensive as well as hypertensive volunteers and experimental animals. It is believed that the increase in PRA is primarily a result of the inhibition of a negative feedback mechanism of AII on the juxtaglomerular apparatus. Reduction of circulating AII caused by ACE inhibition with captopril probably results in an increased renal secretion of renin in an attempt to restore reduced AII levels.
7. Plasma aldosterone and urinary kallikrein excretion are decreased, while urinary sodium level and plasma kinin activity are increased during captopril administration. Serum potassium levels are not significantly affected.

ANGIOTENSIN II, ANGIOTENSIN III, AND ALDOSTERONE

Space constraints do not permit a comprehensive review of the many facets of AII. However, more than 14 review chapters have recently been devoted to the biochemistry, physiology, pathophysiology, and assay of AII (Page and Bumpus, 1974). The following discussion will be limited to a brief review of the physiological effects of AII, followed by some current thoughts regarding AII and suggestions for future study.

Some of the more important effects of AII are (1) potent vasoconstriction, (2) sodium retention (low concentrations) and natriuresis (high concentrations), (3) stimulation of adrenal cortex causing aldosterone biosynthesis and secretion, (4) dipsogenesis, (5) catecholamine release, and (6) prosta-

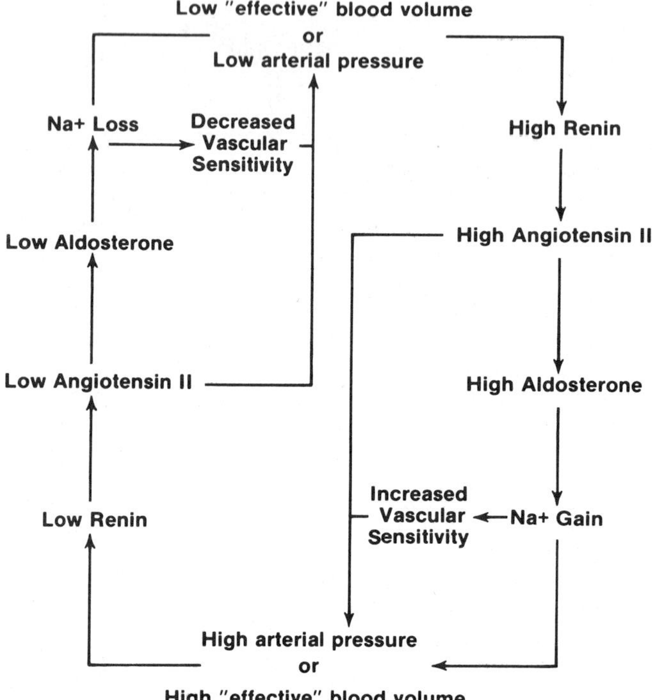

FIG. 3. Simplified RAA feedback loop for regulating sodium balance and arterial pressure. (Modified from Laragh and Sealey, 1973).

glandin release. A summary of these effects leads to the conclusion that AII exerts considerable control over sodium and potassium balance, fluid volume, and blood pressure. Obviously, significant aberrations of the RAAS thus lead to pathophysiological alterations of blood pressure and may be correlated with PRA and plasma aldosterone levels (see the tables compiled by Priest et al., 1976, and Vecsei et al., 1978).

For several years, most of the effects of AII were explained by a simple diagram of the renin-angiotensin-aldosterone feedback loop for regulating sodium balance and arterial pressure (Fig. 3). However, recent studies of the AII heptapeptide fragment Des-Asp^1-angiotensin II indicate that major revisions at the II effector level must be made to include AIII (Blair-West et al., 1971; Chiu and Peach, 1974; Campbell et al., 1974) and prostaglandins (Itskovitz and McGiff, 1974).

It has been considered for 20 years that the RAAS was of prime importance in the control of aldosterone secretion by the action of AII on the adrenal cortex. However, now there is much controversy regarding the relative importance of AII. Oelkers et al. (1975) recently affirmed their notion that AII exerts a powerful influence on aldosterone secretion, while McCaa et al. (1975) assert their reasons why the primacy of the renin-angiotensin system in the control of aldosterone secretion has been justifiably questioned.

Studies utilizing the antagonist [Sar^1, Ala^8]AII and measuring pressor responses in dogs and rats showed that Des-Asp^1-AII may mediate the response of the RAAS at both the adrenal and renal receptors (Freeman et al., 1976). The heptapeptide fragment and AII seem to be qualitatively similar both in steroidogenic potency and in their action on the kidney to inhibit renin release and reduce renal blood flow. However, the pressor activity of the heptapeptide is only about one-half that of AII. Observations by Bravo et al. (1976) provide additional evidence for the theory that the heptapeptide has an important role in the regulation of aldosterone production in dogs and sodium-deprived rats (Peach et al., 1976). A brief summary of the current information of AII- and AIII-induced aldosterone release has been published (Meyer, 1976).

A report on the comparison of the effects of infusions of AII and AIII on blood pressure, plasma aldosterone, and PRA in intact, conscious rabbits has provided important conclusions regarding receptors (Steele et al., 1976). These investigators suggest that (1) those receptors which mediate vasoconstriction show a greater response to AII than to AIII, (2) those mediating the secretion of aldosterone show a lesser response to AII than to AIII, and (3) those mediating the suppression of renin release do not discriminate between AII and AIII. These conclusions hint that AIII may be the ultimate peptide controlling aldosterone release. Excellent reviews of vascular AII receptors are available (Devynck and Meyer, 1976; Thurston, 1976).

A review by Goodfriend and Peach (1975) considered the evidence that the AI nonapeptide [Des-Asp^1]AI, as well as the three other peptides formed from renin substrate (AI, AII, and AIII), have biological activity. It was suggested that the nonapeptide might be formed as an intermediate of the sequential action of an aminopeptidase on the decapeptide AI, leading to the formation of AIII via the action of ACE on [Des-Asp^1]-AI. Tsai et al. (1975) and Chiu et al. (1976) found that AIII can indeed be formed by hog ACE in vitro and that AIII may be acting as an inhibitor of ACE by a feedback mechanism. The results of inhibitor studies are in keeping with previous studies which showed that pentapeptide, hexapeptide, and heptapeptide metabolites of AII inhibit human lung ACE (Fitz et al., 1974).

A recent study of the in vitro angiotensin-induced prostaglandin release showed that the in vitro angiotensin-induced prostaglandin release showed that the order of potency of the peptides examined was AIII $>$ AII $>$ AI [Des-Asp^1]AI (Blumberg et al., 1976). Thus, while it is well documented that prostaglandin release can be induced by AII, it appears that AIII may be the most potent mesenteric prostaglandin (PG) stimulant. Blumberg et al. (1976) speculated that the action of AIII is mediated by PGs.

All of the studies previously discussed involved the measurement of AIII dose responses; i.e., none correlated intrinsic circulating levels of

AIII. Semple and Morton (1976), using a sequence of ion-exchange chromatography (Dowex AG 50W-X2, H^+ form), paper chromatography, and radioimmunoassay, reported on the measurement of AII and its metabolites [Des-Asp^1]AII(AIII), [Des-(Asp^1, Arg^2)]AII, and [Des-(Asp^1, Arg^2, Val^3)]AII in arterial and venous plasma from normal rats. They found slightly more AIII than AII in rat blood, which is in contrast to their previous observations of human blood (Semple and Morton, 1975). The technique for measuring AII and AII metabolites, although cumbersome, provides the means for measuring intrinsic peptide levels in response to various stimuli and perhaps will show some direct physiological consequences of them. Additionally, with the means to measure circulating AII metabolites, it is now possible to elucidate the sites and mechanisms of AIII formation in the circulation. It is clear that before physiological roles can definitely be ascribed to actions of the heptapeptide, it must be demonstrated to occur in plasma commensurate with its physiologically predicted consequence.

The role of vasoactive agents, including AII and chemical mediators of inflammation and/or injury, in increasing atherosclerosis and hypertensive vascular disease has received attention (Kincaid-Smith et al., 1974; Robertson and Khairallah, 1974; Goodfriend et al., 1974). The interest stems from the established evidence that changes in permeability and morphology of arterial endothelium influence the development of the initial states of atherogenesis and other vascular diseases. Many natural substances are known to be involved with the pathogenesis of hypertension and include catecholamines, renin, and angiotensin. For example, there are studies which indicate that high plasma levels of catecholamines, renin, and angiotensin alter the arterial wall metabolism and produce vascular damage and the effects are potentiated by mineralocorticoids and high-sodium diets (Masson et al., 1962; Giese, 1964; Hollander et al., 1964). It has been shown, for instance, that intracardiac or intraortic injections of AII increase the permeability of the arterial intima by causing contraction of the endothelial cells and opening of the interendothelial junctions (Robertson and Khairallah, 1972, 1973). Other studies have suggested that several antihypertensive drugs which are currently in use have a protective effect against hypertensive vascular disease and atherosclerosis (Carrier et al., 1968; Freis et al., 1972). In humans, however, there is only scant evidence that atherosclerotic complications of hypertension are influenced by drug regimens.

Accelerated hypertensive vascular disease has been associated for many years with the kidney and kidney extracts (review by Giese, 1973). The majority of the studies have been performed by Giese and Masson and involved the effects of crude kidney-renin extracts in nephrectomized rats and dogs, or rats pretreated with adrenocortical hormones and sodium chloride. From these studies, performed largely from 1952 to 1964, it was clearly shown that acute arteriolar lesions which were morphologically similar, if not identical to the lesion of malignant hypertension can be induced by the administration and/or the endogenous release of renin and AII.

Similarly, the effect of renin on vascular permeability has been known for many years. It has been demonstrated many times that the injection of crude renin into bilaterally nephrectomized animals produces a syndrome of serious effusion, edema, and necrotic vascular lesions which resemble those present in malignant hypertension. One study, using single bolus injections of purified rat renin into nephrectomized rats, provided strong evidence that renin did enhance vascular permeability along with a sustained rise in blood pressure (Cuthbert and Peart, 1970). An increase in vascular permeability was evidenced only in rats in which a substantial and prolonged rise of blood pressure occurred, the likelihood being that blood pressure and permeability were causally related in these acute experiments.

Important clinical work relative to the previous studies was done by Laragh and colleagues beginning in 1972. It was their series of studies which regenerated keen interest in the phenomena of "renin vasculotoxicity, hypertension and vascular complication." A tenet which they proposed is that the chances of the major vascular complications of essential hypertension (i.e., myocardial infarction and stroke) developing in patients were directly related to the renin status of the patients. This thesis was based on the absence of vascular complications, over a 10-year study period, among 59 of 219 hypertensive patients who had low plasma renin levels. These results were compared to an incidence of vascular disease of 11-14% of the patients with normal or high levels of renin. The major differences between the two groups were that the 59 low-renin hypertensive patients were generally older and the high renin patients had higher blood pressures.

Laragh and colleagues have since maintained that low renin levels seem to protect against heart attack and stroke (Brunner et al., 1972; Laragh et al., 1972a; Brunner et al., 1973; Laragh, 1973). From these studies they arrived at two conclusions: (1) antihypertensive drugs, such as diuretics that increase renin activity, may be harmful; and (2) only modest therapy is desirable in low-renin hypertensives. That is, diuretic-induced hyperreninemia is undesirable in view of the probable relationships between increased plasma renin activity and the development of strokes and heart attacks. It has recently been shown that long-term diuretic therapy can produce small but significant increases in serum cholesterol and triglyceride levels (Ames and Hill, 1976).

The observations and conclusions of Laragh's group stimulated numerous retrospective clinical studies (reviews by Kaplan, 1975; Kirkendall et al., 1978). Only one study indicated concurring results; i.e., the incidence of cardiovascular events in patients with low plasma renin activity was significantly lower than in the normal and high-renin groups (Christlieb et al., 1974). None of the studies was able to provide unequivocal conclusions due to the shortcomings inherent in retrospective studies. Moreover, because of differences in cohort composition (age, sex, race, preexisting vascular disease, etc.) as well as technical variability (drug regimens, renin assay procedures, etc.), few direct comparisons of the data between the various studies could be made.

ANGIOTENSIN II INHIBITORS

The relatively recent development of AII blocking agents has provided much information regarding AII receptor sites, physiological actions of AII, and overall advances in our knowledge of the RAAS. Turker et al. (1974) reviewed those agents that block the indirect actions of AII, such as hexamethonium, and those compounds that antagonize the direct physiologic effects of AII, such as compounds that have opposite effects, e.g., bradykinin and prostaglandin E_1. Although considerable work has been done with noncompetitive antagonists of AII such as hydralazine, the most recent effort has been directed at developing competitive antagonists. An excellent discussion and a comprehensive listing of the structure-activity relationships of the nearly 200 AII analogs which have been prepared is available (Khosla et al., 1974). As summarized by Turker et al. (1974), all the competitive antagonists of AII are specific, and all are analogs of AII with modifications in the 8-position, with or without other positional changes.

The AII analog which has received the most attention is a modification of the 8-alanine-AII analog, 1-sarcosine-8-alanine-AII, which is also known as saralasin or P-113 (Pals et al., 1971). Discussions of the clinical uses of this compound are available (Guthrie et al., 1976; Pettinger, 1976; Horne et al., 1979). An extensive review of experimental studies that have used P-113 to define the action of AII has also been published (Davis, 1975).

A recent study by Munoz-Ramirez et al. (1976) using [Sar^1, Thr^8]AII found that it was a potent antagonist of AII and had less agonistic activity than either [Sar^1, Ala^8]AII or [Sar^1, Ile^8]AII in adrenalectomized and acute two-kidney hypertensive rats. It can be anticipated that there will be continued interest in identifying specific AII competitive inhibitors that lack agonistic activity.

ANGIOTENSINASES

There are numerous enzymes that hydrolyze AII, referred to collectively as "angiotensinases." No enzyme has been described that is specific for AII. Therefore, any hydrolase that can split any of the seven bonds of AII is considered to be an angiotensinase. Two reviews have dealt with the subject of "angiotensinases" (Ryan, 1974; Ledingham and Leary, 1974). Even the problems of studying the hydrolytic degradation of AII in vitro are enormous because there are 35 possible homologs of AII.

Khairallah et al. (1963) purified four plasma angiotensinases. They reported that at physiological pH, most AII is hydrolyzed by an aminopeptidase fraction (angiotensinase A). Khairallah and Page (1967) subsequently separated angiotensinase A into two components: A_1, which hydrolyzes Asn^1-AII; and A_2, which hydrolyzes Asp^1-AII. Both enzymes require Ca^{2+} and are inhibited by chelating agents. A third enzyme, an endopeptidase with a pH optimum of 5.8, cleaved both substrates and was called angiotensinase B. A pancreatic (Lentz et al., 1956) and liver (Johnson and Ryan, 1968) carboxypeptidase A that hydrolyzes Phe^8 from AII has described, and Yang et al. (1968) described a carboxypeptidase (angiotensinase C) that hydrolyzed the terminal bond of AII when Pro^7 was the terminal amino acid. The molecular weight of angiotensinase C has been estimated to be 115,000 by gel filtration (Odya et al., 1978).

Although there is peptidase activity in plasma, the major site of AII hydrolysis occurs in tissue vascular beds. Ledingham and Leary (1974) have compiled data regarding the occurrence of angiotensinases in homogenates and microsome and lysosome fractions of kidney. A comprehensive comparative study of angiotensinase activities from various tissue extracts indicates that activity is highest in intestinal mucosa, kidney cortex, and liver; lesser angiotensinase activity is present in extracts of lung and cardiac tissue. Results obtained from intact-organ studies, using both isolated organ perfusion techniques and in vivo perfusion techniques, have mirrored the results obtained with tissue homogenates.

Although there have been numerous studies designed to correlate changes in plasma angiotensinase activity with various diseases and physiological states, the results have been equivocal. The lack of strong correlations would be expected in view of the relatively minor importance of plasma angiotensinases compared to tissue enzymic activity. There is, however, good evidence from experimental renovascular hypertension studies using perfusion techniques that a decreased catabolism of AII contributes to both one- and two-kidney Goldblatt hypertension, inasmuch as the ability to hydrolyze AII was reduced in both models (Ledingham and Leary, 1974).

As it has recently been shown that angiotensinase A acting on either AI or AII leads ultimately to AIII, it is anticipated that renewed interest in angiotensinases will occur.

RENIN-ANGIOTENSIN SYSTEM, PROSTAGLANDINS, AND KALLIKREIN-KININ SYSTEM

There is much interest in defining the interactions of two renal hormonal systems, renin-angiotensin and prostaglandins (PGs), and their effects on blood pressure control (reviews and symposia: McGiff et al., 1976; Lee, 1976; Terragno et al., 1976; Tobian and O'Donnell, 1976; Heinemann and Lee, 1976; Dunn and Hood, 1977; Vapaatalo and Parantainen, 1978; McGiff, 1979). Rapid developments have occurred regarding prostaglandins during the last half decennium. New intermediates of prostaglandin synthesis, prostaglandin derivatives, cyclic endoperoxides, thromboxanes, and prostacyclin have been identified. The chemistry and physiology pertaining to these substances will be considered in detail in other chapters. The following discussion will, in the main, be limited to a review of the interactions of PG and components of the RAAS.

The earliest evidence for an association of PGs and the RAAS was obtained from observations of patients with renovascular hypertension. It was found that these patients had high levels of PGs and renin activity in the ischemic kidney and renal venous blood (Strong et al., 1966; Edwards et al., 1969). To the contrary, however, data from experimental studies seemed to weaken the association between the RAAS and PGs. Infusions of either PGE_1 or PGE_2 into the right renal artery of dogs failed to induce any consistent effect in renin release, mean or pulsatile arterial pressure, heart rate, or plasma sodium levels (Vander, 1968). Significant increases in urine flow, sodium excretion, and total renal plasma flow did occur.

The early studies of McGiff et al. (1970a, b) provided the major impetus for many studies concerning the interaction of PGs and the RAAS. They found that when AII was infused into the renal artery of dogs, a substance was released into the renal venous blood which was indistinguishable from PGE_2. They suggested that renal PGE_2 serves to regulate renal blood flow and urine formation when circulating levels of AII are elevated. It was subsequently found that AI has similar but less potent effects (Needleman et al., 1973). The studies of Saruta and Kaplan (1972) further implicated the interaction of the RAAS and PGs by demonstrating that PGE_1 and PGE_2 stimulated aldosterone formation by bovine outer adrenal slices; other PGs (PGA, $PGF_{1\alpha}$, $PGF_{2\alpha}$) had no such effects. Later studies demonstrated that systemic or intrarenal infusions of AII resulted in increases of venous PGF (Dunn et al., 1978) and increases in urinary excretion of PGE_2 and PGF_2 in humans (Frölich et al., 1975) and dogs (Dunn et al., 1978).

There have been relatively few experimental studies regarding the effects of AII on PGE levels in humans. Hornych and Papanicolaou (1974) found that infusions of AII increased renal venous concentrations of both PGE and PGA in two of four essential hypertensive patients. Frölich et al. (1975) found that PGE content of urine doubled, with no change in urine flow rate, in six normal subjects infused with AII. A recent study of Speckart et al. (1976) reported that peripheral plasma "immunoreactive PGE" concentrations of normal volunteers rose in response to pressor doses of AII, and that the rise was exaggerated by a low-salt diet and abolished by the administration of indomethacin.

Evidence for a direct effect of AI and AII on renal PG synthetase activity has been obtained by some workers (Itskovitz et al., 1973; Danon and Chang, 1973), while evidence against a direct effect is also available (Sirois and Gagnon, 1974). Studies by Mimran et al. (1975) have provided data from rat studies showing that inhibition of PG synthesis enhances the systemic and renal vascular effects of endogenous circulating AII and noradrenaline. Limas (1974) found that AII and norepinephrine produced a marked stimulation of PG synthetase activity when heart slices from adult male rats were incubated with AII. However, the omission of tyrosine from the incubation medium eliminated the AII-induced stimulation. Thus it appears that the major mechanism of AII-induced stimulation of myocardial PG biosynthesis depends on the ability of AII to stimulate the release of newly synthesized norepinephrine.

Studies designed to correlate plasma renin activity levels with PGE infusions presented discordant results. Infusions of PGE produced a rise of PRA in two of seven dogs (Vander, 1968), a rise in PRA in two of four human subjects (Carlson et al., 1969), and an invariable rise in PRA in dogs (Werning et al., 1971). A more recent experiment has shown that the infusion of either PGE_1 or PGA_1 into the stenosed renal artery of anesthetized hypertensive dogs caused an increase in renin activity in renal vein effluent of the infused kidney (Varkarakis et al., 1975). This study suggested several possible explanations for the apparent PG-enhanced renin release, including (1) the decreased aortic pressure that was found close to the level of the renal artery acting according to the baroreceptor theory of renin release, (2) a direct effect of PGs on the JG cells, (3) changes in tubular sodium concentration of sodium load due to the increased diuresis, and (4) the occurrence of kaliuresis.

Clinical observations have recently been made concerning the response to intravenous infusion of PGA of low-, normal-, and high-renin hypertensives (Krakoff et al., 1975). In this study all patients were maintained on a similar electrolyte intake. The low-renin subgroup showed the greatest decrease in arterial pressure and the greatest increase in sodium excretion; PRA was unaffected. The normal-renin group showed a lesser reduction in pressure and sodium excretion; however, PRA rose significantly. The high-renin group did not show a significant change in either blood pressure or sodium excretion, but there were striking increases in PRA. Various interpretations of the apparent differing actions of PGA_1 in the three renin subgroups were suggested.

Undoubtedly, much of the confusion regarding the effects of PGs on renin activity reflects differences in the sodium balance of the individuals and experimental animals. Certainly, the condition of sodium balance alone is a potent regulator of renin activity. Thus when sodium balance is altered, renin release will change regardless of the stimulus. For example, McGiff and Itskovitz (1973) found that the amount of PGE released into renal venous blood was not related to the dose of norepinephrine, but it was inversely related to PRA. That is, they found that norepinephrine induced the greatest release of PGE when there was a condition of positive sodium balance ("low" PRA activity). Norepinephrine induced the smallest release of PGE when there was a condition of negative sodium balance ("high" PRA). There is, however, some recent evidence which tends to refute the notion that PGE release is volume dependent. Jubiz et al. (1976) measured the concentration of PGE in renal venous blood of dogs before and after injections of NaCl into the renal arterial circulation. They found an increase in renal venous PGE which was independent of either changes in serum osmolality or total renal blood flow; indomethacin blocked the rise in PGE. The importance of sodium balance on the cybernetics of PGs and AII was emphasized by Tobian et al. (1974), who found that rats maintained on a high-sodium diet had significantly reduced renal PGE_2 levels. Since a high sodium intake reduces PRA, AII, and catecholamine levels, it was anticipated that a reduced amount of PGE_2 would result.

There have been several clinical studies which demonstrate that dietary sodium intake significantly affects plasma PGA, PRA, and aldosterone levels (Fichman et al., 1972, Zusman et al., 1973a; Payakkapan et al., 1975). These studies of normotensive subjects generally showed that (1) there was a progressive decrease in plasma PGA with increasing sodium intake, (2) there was less of a rise in PRA than there was in PGA levels during changes from high- to low-sodium diets, and (3) there was an increase in both plasma and urinary aldosterone during low sodium intake. Surprisingly, that data indicated that PGA has little natriuretic activity in normotensive individuals. Indeed, it appears that volume depletion which results in a rise in PRA (AII) followed by an increase in aldosterone release with sodium retention also leads to a rise in PGA, which in turn stimulates aldosterone release and sodium retention.

Infusions of PGA_1 have been shown to antagonize the pressor effect of AII, whereas it increased the aldosterone-stimulating effect of AII (Golub and Horton, 1974). This study also presented data which indicate that PGE and PGA infusions stimulate renin secretion, and that AII infusions increase PG synthesis. As suggested by Lee (1976), it would seem that the benefits of a salt-restricted diet for essential hypertensive patients are gained not only through volume depletion but also through a rise in peripheral vasodilating PGA levels. In patients with essential hypertension it is well documented that infusions of PGA_1 or PGA_2 lead to an initial increase in renal blood flow and marked natriuresis and diuresis. When the infusion rate is increased, there is a fall in blood pressure due to peripheral arteriolar dilation. Concurrently, the elevated blood flow, natriuresis, and diuresis is normalized.

Since diuretic therapy is a cornerstone therapeutic measure for the treatment of many hypertensives it is important to learn its effect on PGA levels. Preliminary data indicate that the beneficial effects of a low-sodium diet and diuretic therapy in patients with essential hypertension may be mediated by the increase in plasma PGA.

The direct effects of indomethacin, which has often been used as a PG blocking agent on renin activity has often been neglected in many studies concerning the effects of PGE on renin activity. Various studies have shown that indomethacin suppresses PRA in normotensive and hypertensive states, and inhibits the normal increase in PRA after the administration of either diuretics or a low-sodium diet (Rumpf et al., 1975; Romero et al., 1975; Patak et al., 1976). Frölich et al. (1976) obtained evidence that indomethacin significantly lowers PRA, aldosterone levels, 24-hr sodium excretion, and urinary PGE excretion in essential and postmalignant hypertensives and normal subjects. Indomethacin also causes sodium retention and reduces the natriuretic response to furosemide. Since the changes in PRA were accompanied by some degree of sodium retention, it could not be concluded whether indomethacin lowered PRA by a direct renal PGE mechanism, or by increasing plasma volume, or both.

Romero et al. (1976) studied the effects of indomethacin, meclofenamate, and aspirin on renin release in rabbits which were bled to stimulate renin activity. They found that all three compounds lowered PRA and concluded that the lowering was due to interference with renal renin release. They found no evidence for in vitro renin inhibition by indomethacin. There is, nevertheless some evidence which indicates that indomethacin can inhibit PRA directly. In vitro studies have shown that PGE and PGA inhibit AI production (Kotchen et al., 1974). Eggena et al. (1975) found that PGE_2 was more significant in normotensive than in hypertensive plasma, and suggested that the results obtained from the hypertensive plasma might be due to the presence of an unidentified modifier (activator?).

There are considerable data which support the concept that PGE_2 can act as a physiological antagonist to AII. The administration of the prostaglandin biosynthesis inhibitors indomethacin and meclofenamate has been shown to cause a decrease in renal blood flow and a decrease in PGE_2 levels (Aiken and Vane, 1973; Lonigro et al., 1973a), a decrease in autoregulatory vasodilatation as a result of decreased perfusion pressure (Herbaczynska-Cedro and Vane, 1973), and potentiation of the renal vasoconstrictor actions of AII (Aiken and Vane, 1973). Conversely, the antidiuretic and vasoconstrictor actions of AII and renal nerve stimulation have also been shown to be reduced by PGE_2 infusions (Lonigro et al., 1973b). Together these observations suggest that a decrease in PG synthesis might be a factor in the etiology of some types of hypertension.

Since it was first suggested that PGA_2 might serve as an antihypertensive hormone (Lee et al., 1965) there have been numerous studies performed in an attempt to provide evidence that PG deficiencies are associated with essential hypertension and/or the RAAS (review by Lee, 1976). Lee et al. (1971) reported an increase in renal blood flow which was accompanied by an increase in renal venous renin content in five of six essential hypertensive patients who were infused with PGA_1 for 1 hr. Conclusions regarding the direct effect of the PGA_1 infusions upon renin activity were, however, obscured by natriuresis and the hypokalemia that occurred concurrently in all six patients. Interestingly, Fichman et al. (1972) reported a slight, but insignificant rise in PRA in 4 of 10 normal subjects during infusion with PGA. Similarly, a more recent study of normotensives demonstrated a significant positive linear regression of plasma PGA on urinary aldosterone, whereas the correlation between plasma PGA and PRA was much less striking (Lee, 1975). Zusman et al. (1973a) found a PGA deficiency in the plasma of essential as well as renovascular hypertensive patients. However, plasma and renal concentrations of PGA were higher in spontaneously hypertensive rats (Zusman et al., 1973b), which have served as experimental models of essential hypertension for numerous investigators. These results contribute positively to other data which suggest that these rats may not be valid models for studies concerning PGs (Terragno et al., 1976). Other clinic evidence has recently been provided by a case report that a renal cell carcinoma was secreting a PGA-like material which was normalizing blood pressure in a patient who had severe hypertension for some time before the tumor was detected. Upon removal of the tumor the PGA level was sharply reduced and the hypertension was established (Zusman et al., 1974).

An investigation has been performed to evaluate the involvement of PGs in a one-kidney hypertension model (Romero et al., 1975). This study concerned the effect of the release of a renal arterial constriction on the blood pressure of one-kidney (renin-independent) hypertensive rabbits after PG synthesis had been blocked by indomethacin. It was concluded that there is no major participation of PGs in the reversal of one-kidney hypertension, because 8-9 hr after releasing the renal artery clip there was no difference in the blood pressure of the treated versus the untreated group. Evidence was obtained, however, that PGs may have a facilitatory role in reversing one-kidney hypertension. This conclusion was supported by observations from untreated rabbits which showed (1) increased renal blood flow, (2) increased glomerular filtration rate, (3) increased urinary output, and (4) a more abrupt decrease in blood pressure in response to the release of the arterial clip.

There are several studies which demonstrate direct feedback mechanisms involving PGA and the RAAS. Hemodynamic studies in dogs have been performed to assess the effect of PGs on the renal vasculature and the RAAS in a modified two-kidney hypertension model (Satoh and Zimmerman, 1975). Contrary to the results of other workers, neither meclofenamate nor indomethacin altered renal blood flow or renal vascular resistance under basal conditions. They did, however, obtain a significant renal vasoconstrictor effect during renal ischemia (Goldblatt clamp) with the concentrations of meclofenamate and indomethacin used in the control studies. Arterial and renal venous PRA was increased by the compromised renal blood flow that was produced by the clamp. It was concluded, therefore, that the ability of PG synthesis inhibitor to cause renal vasoconstriction depends on the stimulation of renin release by renal ischemia. These results are difficult to interpret, for it was not determined whether the increased AII, as the result of increased PRA, stimulated PG synthetase directly, or indirectly through its renal hemodynamic effects. However, it was observed that the AII antagonist P-113 significantly blocked the renal vasoconstriction induced by the PG synthesis inhibitor during renal ischemia. It was not clear, however, whether AII was stimulating the synthetase enzyme in the kidney directly or whether it was acting through a hemodynamic effect.

Other studies designed to evaluate the contribution of prostaglandins to the severity of two-kidney Goldblatt hypertension and acute and chronic renal hypertension have provided additional observations. Pugsley et al. (1975) found that (1) systolic blood pressures were higher in indomethacin-treated clipped rats, (2) PG synthesis in vitro was suppressed in the hypertensive animals regardless of whether they had received indomethacin, and (3) PG synthesis was equal in the clipped and nonclipped kidneys of hypertensive rats. Reliable explanations for these interesting observations await further studies. The studies do not indicate that PG act as an inhibitory mechanism to counter hypertensive mechanisms of the RAAS that operate when renal blood flow is reduced. This conclusion is in contrast to the notion that a deficiency of PGs in animals with normal kidneys results in hypertension. Scholkens and Steinbach (1975) similarly found that PG biosynthesis inhibition with indomethacin, mefenamic acid, or acetylsalicylic acid significantly increased acute and chronic renal hypertension in the rat, and AII-stimulated decrease of blood flow in the dog.

Pugsley et al. (1976) reported that indomethacin exacerbates renal clip two-kidney hypertension in rats. They concluded that PGE is associated with blood pressure regulation in two-kidney (renin-dependent) Goldblatt hypertension and suggested that PGs act as a "braking" mechanism against the "hypertensive" mechanisms that operates when renal blood flow is significantly reduced.

Clinical studies have provided evidence for the participation of PGs in the etiology of Bartter's syndrome. This renal syndrome apparently results from hyperplasia of renomedullary interstitial cells and is characterized by (1) normal blood pressure, (2) an obligatory renal tubular loss of sodium and potassium, (3) hypovolemia, (4) increased PRA and aldosterone, and (5) a loss of sensitivity to the pressor effect of AII. It has recently been shown that Bartter's syndrome can be successfully treated with indomethacin (Verberckmoes et al., 1976; Gill et al., 1976). From these studies it would appear that an inappropriate release of PGs from the kidney induces reduced sodium reabsorption, volume depletion, AII insensitivity, elevated renin secretion, and secondary hyperaldosteronism. Thus, by blocking the overproduction of PGs with indomethacin, the patient becomes normalized. Utilizing PG synthetase inhibitors, results have been obtained which suggest that, in Bartter's syndrome, PG mediates the low urinary kinins and the high plasma bradykinins, and that urinary kallikrein, which is aldosterone dependent, does not control kinin formation (Vinci et al., 1978). Furthermore, it appears that the high plasma bradykinin may be the cause of the pressor hyporesponsiveness to AII which characterizes the syndrome.

Much of the controvertible data regarding the actions of PGs undoubtedly are due to the various abilities to measure them. For example, despite new techniques and advanced instrumentation, there is still controversy concerning the detection of PGA in human peripheral plasma. Using a combination of gas chromatography and mass spectrometry, Frölich et al. (1975) were unable to detect prostaglandins A, while measurable levels had been reported using radioimmunoassay procedures (Zusman et al., 1974; Pletka and Hickler, 1974; Payakkapan et al., 1975; Speckart et al., 1976). Because of the similarities in the concentration found by various laboratories, it is difficult to conclude that PGA is not present in human plasma.

The recent discoveries of thromboxane A_2 (TxA_2), which aggregates platelets and constricts smooth muscle (Hamberg et al., 1975), and prostacyclin (PGI_2), which inhibits platelet aggregation and is a vasodilator agent (Gryglewski et al., 1976), have added new dimensions to PG research (reviewed by Moncada and Vane, 1979). Since prostacyclin occurs primarily in vascular tissues, and thromboxanes in platelets and injured tissue, their relationship with the components of the RAAS have not received much attention. However, with the recent studies which indicate that the various substances of the RAAS are also distributed throughout various organs and vessels, there is reason to believe that they could interact in situ, thus negating the necessity of their presence in the circulation.

Since renin is synthesized in the juxtaglomerular apparatus, and the probable site of kallikrein synthesis is the macula densa area of the distal nephron, it is expected that the RAAS and the kallikrein-kinin system interact. These interactions have been discussed in several recent reviews (Obika, 1978; Levinsky, 1979; Mills, 1979). There are at least three possible mechanisms by which the RAAS can stimulate the activity of the kallikrein-kinin system (KKS): (1) aldosterone can stimulate kallikrein synthesis or secretion (Margolius et al., 1974; (2) the renin-angiotensin system stimulates aldosterone secretion and thus kallikrein synthesis; and (3) AII stimulates kallikrein release directly (MacFarlane et al., 1974). In addition, AII increases PG synthesis, which in turn, via increased PGE levels, leads to increased urinary kallikrein excretion (Terragno et al., 1976). Correspondingly, there is much evidence that the KKS can evoke responses from the RAAS and PG mechanisms (reviews by Mills, 1979; Nasjletti and Malik, 1979).

RENIN AND CLINICAL HYPERTENSION

It has long been held that the RAAS is involved in some hypertensive syndromes as a result of its effects on effective blood volume via aldosterone, and arteriolar constriction via angiotensin II. Because of this, measurements of plasma renin activity (PRA) and urinary sodium excretion have been used to determine the involvement of renin in the vasoconstriction etiology of hypertension. Laragh et al. (1979) have prepared a vasoconstriction volume analysis scheme to aid in the understanding and treatment of hypertension. He concluded that hypertension is the result of either arteriolar constriction without increased volume (vasoconstriction hypertension), arterial overfilling (volume hypertension), or a disturbed interaction of the two. Since the RAAS is involved in the cybernetics of these activities, Laragh and his colleagues have recommended grouping hypertensive patients according to PRA levels (i.e., low, normal, and high PRA). They have proposed that PRA can thus be used to dictate therapeutic regimens and forecast prognosis based on the assumption that high-PRA aggravates and accelerates cardiovascular problems leading to heart attack and stroke

(Brunner et al., 1972). Although it is generally agreed that β-blocking drugs, propranolol in particular, suppress renin release in normal- and high-renin patients, there are disagreements as to the cause-and-effect relationship between renin-suppressive and hypotensive activities (review by Guthrie et al., 1976).

The recent development of inhibitors of the RAAS such as saralasin, a competitive antagonist of AII, and inhibitors of AII-converting enzyme, has provided a means for determining the renin dependence of hypertension. Brunner et al. (1973), using saralasin, [Sar^1, Ala^8]-angiotensin II, and Gavras et al. (1974) and Johnson et al. (1975), using SQ 20,881, a converting enzyme inhibitor, have reported significant reductions in blood pressure in hypertensive patients with high PRA levels; normal- and low-renin patients showed little and no response, respectively. Both drugs gave greater blood pressure reductions when the patients were salt depleted. The studies provide apparent support for the theory that hypertension in patients with high PRA is the result of high levels of circulating AII, and that AII has little if any pressor role in low-renin hypertensives. Conclusions are more difficult to obtain regarding the role of renin in normal-renin hypertensives.

A publication by Streeten et al. (1976) reviewed much of the available data regarding saralasin (P-113) infusions and reported on a study which they performed. Briefly, they gave an unselected group of 300 hypertensives intravenous injections of furosemide prior to infusion of P-113. They found that the blood pressure level fell an average of more than 10/8 mmHg in 31 patients. All 31 patients had elevated peripheral plasma renin levels and/or renal vein plasma renin activity ratios greater than 1.5. Radiographic evidence of renal or renovascular disease was subsequently obtained in the majority (20) of these patients. This group of 31 patients who demonstrated angiotensinogenic hypertension, at least in part, had the following recognizable renal lesions: (1) 11 patients (36%) had unilateral renal artery stenosis, (2) three patients (10%) had unilateral renal artery stenosis with renal insufficiency, (3) three patients (10%) had bilateral renal artery stenosis, and (4) three patients (10%) had bilateral renal parenchymal disease. Unfortunately, 11 patients (36%) had no renal abnormality by the radiographic studies performed, but had elevated renin measurements. Contrary to earlier reports by others, only half of the patients with high renin levels showed a fall in blood pressure during saralasin infusion. In approximately one-third of the patients (97 of 300) agonistic blood pressure response was induced by P-113 infusions. This response was commonly, but not solely, seen in patients who had low-renin levels.

According to Streeten et al. (1976), no serious side effects were occasioned by infusions of P-113 in over 800 patients demonstrating various types of hypertension. The only potentially serious side effect of P-113 which they encountered with the agonistic effect on blood pressure. Saralasin infusion induced a precipitous hypotensive response in only one of the more than 800 patients.

Streeten and colleagues concluded that (1) saralasin is a highly specific antagonist of AII, (2) it has a mild agonistic action which is seldom of clinical significance, and (3) it has great potential as a pharmacologic tool for investigating hypertensive phenomena. They proposed that P-113 is quite valuable as a means of recognizing, rapidly and reliably, the occurrence of an angiotensinogenic component of hypertension. A similar study of 52 untreated hypertensive patients by Case et al. (1976a) reaffirmed the conclusion that P-113 infusion consistently and reliably identified an AII pressor response associated with high-renin forms of hypertension. To the contrary, however, they observed that P-113 infusions caused transient small, but striking pressor responses in more than 94% of their patients. Because of this response, predominantly in the low-renin hypertensives, they concluded that saralasin should be viewed as a weak competitive agonist rather than as a true antagonist of AII. Counter to the conclusions of Streeten and colleagues, Case et al. (1976a) concluded that renin measurements using a renin-sodium index more accurately reflect the renin involvement in the hypertensive state than does P-113 testing; and that prior sodium depletion recommended to increase the frequency of depressor response is not desirable, since the response then becomes an index of the reactivity of the system to sodium depletion. They suggested that perhaps another type of drug, such as the AI-converting enzyme inhabitor SQ 20,881, would be more effective for identifying a renin factor in hypertension. A later study substantiated this idea (Case et al., 1976b).

A large cooperative study, involving 13 hypertension centers, concerning the value of P-113 was reported in 1979 (Horne et al., 1979). The results indicate that saralasin testing of hypertensives is relatively safe, accurate, and simple and may have clinical utility as a screening agent for angiotensin-dependent hypertension.

CLASSIFICATION OF HYPERTENSIVE PATIENTS BY PLASMA RENIN ACTIVITY

Plasma renin determinations are of value in defining subpopulations of hypertensive patients with certain physiologic traits. Two factors, however, have limited the widespread clinical use of the PRA as a diagnostic tool for the hypertensive patient. First, the proper conditions for reproducible measurements are difficult to achieve. For instance, to demonstrate that patients have a PRA level that is not responsive to appropriate stimuli, such variables as posture, dietary sodium intake, diurnal variation of PRA, and the effects of a variety of drugs on renin release must be controlled. In addition, it is difficult to obtain a reproducible, sensitive, and accurate laboratory determination of PRA in many localities. Second, correctable forms of low-renin hypertension secondary to correctable causes will have hypokalemia in the majority of instances. High-renin hypertensives with correctable causes, except for those with renin-producing tumors, can usually be identified by information from the history or physical examination.

Low-renin hypertensive patients may be grouped into those with or without a cause for the renin suppression. There is considerable evidence that 20-30% of hypertensives have low renin levels when tested under standardized conditions. It is not yet certain, however, that these individuals represent a stable, well-defined group, since Crane et al. (1972), Brunner et al. (1972), and others have noted many patients who have low-renin hypertension on occasion and will have normal-renin responsiveness on retesting. It is known that prolonged diuretic therapy and treatment with other antihypertensive drugs, including spironolactone, may alter PRA for weeks and months (Lowder and Liddle, 1974). Age, sex, and race also influence renin levels. Several studies have shown that low-renin hypertension is correlated with age of the patient. Some believe that renin responsiveness even in normal individuals declines with advancing age. Most studies have found the majority of low-renin hypertensive patients to be female (Crane et al., 1972). A number of studies have found that black patients have a much higher incidence of low-renin hypertension than do whites. The frequency is found to be about 42% among blacks, in contrast to a frequency of 9-30% in white populations (Brunner et al., 1972; Mroczek et al., 1973).

Secondary hypertensive states when characterized by excessive expansion of extracellular fluid volume have chronic renin suppression. One common form occurs with mineralocorticoid induced sodium and water retention, and is usually associated with hypokalemia; a second type is associated with volume expansion due to renal failure. Known causes of low-renin hypertionsion from mineralocorticoid excess include those conditions listed in Table 1.

TABLE 1 Known Causes of Low-Renin Hypertension

1. Aldosterone overproduction from an adrenal adenoma (primary aldosteronism)
2. Aldosterone overproduction from bilateral nodular hyperplasia (tertiary aldosteronism)
3. 11-Deoxycorticosterone (DOC) from 17α-hydroxylation defect or from non-ACTH-dependent overproduction
4. 11β-Hydroxylation deficiency (children) with DOC and 11-deoxycortisol overproduction
5. Mixtures of mineralocorticoids associated with adrenal carcinoma or ectopic ACTH-producing tumors
6. 18-Hydroxy-DOC excess
7. 16β-Hydroxydehydroepiandrosterone (DHEA) excess
8. Medicaments such as licorice and sodium carbenoxalone

The majority of patients with primary and tertiary aldosteronism have hypokalemia. Low-renin hypertensive states arising from mineralocorticoid excesses also are associated with hypokalemia. On the other hand, many patients with low-renin hypertension do not present with hypokalemia and cannot be identified by this means. At the moment, evidence that one can predict prognosis on the basis of the renin state is controversial and there is not yet clear evidence that one can better outline appropriate antihypertensive therapy by knowing the renin level (Woods et al., 1976).

The cause of the low PRA in those hypertensives who do not have evident mineralocorticoid excess have been a topic of considerable interest. Several theories have been suggested but none of these have adequate support to explain the phenomenon fully. The most commonly expressed thought is that there is an excess of an "abnormal" steroid or excessive mineralocorticoid activity in these patients (Spark, 1972). Others have suggested a disordered regulation of aldosterone metabolism or decreased metabolic clearance of aldosterone as contributing factors (Brown et al., 1978). Laragh et al. (1972b) have suggested an impairment of the ability to normally secrete potassium. An impaired peripheral β-adrenergic responsiveness has also been proposed. In this formulation, the suppression of renin release reflects inadequate β-adrenergic renin release and the hypertension results from unopposed α-adrenergic activity. Some have proposed that a low-renin state may simply be the late manifestation of the hypertensive condition itself, i.e., a long-term effect of elevated blood pressure on the kidney or a primary renal abnormality in renin secretion (Taylor, 1977). Because of the importance of this group of hypertensive patients, a better understanding of the factors causing the low-renin state is important.

High PRA values are found commonly in patients with (1) malignant or accelerated hypertension, (2) unilateral renal artery stenosis, (3) bilateral renal artery stenosis, and (4) end-stage renal parenchymal disease. Patients with renin-secreting kidney tumors also have high PRA, as do some patients who take oral contraceptives. Certain drugs, particularly the vasodilator antihypertensive agents, also cause PRA to rise. Some patients with hypokalemia may have high PRA measurements without increased secretion of aldosterone. A number of other patients without recognized causes for hypertension have relatively high peripheral plasma renin activity.

The classification of hypertensive patients by PRA has been justified on the basis that such a classification improves information concerning prognosis and the ability to treat with more appropriate drugs. At the moment, evidence does not support the view that renin is an independent risk factor and that it may predict morbidity in hypertensives. Information presented to support this hypothesis is provocative and indicates the need for better controlled studies of the subject.

The presence of elevated PRA has been suggested as a guide for the selection of specific drugs for the treatment of hypertension (Laragh, 1973).

It is known that certain agents, particularly propanolol and other drugs that affect activity of the sympathetic nervous system, tend to reduce PRA, and others, particularly the vasodilators and diuretics, tend to increase plasma renin activity. There is not yet proof, however, that the utilization of such an index provides better therapy despite a number of articles which suggest that it does. The evidence to this point does not weigh heavily in support of the concept that the lowering of PRA itself actually does much to lower blood pressure, except that drugs that block angiotensin receptors and with converting enzyme inhibitors. Rather, the evidence suggests that both the lowering of blood pressure and the lowering of PRA represent dual actions of the β-blocking drugs and those that affect sympathetic activity.

Because many low-renin hypertensives respond well to β-blocking drugs and because most patients with normal or high renins respond with a fall in blood pressure in response to diuretics, renin profiling is less specific than one would like. When one adds to this indecisiveness the expense of several office visits, withholding of drugs before renin profiling, the imposition of a low-salt diet or diuretic program to set the stage, and the measurement of a 24-hr urine collection and PRA, the expense becomes considerable. These two problems, the nonspecificity and the expense of renin profiling, plus the ease with which one can generate a treatment program by other means make it impractical in the routine management of the hypertensive.

In summary, there are certain clinical situations in which the examination of PRA has critical diagnostic importance. The PRA is essential for the diagnosis of primary aldosteronism, for the diagnosis of selective hypoaldosteronism due to renin deficiency, and for the detection of primary renin excess due to renin-secreting tumors. The measurement of plasma renin is also helpful in separating patients with aldosteronism and other mineralocorticoid excess into proper categories. The measurement of renin activity from the two renal veins is also essential in the evaluation of the patient with renal artery hypertension and those with unilateral renal disease hypertension. Measurement of PRA is of importance in certain patients with end-stage kidney disease and intractable hypertension since it may provide information to support bilateral nephrectomy.

Because the clinical situations in which the PRA measurement is needed are quite specific and for the most part can be detected by either hypokalemia, severe hypertension, or other clinical clues, it is not appropriate to apply the measurement of PRA to the evaluation of all hypertensives. Only the extremely rare patient with a renin-secreting tumor may be overlooked if one uses PRA as a selective diagnostic tool rather than as a screening one.

Thus classification of hypertensives by PRA is of considerable epidemiologic and clinical interest. At the moment, however, there is no clear advantage in using this measurement for routine screening of hypertensive patients.

ACKNOWLEDGMENT

This work was supported in part by the Lillian and Charles Duncan Foundation and the National Heart, Lung and Blood Institute, Grant HL-20189.

REFERENCES

Aiken, J. W., and Vane, J. R. (1973). Intrarenal prostaglandin release attenuates the renal vasoconstrictor activity of angiotensin. J. Pharmacol. Exp. Ther. 184:678-687.

Allison, D. J., Tanigawa, H., and Assaykeen, T. A. (1972). The effects of cyclic nucleotides on plasma renin activity and renal functions in dogs. In Control of Renin Secretion. T. A. Assaykeen (Ed.). Plenum Press, New York, pp. 33-47.

Ames, R. P., and Hill, P. (1976). Elevation of serum lipid levels during diuretic therapy of hypertension. Am. J. Med. 61:748-757.

Aoi, W., Wade, M. B., Rosner, D. R., and Weinberger, M. H. (1974). Renin release by rat kidney slices in vitro: effects of cations and catecholamines. Am. J. Physiol. 227:630-634.

Aoi, W., Henry, D. P., and Weinberger, M. H. (1976). Evidence of a physiological role of renal sympathetic nerves in adrenergic stimulation of renin release in the rat. Circ. Res. 28:123-126.

Aoyagi, T., and Umezawa, H. (1975). Structures and activities of protease inhibitors of microbial origin. In Proteases and Biological Control, E. Reich, D. B. Rifkin, and E. Shaw (Eds.). Cold Spring Harbor Laboratory, Cold Spring Harbor, New York, pp. 429-454.

Aoyagi, T., Morishima, H., Nishizawa, R., Kunimoto, S., Takeuchi, T., and Umezawa, H. (1972). Biological activity of pepstatins, pepstanone A and partial peptides on pepsin, cathepsin D and renin. J. Antibiot. 15:690-694.

Baggio, B., Favaro, S., Antonello, A., Todesco, S., Campanacci, L., and Borsatti, A. (1973). A procedure for the determination of a renin inhibitor in human plasma. Clin. Chim. Acta 45:67-71.

Bakhle, Y. S. (1972). Inhibition of converting enzyme by venom peptides. In Hypertension '72, J. Genest and E. Koiw (Eds.). Springer-Verlag, New York, pp. 541-549.

Bakhle, Y. S. (1974). Converting enzyme in vitro measurement and properties. In Angiotensin, I. H. Page and F. M. Bumpus (Eds.). Springer-Verlag, New York, pp. 41-80.

Bakhle, Y. S., Reynard, A. M., and Vane, J. R. (1969). Metabolism of the angiotensins in isolated perfused tissues. Nature (Lond.) 222:956-959.

Barrett, A. J. (1973). Human cathepsin Bl. Purification and some properties of the enzyme. Biochem. J. 1231:809-822.

Bath, N. M., and Gregerman, R. I. (1972). Labeled polymeric substrate for renin. Synthesis of N-acetylpoly(L-glutamyl)-[I^{125}]tridecapeptide and use for enzyme assay. Biochemistry 11:2845-2853.

Beck, N., Reed, S. W., Murdaugh, V. H., and Davis, B. B. (1972). Effect of catecholamines and their interaction with other hormones on cyclic 3',5'-aldenosine monophosphate of the kidney. J. Clin. Invest. 51:939-944.

Beck, N., Kim, K. S., and Davis, B. B. (1975). Catecholamine-dependent cyclic adenosine monophosphate and renin in the dog kidney. Circ. Res. 36:401-405.

Bell, C., and Bakhle, Y. S. (1975). Effects of chronic oral contraceptive treatment on the conversion of A-I to A-II in the rat. J. Pharmacol. Exp. Ther. 193:160-165.

Berman, L. B., Vertes, V., Mitra, S., and Gould, A. B. (1972). Renin-angiotensin system in anephric patients. N. Engl. J. Med. 286:58-61.

Biron, P., and Huggins, C. G. (1968). Pulmonary activation of synthetic angiotensin I. Life Sci. 7:965-970.

Blair-West, J. R., Coghlan, J. P., Denton, D. A., Funder, J. W., Scoggins, B. A., and Wright, R. D. (1971). The effect of the heptapeptide (2-8) and hexapeptide (3-8) fragments of angiotensin II on aldosterone secretion. J. Clin. Endocrinol. Metab. 32:575-578.

Blumberg, A., Denny, S., Nishikawa, K., Pure, E., Marshall, G. R., and Needleman, P. (1976). Work in progress—angiotensin III-induced prostaglandin (PG) release. Prostaglandins 11:195-197.

Boaz, D., Wyatt, S., and Fitz, A. (1975). Angiotensin I [Phe^8-His^9] hydrolase: studies with renin substrates. Biochem. Biophys. Res. Commun. 63:490-495.

Boucher, R., Saidi, M., and Genest, J. (1972). A new "angiotensin I converting enzyme" system. In Hypertension '72, J. Genese and E. Koiw (Eds.). Springer-Verlag, New York, pp. 512-523.

Boucher, R., Asselin, J., and Genest, J. (1974). A new enzyme leading to the direct formation of angiotensin II. Circ. Res. 34/35(Suppl. I):203-209.

Boyd, G. W. (1974). A protein-bound form of porcine renal renin. Circ. Res. 35:426-438.

Braverman, B., Freeman, R. H., and Rostorfer, H. H. (1971). The influence of dietary sodium chloride on in vitro renin release from rat kidney slices. Proc. Soc. Exp. Biol. Med. 138:81-88.

Bravo, E. L., Tarazi, R. C., Dustan, H. P., and Lewis, J. W. (1975). Dissociation between renin and arterial pressure responses to beta-adrenergic blockade in human essential hypertension. Circ. Res. 36/37(Suppl. I):241-247.

Bravo, E. L., Khosla, M. C., and Bumpus, F. M. (1976). The role of angiotensins in aldosterone production. Circ. Res. 38(Suppl. II):104-107.

Brown, R. D., Tucker, R., Tue, K., Wisgerhof, M., and Salassa, R. (1978). Effect of saralasin on plasma aldosterone in hypertensive man. J. Lab. Clin. Med. 91:473-479.

Brunner, H. R., Laragh, J. H., Baer, L., Newton, M. A., Goodwin, F. T., Krakoff, L. R., Bard, R. H., and Buhler, F. R. (1972). Essential hypertension: renin and aldosterone, heart attack and stroke. N. Engl. J. Med. 286:441-449.

Brunner, H. R., Gavras, H., Laragh, J. H., and Keenan, R. (1973). Angiotensin II blockade in man by Sar^1-Ala^8-angiotensin II for understanding and treatment of high blood pressure. Lancet 2:1045-1048.

Buckley, J. P., and Ferrario, C. (1977). The Central Actions of Angiotensin and Related Hormones. Pergamon Press, Elmsford, N. Y.

Buhler, F. R., Laragh, J. H., Vaughan, E. D., Brunner, H. R., Gavras, H., and Baer, L. (1973). Antihypertensive action of propanolol. Specific antirenin responses in high and normal renin forms of essential, renal, renovascular, and malignant hypertension. Am. J. Cardiol. 32: 511-522.

Caldwell, P. R. B., Seegal, B. C., Hsu, K. C., Das, M., and Soffer, R. L. (1976). Angiotensin-converting enzyme: vascular endothelial localization. Science 191:1050-1051.

Campbell, W. B., Brooks, S., and Pettinger, W. A. (1974). Angiotensin II- and angiotensin III-induced aldosterone release in vivo in the rat. Science 184:994-996.

Carlson, L. A., Ekelund, L. G., and Oro, L. (1969). Circulatory and respiratory effects of different doses of prostaglandin E_1 in man. Acta Physiol. Scand. 75:161-169.

Carrier, O., Clower, B. R., and Whittington, P. J. (1968). Inhibition of cholesterol-induced vascular lesions by dietary reserpine. J. Atheroscler. Res. 8:229.

Case, D. B., Wallace, J. M., Keim, H. J., Sealey, J. E., and Laragh, J. H. (1976a). Usefulness and limitations of saralasin, a partial competitive agonist of angiotensin II, for evaluating the renin and sodium factors in hypertensive patients. Am. J. Med. 60:825-836.

Case, D. B., Wallace, J. M., Keim, H. J., Weber, M. A., Drayer, J. I. M., White, R. P., Sealey, J. E., and Laragh, J. H. (1976b). Estimating renin participation in hypertension: superiority of converting enzyme inhibitor over saralasin. Am. J. Med. 61:790-796.

Chiu, A. T., and Peach, M. J. (1974.) Inhibition of induced aldosterone biosynthesis with a specific antagonist of angiotensin II. Proc. Natl. Acad. Sci. USA 71:341-344.

Chiu, A. T., Ryan, J. W., Stewart, J. M., and Dorer, F. E. (1976). Formation of angiotensin III by angiotensin-converting enzymes. Biochem. J. 155:189-192.

Chonko, A. M., Stein, J. H., and Ferris, T. F. (1975). Renin and the kidney. Nephron 15:279-305.

Christlieb, A. R., Gleason, R. E., Hickler, R. B., and Lauler, D. P. (1974). Renin: a risk factor for cardiovascular disease. Ann. Intern. Med. 81:7-10.

Cohen, S., Taylor, J. M., Murakami, K., Michelakis, A. M., and Inagami, T. (1972). Isolation and characterization of renin-like enzymes from mouse submaxillary glands. Biochemistry 11:4286-4293.

Collier, J. G., Robinson, B. F., and Vane, J. R. (1973). Reduction of pressor effects of angiotensin I in man by synthetic nonapeptide (B. P. P. 92 or SQ 20, 881) which inhibits converting enzyme. Lancet 1:72-77.

Cooper, R. M., Osmond, D. H., Scaiff, K. D., and Ross, L. J. (1974). Increase in angiotensin I (AI) production upon incubation of human plasma with trypsin. Fed. Proc. 33:584.

Cooper, R. M., Murray, G. F., and Osmond, D. H. (1977). Trypsin-induced activation of renin precursor in plasma of normal and anephric man. Circ. Res. 40(Suppl. I):171-179.

Corsini, W. A., Crosslan, K. L., and Bailie, M. D. (1974). Renin secretion by rat kidney slices in vitro. Proc. Soc. Exp. Biol. Med. 145: 403-406.

Crane, M. G., Harris, J. J., and Johns, V. J., Jr. (1972). Hyporeninemic hypertension. Am. J. Med. 52:457-466.

Cushman, D. W., and Cheung, H. S. (1971). Spectrophotometric assay and properties of the angiotensin-converting enzyme of rabbit lung. Biochem. Pharmacol. 20:1637-1648.

Cushman, D. W., and Cheung, H. S. (1972). Studies in vitro of angiotensin-converting enzyme of lung and other tissues. In Hypertension '72, J. Genest and E. Koiw (Eds.). Springer-Verlag, New York, pp. 532-541.

Cushman, D. W., Cheung, H. S., Sabo, E. F., and Ondetti, M. A. (1977). Design of potent competitive inhibitors of angiotensin-converting enzyme. Carboxyalkanoyl and mercaptoalkanoyl amino acids. Biochemistry 16: 5484-5491.

Cuthbert, M. F., and Peart, W. S. (1970). Studies on the identity of a vascular permeability factor of renal origin. Clin. Sci. 38:309-325.

Danon, A., and Chang, L. C. T. (1973). Release of prostaglandins from rat renal papilla in vitro: effects of arachidonic acid and angiotensin II. Fed. Proc. 32:788.

Das, M., and Soffer, R. L. (1975). Pulmonary angiotensin-converting enzyme. J. Biol. Chem. 250:6762-6768.

Davis, J. O. (1975). The use of blocking agents to define the functions of the renin-angiotensin system. Clin. Sci. Mol. Med. 48(Suppl. II):3-14.

Davis, J. O. (1977). Advances in our knowledge of the renin-angiotensin system. Fed. Proc. 36:1753-1787.

Davis, J. O., and Freeman, R. H. (1976). Mechanisms regulating renin release. Physiol. Rev. 56:1-56.

Day, R. P., and Luetscher, J. A. (1974). Big renin: a possible prohormone in kidney and plasma of a patient with Wilms' tumor. J. Clin. Endocrinol. Metab. 38:923-926.

Day, R. P., and Luetscher, J. A. (1975). Biochemical properties of big renin extracted from human plasma. J. Clin. Endocrinol. Metab. 40: 1085-1093.

Day, R. P., and Reid, I. A. (1976). Renin activity in dog brain: enzymological similarity to cathepsin D. Endocrinology 99:93-100.

Day, R. P., Luetscher, J. A., and Gonzales, C. M. (1975). Occurrence of big renin in human plasma, amniotic fluid and kidney extracts. J. Clin. Endocrinol. Metab. 40:1078-1084.

Day. R. P., Luetscher, J. A., and Zager, P. G. (1976). Big renin: identification, chemical properties and clinical implications. Am. J. Cardiol. 37:667-674.

deLeiva, A., Christlieb, A. R., Melby, J. C., Graham, C. A., Day, R. P., Luetscher, J. A., and Zager, P. G. (1976). Big renin and biosynthetic defect of aldosterone in diabetes mellitus. N. Engl. J. Med. 295:639-643.

Depierre, D., and Roth, M. (1972). Activity of a dipeptidyl carboxypeptidase (angiotensin converting enzyme) in lungs of different animal species. Experimentia 28:154-155.

Derkx, F. H. M., Wenting, G. J., Man in't Veld, A. J., v. Gool, J. M. G., Verhoeven, R. P., and Schalekamp, M. A. D. H. (1976). Inactive renin in human plasma. Lancet 2:495-498.

Devaux, C., Rebourcet, M. C., Ducloux, J., Corvol, P., and Menard, J. (1975). Application de la chromatographie d'affinité à l'étude de la rénine. Pathol. Biol. 23:805-808.

Devynck, M. A., and Meyer, P. (1976). Angiotensin receptors in vascular tissue. Am. J. Med. 61:758-767.

Dorer, F. E., Kahn, J. R., Lentz, K. E., Levine, M., and Skeggs, L. T. (1975). Formation of angiotensin II from tetradecapeptide renin substrate by angiotensin II from tetradecapeptide renin substrate by angiotensin-converting enzyme. Biochem. Pharmacol. 24:1137-1139.

Dorer, F. E., Kahn, J. R., Lentz, K. E., Levine, M., and Skeggs, L. T. (1976). Kinetic properties of pulmonary angiotensin-converting enzyme. Hydrolysis of hippurylglycylglycine. Biochim. Biophys. Acta 492:220-228.

Dorer, F. E., Lentz, K. E., Kahn, J. R., Levine, M., and Skeggs, L. T. (1978). Purification of human renin substrate. Anal. Chem. 87:11-18.

Douglas, J. R., Jr., Johnson, E. M., Jr., Marshall, G. R., Heist, J., Hartman, B. K., and Needleman, P. (1975). Development and maintenance of renal hypertension in normal and guanethidine sympathectomized rats. Circ. Res. 36/37(Suppl. I):171-178.

Druilhet, R. E., Overturf, M. L., Hinshaw, R. A., and Kirkendall, W. M. (1979). Evidence against acetone-soluble renin inhibitors in normal human plasma. Hypertension 1:98-105.

Dunn, M. J., and Hood, V. L. (1977). Prostaglandins and the kidney. Am. J. Physiol. 233:169-184.

Dunn, M. J., Liard, J. F., and Dray, F. (1978). Basal and stimulated rates of renal secretion and excretion of prostaglandins E_2, F_α, and 13,14-dihydro-15-keto F_α in the dog. Kidney Int. 13:136-143.

Edwards, W. G., Strong, C. G., and Hunt, J. C. (1969). A vasodepressor lipid resembling prostaglandin E_2 (PGE_2) in the renal venous blood of hypertensive patients. J. Lab. Clin. Med. 74:389-399.

Eggena, P., Barrett, J., and Sambhi, M. (1975). Effects of prostaglandins (E_2 and A_2) on the enzymatic reaction of human renin in isolated homologous system and with added normal and hypertensive plasma. Clin. Sci. Mol. Med. 48:307-309.

Eggena, P., Barrett, J., and Sambhi, M. P. (1979). The influence of plasma lipoproteins on the renin reaction in normal human plasma. Biochem. Med. 21:347-351.

Epstein, N., Fitzsimons, J. T., and Johnson, A. K. (1974). Peptide antagonists of the renin-angiotensin system and the elucidation of the receptors for angiotensin-induced drinking. J. Physiol. 238:34-35.

Erdös, E. G. (1976). Conversion of angiotensin I to angiotensin II. Am. J. Med. 60:749-759.

Erdös, E. G. (1977). The angiotensin I converting enzyme. Fed. Proc. 36: 1760-1766.

Erdös, E. G., and Massion, W. H., Downs, D. R., and Gecse, A. (1974). Effect of the inhibition of angiotensin I converting enzyme in endotoxin and hemorrhagic shock. Proc. Soc. Exp. Biol. Med. 145:948-951.

Erdös, E. G., and Yang, H. Y. T. (1967). An enzyme in microsomal fraction of kidney that inactivates bradykinin. Life Sci. 6:569-574.

Faiers, A. A., Loh, A. Y., and Osmond, D. H. (1977). Resolution of rat renin substrates by isoelectric focusing. Can. J. Biochem. 55:869-875.

Fichman, M. P., Littenburg, G., Brooker, G., and Horton, R. (1972). Effect of prostaglandin A_1 on renal and adrenal function in man. Circ. Res. 30/31(Suppl. II):19-35.

Fischer, H., Flugel, R. M., Schelling, P., and Ganten, D. (1975). Differences in endogenous iso-renin in normal and SV 40 transformed 3T3 mouse cells: correlation with cell growth. Int. Res. Commun. Med. Sci. 3:328.

Fitz, A., and Overturf, M. (1970). Human lung converting enzyme. J. Lab. Clin. Med. 76:1035.

Fitz, A., and Overturf, M. (1972a). Molecular weight of human angiotensin I converting enzyme. J. Biol. Chem. 247:581-584.

Fitz, A., and Overturf, M. (1972b). Human lung converting enzyme. In Hypertension '72, J. Genest and E. Koiw (Eds.). Springer-Verlag, New York, pp. 507-511.

Fitz, A., Boyd, G. W., and Peart, W. S. (1971). Converting enzyme activity in human plasma. Circ. Res. 28:246-253.

Fitz, A., Boaz, D., and Wyatt, S. (1974). Studies of human lung angiotensin I converting enzyme. Circulation 49/50(Suppl. III):30.

Freeman, R. H., Davis, J. O., Lohmeier, T. E., and Speilman, W. S. (1976). Evidence that Des-Asp-angiotensin II mediates the renin-angiotensin response. Circ. Res. 38(Suppl. II):99-103.

Freis, E. D., Ragan, D., Pillsbury, H., and Mathews, M. (1972). Alteration of the course of hypertension in the spontaneously hypertensive rat. Circ. Res. 31:1-7.

Frölich, J. C., Sweetman, B. J., Carr, K., Hollifield, J. W., and Oates, J. A. (1975). Assessment of the levels of PGA_2 in human plasma by gas chromatography-mass spectrometry. Prostaglandins 10:185-195.

Frölich, J. C., Hollifield, J. W., Dormois, J. C., Frolich, B. L., Seyberth, H., Michelakis, A. M., and Oates, J. A. (1976). Suppression of plasma renin activity by indomethacin in man. Circ. Res. 39:447-452.

Ganong, W. F. (1972). Sympathetic effects on renin secretion: mechanism and physiological role. In Control of Renin Secretion, T. A. Assaykeen (Ed.). Plenum Press, New York, pp. 17-32.

Ganten, D., and Speck, G. (1978). The brain renin-angiotensin system: a model for the synthesis of peptides in the brain. Biochem. Pharmacol. 27:2379-2389.

Ganten, D., Marquez-Julio, A., Granger, P., Hayduk, K., Karsunky, K. P., Boucher, R., and Genest, J. (1971). Renin in dog brain. Am. J. Physiol. 221:1733-1737.

Ganten, D., Hutchinson, J. S., and Schelling, P. (1975a). The intrinsic brain iso-renin-angiotensin system in the rat; its possible role in central mechanisms of blood pressure regulation. Clin. Sci. Mol. Med. 48:265-268.

Ganten, D., Schelling, P., Flugel, R. M., and Fischer, H. (1975b). Effect of angiotensin and an angiotensin antagonist on iso-renin and cell growth in 3T3 mouse cells. Int. Res. Commun. Med. Sci. 3:327.

Ganten, D., Schelling, P., Vecsei, P., and Ganten, U. (1976). Iso-renin of extrarenal origins. The tissue angiotensinogenase systems. Am. J. Med. 60:760-772.

Ganten, D., Hackenthal, F., and Vecsei, P. (1978). Symposium: Renin-Angiotensin Aldosterone System and Hypertension. Springer-Verlag, Berlin.

Gavras, H., Brunner, H., Laragh, J. H., Sealey, J. E., Gavras, I., and Vukovich, R. A. (1974). An angiotensin converting-enzyme inhibitor to identify and treat vasoconstrictor and volume factors in hypertensive patients. N. Engl. J. Med. 291:817-821.

Genest, J., Rojo-Ortega, J. M., Kuchel, O., Boucher, R., Nowaczynski, W., Lefebvre, R., Chretien, M., and Cantin, M. (1975). Malignant hypertension with hypokalemia in a patient with renin-producing pulmonary carcinoma. Clin. Res. 23:448.

Genest, J., Koiw, E., and Kuchel, O. (1977). Hypertension: Physiopathology and Treatment. McGraw-Hill, New York.

Giese, J. (1964). Acute hypertensive vascular disease: I. Relation between blood pressure changes and vascular lesions in different forms of acute hypertension. Acta Pathol. Microbiol. Scand. 62:481-496.

Giese, J. (1973). Renin, angiotensin and hypertensive vascular damages a review. Am. J. Med. 55:315-332.

Gill, J. R., Frölich, J. C., Bowden, R. E., Taylor, A. A., Keiser, H. R., Seyberth, H. W., Oates, J. A., and Bartter, F. C. (1976). Bartter's syndrome: a disorder characterized by high urinary prostaglandins and a dependence of hyperreninemia on prostaglandin synthesis. Am. J. Med. 61:43-51.

Golub, M., and Horton, R. (1974). Hypothesis: dual hormonal regulation of sodium balance. Prostaglandins 6:91-95.

Goodfriend, T. L., and Peach, M. J. (1975). Angiotensin III: (Des-aspartic acid[1])-angiotensin II. Evidence and speculation for its role as an important agonist in the renin-angiotensin system. Circ. Res. 36/37(Suppl. I): 38-48.

Goodfriend, T. L., Fyhrquist, F., and Allmann, D. (1974). Biochemical effects of angiotensin in angiotensin. I. H. Page and F. M. Bumpus (Eds.). Springer-Verlag, New York, pp. 511-517.

Gordon, D. B., and Sachin, I. N. (1975). Renin substrate in plasma of various mammalian species: electrophoresis on polyacrylamide gel. Proc. Soc. Exp. Biol. Med. 150:645-649.

Gould, A. B., and Green, D. (1971). Kinetics of the human substrate reaction. Cardiovasc. Res. 5:86-89.

Gould, A. B., Goodman, S., Dewolf, R., Onesti, G., and Swartz, C. (1979). Measurement of renin and substrate concentrations in human serum. Anal. Biochem. 94:125-139.

Grandino, A., and Paiva, A. C. M. (1974). Isolation of angiotensin-converting enzyme without kininase activity from hog and guinea pig plasma. Biochim. Biophys. Acta 364:113-119.

Gryglewski, R. J., Bunting, S., Moncada, S., Flower, R. J., and Vane, J. R. (1976). Arterial walls are protected against deposition of platelet thrombi by a substance (prostaglandin X) which they make from prostaglandin endoperoxides. Prostaglandins 12:685-713.

Guthrie, G. P., Genest, J., and Kuchel, O. (1976). Renin and the therapy of hypertension. Annu. Rev. Pharmacol. Toxicol. 16:287-308.

Haas, E., and Goldblatt, H. (1967). Kinetic constants of the human renin and human angiotensinogen reaction. Circ. Res. 20:45-55.

Haber, E., Koerner, T., Page, L. B., Kliman, B., and Purnode, A. (1969). Application of a radioimmunoassay for angiotensin I to the physiologic measurements of plasma renin activity in normal human subjects. J. Clin. Endocrinol. Metab. 29:1349-1355.

Haber, E., and Slater, E. E. (1977). Purification of renin: a review. Circ. Res. 40(Suppl. I):36-40.

Hackenthal, E., Hackenthal, R., and Hilgenfeldt, U. (1978a). Purification and partial characterization of rat brain proteinase (isorenin). Biochim. Biophys. Acta 522:561-573.

Hackenthal, E., Hackenthal, R., and Hilgenfeldt, U. (1978b). Isorenin pseudorenin, cathepsin D and renin. A comparative enzymatic study of angiotensin-forming enzymes. Biochim. Biophys. Acta 522:574-588.

Hamberg, M., Svensson, J., and Samuelsson, B. (1975). Thromboxanes: a new group of biologically active compounds derived from prostaglandin endoperoxides. Proc. Natl. Acad. Sci. USA 72:2994-2998.

Heinemann, H. O., and Lee, J. B. (1976). Prostaglandins and blood pressure control. Am. J. Med. 61:681-695.

Herbaczynska-Cedro, K., and Vane, J. R. (1973). Contribution of intrarenal generation of prostaglandin to autoregulation of renal blood flow in the dog. Circ. Res. 33:428-436.

Hiwada, K., Kokubu, T., and Yamamura, Y. (1969). Inhibitory effect of bile on renin angiotensinogen reaction system. Jap. Circ. J. 33:1231-1236.

Hiwada, K., Kokubu, T., and Yamamura, Y. (1971). Inhibition of renin by sodium deoxycholate. Biochem. Pharmacol. 20:914-916.

Hofbauer, K. G., Zschiedrich, H., Hackenthal, E., and Gross, F. (1974). Function of the renin-angiotensin system in the isolated perfused rat kidney. Circ. Res. 34/35(Suppl. I):193-201.

Hollander, W., Yagi, S., and Kramsch, D. M. (1964). In vitro effects of vasopressor agents on the metabolism of the vascular wall. Circulation 30(Suppl. II):1-10.

Horne, M. L., Conklin, V. M., Keenan, R., Varady, P. D., and DiNardo, J. (1979). Angiotensin II profiling with saralasin: summary of Eaton collaborative study. Kidney Int. 15:115-122.

Hornych, A., and Papanicolaou, W. (1974). Prostaglandins in renal venous blood of essential hypertensive patients. Prostaglandins 7:383-386.

Igic, R., Erdös, E. G., Yeh, H. S. J., Sorrells, K., and Nakajima, T. (1972). Angiotensin I converting enzyme of the lung. Circ. Res. 30/31 (Suppl. II):51-61.

Imbs, J. L., Schmidt, M., and Schwartz, J. (1975). Effect of dopamine on renin secretion in the anesthetized dog. Eur. J. Pharmacol. 33:151-157.

Inagami, T., Murakami, K., Takahashi, N., Michelakis, A. M., Oreshi, A., and Haas, E. (1976). Purification of human renin. Fed. Proc. 35:1696.

Inagami, T., Takahashi, N., Yokosawa, N., and Takii, Y. (1978). Affinity chromatographic isolation of inactive renin from human plasma and activation by kallikrein. A possible new link between renin-angiotensin system and kallikrein-kinin system. Proc. Int. Renin Symp., Tokyo, Nov. 1978, p. 79.

Itskovitz, H. D., and McGiff, J. C. (1974). Hormonal regulation of the renal circulation. Circ. Res. 34/35(Suppl. I):65-73.

Itskovitz, H. D., Hebert, L. A., and McGiff, J. C. (1973). Angiotensin as a possible intrarenal hormone in isolated dog kidneys. Circ. Res. 32:550-555.

Johnson, D. C., and Ryan, J. W. (1968). Degradation of angiotensin II by a carboxypeptidase of rabbit liver. Biochim. Biophys. Acta 160:196-203.

Johnson, J. G., Black, W. D., Vukovich, R. A., Hatch, F. E., Jr., Friedman, B. I., Blackwell, C. F., Shenouda, A. N., Share, L., Shade, R. E., Acchiardo, S. R., and Muirhead, E. E. (1975). Treatment of patients with severe hypertension by inhibition of angiotensin-converting enzyme. Clin. Sci. Mol. Med. 48:53-56.

Johnson, J. A., Davis, J. E., Gotshall, R. W., Lohmeier, T. E., Davis, J. L., Braverman, B., and Tempel, G. E. (1976). Evidence for an intrarenal beta receptor in control of renin release. Am. J. Physiol. 230:410-418.

Johnson, R. L., Poisner, A. M., and Crist, R. D. (1979). Partial purification and chromatographic properties of inactive renin from human amniotic fluid. Biochem. Pharmacol. 28:1791-1999.

Jubiz, W., Terashima, R., and Anderson, F. (1976). Effect of sodium on prostaglandin E output by the canine kidney. Adv. Prostaglandin Thromboxane Res. 2:603-607.

Kaplan, N. M. (1975). The prognostic implications of plasma renin in essential hypertension. J. Am. Med. Assoc. 231:167-170.

Keeton, T. K., Pettinger, W. A., and Campbell, W. B. (1976). The effects of altered sodium balance and adrenergic blockade on renin release induced in rats by angiotensin antagonism. Circ. Res. 38:531-539.

Khairallah, P. A., and Page, I. H. (1967). Plasma angiotensinases. Biochim. Med. 1:1-8.

Khairallah, P. A., Bumpus, F. M., Page, I. H., and Smeby, R. R. (1963). Angiotensinase with a high degree of specificity in plasma and red cells. Science 140:672-674.

Khairallah, P. A., Robertson, A. L., and Davila, D. (1972). Effects of angiotensin II on DNA, RNA and protein synthesis. In Hypertension '72, J. Genest and E. Koiw (Eds.). Springer-Verlag, New York, pp. 212-220.

Khosla, M. C., Smeby, R. R., and Bumpus, F. M. (1974). Structure-activity relationship in angiotensin II analogs. In Angiotensin, I. H. Page and F. M. Bumpus (Eds.). Springer-Verlag, New York, pp. 126-161.

Kincaid-Smith, P., Friedman, A., and Hobbs, J. B. (1974). Morphological effects of angiotensin in arteries. In Angiotensin, I. H. Page and F. M. Bumpus (Eds.). Springer-Verlag, New York, pp. 490-499.

Kirkendall, W. M., Overturf, M., Druilhet, R. E., and Arnold, P. (1975). Problems of the radioimmunoassay of renin activity. In Epidemiology and Control of Hypertension, O. Paul (Ed.). Symposia Specialists, Miami, Fla., pp. 207-219.

Kirkendall, W. M., Hammond, J. J., and Overturf, M. L. (1978). Renin as a predictor of hypertensive complications. Ann. N.Y. Acad. Sci. 304:147-160, 1978.

Knight, C. G., and Barrett, A. J. (1976). Interaction of human cathepsin D with the inhibitor pepstatin. Biochem. J. 155:117-125.

Kokubu, T., Hiwada, K., Taketoshi, I., Ueda, E., Yamamura, Y., Mizoguchi, T., and Shigezane, K. (1973). Peptide inhibitors of renin angiotensinogen reaction system. Biochem. Pharmacol. 22:3217-3223.

Kokubu, T., Kato, I., Nishimura, K., Hiwada, K., and Ueda, E. (1978). Angiotensin I converting enzyme in human urine. Clin. Chem. Acta 89:375-379.

Kotchen, T. A., Hedrick, J. L., Miller, M. C., and Talwalker, R. T. (1974). Effect of prostaglandins on the velocity of the reaction between human renin and homologous renin substrate. J. Clin. Endocrinol. 9: 530-535.

Kotchen, T. A., Talwalker, R. T., Kotchen, J. M., Miller, M. C., and Welch, W. J. (1975). Evidence for the existence of an acetone soluble renin inhibiting factor in normal human plasma. Circ. Res. 36/37 (Suppl. I):17-27.

Kotchen, T. A., Talwalker, R. T., Miller, M. C., and Welch, W. J. (1976). Modification of renin reactivity by lipids extracted from normal, hypertensive and uremic plasma. J. Clin. Endocrinol. Metab. 43: 971-981.

Kotchen, T. A., Talwalker, R. T., and Welch, W. J. (1977). Inhibition of the in vitro renin reaction by circulating neutral lipids. Circ. Res. 41 (Suppl. II):46-48.

Krakoff, L. R., Vlachakis, N., Mendlowitz, M., and Stricker, J. (1975). Differential effect of prostaglandin A_1, in hypertensive patients with low, normal and high renin. Clin. Sci. Mol. Med. 48:311-313.

Laragh, J. H. (1973). Vasoconstriction-volume analysis for understanding and treating hypertension: the use of renin and aldosterone profiles. Am. J. Med. 55:261-275.

Laragh, J. H., and Sealey, J. E. (1973). The renin-angiotensin-aldosterone hormonal system and regulation of sodium potassium and blood pressure homeostasis. In Handbook of Physiology, Sec. 8: Renal Physiology, J. Orloff, R. W. Berliner, and S. R. Geiger (Eds.). American Physiological Society, Washington, D.C., pp. 831-908.

Laragh, J. H., Baer, L., Brunner, H. R., Buhler, F. R., Sealey, J. E., and Vaughan, E. D. (1972a). Renin, angiotensin and aldosterone system in pathogenesis and management of hypertensive vascular disease. Am. J. Med. 52:633-652.

Laragh, J. H., Sealey, J. E., and Brunner, H. R. (1972b). The control of aldosterone secretion in normal and hypertensive man: abnormal renin-aldosterone patterns in low renin hypertension. Am. J. Med. 53:649-663.

Laragh, J. H., Letcher, R. L., and Pickering, T. G. (1979). Renin profiling for diagnosis and treatment of hypertension. J. Am. Med. Assoc. 241:151-156.

Lauritzen, M., Damsgaard, J. J., Rubin, I., and Lauritzen, E. (1976). A comparison of the properties of renin isolated from pig and rat kidney. Biochem. J. 155:317-323.

Lazar, J., Romero, J. C., and Hoobler, S. W. (1971). Renin kinetics in experimental renal hypertension. Am. J. Physiol. 220:191-195.

Leckie, B. (1973). The activation of a possible zymogen of renin in rabbit kidney. Clin. Sci. 44:301-304.

Leckie, B. J., and McConnell, A. (1975). A renin inhibitor from rabbit kidney. Conversion of a large inactive renin to a smaller active enzyme. Circ. Res. 36:513-519.

Ledingham, J. G., and Leary, W. P. (1974). Catabolism of angiotensin II. In Angiotensin, I. H. Page and F. M. Bumpus (Eds.). Springer-Verlag, New York, pp. 112-125.

Lee, H.-J., Larue, J. N., and Wilson, I. B. (1971a). Human plasma converting enzyme. Arch. Biochem. Biophys. 142:548-551.

Lee, H.-J., Larue, J. N., and Wilson, I. B. (1971b.) Angiotensin-converting enzyme from porcine plasma. Biochim. Biophys. Acta 235:521-528.

Lee, H.-J., Larue, J. N., and Wilson, I. B. (1971c). Angiotensin-converting enzyme from guinea pig and hog lung. Biochim. Biophys. Acta 250: 549-557.

Lee, J. B. (1975). Renal prostaglandins and the antihypertensive endocrine function. Med. Clin. N. Am. 59:713-733.

Lee, J. B. (1976). The renal prostaglandins and blood pressure regulation. Adv. Prostaglandin Thromboxane Res. 2:573-585.

Lee, J. B., Covino, B. G., Takman, B. H., and Smith, E. R. (1965). Renomedullary vasodepressor substance, medullin: isolation, chemical characterization and physiological properties. Circ. Res. 17:57-77.

Lee, J. B., McGiff, J. C., Kannegieser, H., Aykent, Y. Y., Mudd, J. G., and Frawley, T. F. (1971). Prostaglandin A_1: antihypertensive and renal effects. Ann. Intern. Med. 74:703-710.

Lentz, K. E., Skeggs, L. T., Woods, K. R., Kahn, J. R., and Shumway, N. P. (1956). The amino acid composition II hypertensin II and its biochemical relationship to hypertension I. J. Exp. Med. 104:183-191.

Lentz, K. E., Skeggs, L. T., Dorer, F. E., Kahn, J. R., and Levine, M. (1976). A new radiolabeled protein renin substrate. Anal. Biochem. 74:1-11.

Levinsky, N. G. (1979). The renal kallikrein-kinin system. Circ. Res. 44:441-451.

Lieberman, J. (1975). Elevation of serum angiotensin-converting-enzyme (ACE) level in sarcoidosis. Am. J. Med. 59:365-372.

Limas, C. J. (1974). Stimulation by angiotensin of myocardial prostaglandin synthesis. Biochim. Biophys. Acta 337:417-420.

Lonigro, A. J., Itskovitz, H. D., Crowshaw, K., and McGiff, J. C. (1973a). Dependency of renal blood flow on prostaglandin synthesis in the dog. Circ. Res. 32:712-717.

Lonigro, A. J., Terragno, N. A., Malik, K. U., and McGiff, J. C. (1973b). Differential inhibition by prostaglandins of the renal actions of pressor stimuli. Prostaglandins 3:595-606.

Lowder, S. C., and Liddle, G. W. (1974). Prolonged alteration of renin responsiveness and spironolactone therapy. A cause of false-negative testing for low-renin hypertension. N. Engl. J. Med. 291:1243-1244.

Loyke, H. F. (1975). The inhibition of angiotensin converting enzyme in chronic renal hypertension by a synthetic peptide (39055). Proc. Soc. Exp. Biol. Med. 150:457-460.

MacFarlane, N. A. A., Adetuyibi, A., and Mills, I. H. (1974). Changes in kallikrein excretion during arterial infusion of angiotensin. J. Endocrinol. 61:72.

Majstoravich, J., Ontjes, D. A., and Roberts, J. C. (1974). Affinity chromatography of renin using inhibitory renin substrate analogs. Proc. Soc. Exp. Biol. Med. 146:674-679.

Mancia, G., Romero, J. C., and Shepherd, J. T. (1975). Continuous inhibition of renin release in dogs by vagally innervated receptors in the cardiopulmonary region. Circ. Res. 36:529-535.

Margolius, H. S., Horwitz, D., Geller, R. G., Alexander, R. W., Gill, J. R., Pisano, J. J., and Keiser, H. R. (1974). Urinary kallikrein excretion in normal man. Relationships to sodium intake and sodium-retaining steroids. Circ. Res. 35:812-819.

Masson, G. M. C., Mikasa, A., and Yasuda, H. (1962). Experimental vascular disease elicited by aldosterone and renin. Endocrinology 71:505-512.

Mattioli, L., Zakheim, R. M., Mullis, K., and Molteni, A. (1975). Angiotensin I-converting enzyme activity in idiopathic respiratory distress syndrome of the newborn infant and in experimental alveolar hypoxia in mice. J. Pediatr. 87:97-101.

McCaa, R. E., McCaa, C. S., and Guyton, A. C. (1975). Role of angiotensin II and potassium in the long-term regulation of aldosterone secretion in intact conscious dogs. Circ. Res. 36/37(Suppl. I):57-67.

McGiff, J. (1979). Symposium: New developments in prostaglandin and thromboxane research. Fed. Am. Soc. Exp. Biol. 38:64-93.

McGiff, J. C., and Itskovitz, H. D. (1973). Prostaglandins and the kidney. Circ. Res. 33:479-488.

McGiff, J. C., Crowshaw, K., Terragno, N. A., and Lonigro, A. J. (1970a). Release of a prostaglandin-like substance into renal venous blood in response to angiotensin II. Circ. Res. 27(Suppl. I):21-30.

McGiff, J. C., Crowshaw, K., Terragno, N. A., Lonigro, A. J., Strand, J. C., Williamson, M. A., Lee, J. B., and Ng, K. K. F. (1970b). Prostaglandin-like substances appearing in canine renal venous blood during renal ischemia. Their partial characterization by pharmacologic and chromatographic procedures. Circ. Res. 27:765-782.

McGiff, J. C., Malik, K. U., and Terragno, N. A. (1976). Prostaglandins as determinants of vascular reactivity. Fed. Proc. 35:2382-2387.

McKenzie, J. K., and Montgomerie, J. Z. (1969). Renin-like activity in the plasma of anephric men. Nature 223:1156.

Mendelsohn, F. A., and Johnston, C. I. (1971). A radiochemical renin assay. Biochem. J. 121:241-244.

Menzie, J. W., Michelakis, A. M., and Yoshida, H. (1974). Sympathetic nervous system and renin release from submaxillary glands and kidneys. Am. J. Physiol. 227:1281-1284.

Meyer, P. (1976). Summary of current studies on angiotensin-induced aldosterone release. Circ. Res. 38(Suppl. II):127-128.

Michelakis, A. M., and McAllister, R. G., Jr. (1972). Renin secretion, adrenergic blockade and hypertension. In Control of Renin Secretion, T. A. Assaykeen (Ed.). Plenum Press, New York, pp. 83-91.

Michelakis, A. M., Yoshida, H., Menzie, J., Marakami, K., and Inagami, T. (1974). A radioimmunoassay for the direct measurement of renin in mice and its application to submaxillary gland and kidney studies. Endocrinology 94:1101-1105.

Miller, E. D., Samuels, A. L., Haber, E., and Barger, A. C. (1975). Inhibition of angiotensin conversion and prevention of renal hypertension. Am. J. Physiol. 228:448-453.

Miller, R. P., Poper, C. J., Wilson, C. W., and DeVito, E. (1972). Renin inhibition by pepstatin. Biochem. Pharmacol. 21:2941-2944.

Mills, I. H. (1979). Kallikrein, kininogen and kinins in control of blood pressure. Nephron 23:61-71.

Mimran, A., Casellas, D., DuPont, M., and Barjon, P. (1975). Effect of a competitive angiotensin antagonist on the renal haemodynamic changes induced by inhibition of prostaglandin synthesis in rats. Clin. Sci. Mol. Med. 48:299-302.

Molteni, A., Zakheim, R. M., Mullis, K. B., and Mattioli, L. (1974). The effect of chronic alveolar hypoxia on lung and serum angiotensin I converting enzyme activity. Proc. Soc. Exp. Biol. Med. 147:263-265.

Moncada, S., and Vane, J. R. (1979). Pharmacology and endogenous roles of prostaglandin endoperoxides, thromboxane A_2 and prostacyclin. Pharmacol. Rev. 30:293-331.

Montague, D. (1968). Kinetics of renin-angiotensinogen reaction in plasma of normal and nephrectomized rats. Am. J. Physiol. 215:78-83.

Montague, D., Riniker, B., Brunner, H., and Gross, F. (1966). Synthesis and biological activities of a tetradecapeptide renin substrate. Am. J. Physiol. 210:591-598.

Morris, B. J. (1978). Activation of human inactive ("pro-") renin by cathepsin D and pepsin. J. Clin. Endocrinol. Metab. 46:153-157.

Morris, B. J., and Johnston, C. I. (1976a). Renin substrate in granules from rat kidney cortex. Biochem. J. 154:625-637.

Morris, B. J., and Johnston, C. I. (1976b). Isolation of renin granules from rat kidney cortex and evidence for an inactive form of renin (prorenin) in granules and plasma. Endocrinology 98:1466-1474.

Morris, B. J., and Lumbers, E. R. (1972). The activation of renin in human amniotic fluid by proteolytic enzymes. Biochim. Biophys. Acta 289: 385-391.

Morris, B. J., and Reid, I. A. (1978). The distribution of angiotensinogen in dog brain by cell fractionation. Endocrinology 103:492-500.

Mroczek, W. J., Finnerty, F. A., and Catt, K. J. (1973). Lack of association between plasma-renin and history of heart-attack or stroke in patients with essential hypertension. Lancet 2:464-469.

Munoz-Ramirez, H., Khosla, M. C., Hall, M. M., Bumpus, F. M., and Khairallah, P. A. (1976). In vitro and in vivo studies of [1-sarcosine,

8-threonine]-angiotensin II. Res. Commun. Chem. Pathol. Pharmacol. 13:649-663.

Murakami, K., and Inagami, T. (1975). Isolation of pure and stable renin from hog kidney. Biochem. Biophys. Res. Commun. 62:757-763.

Murakami, K., Matoba, T., and Inagami, T. (1976). Big and big big renin from hog kidneys: proof for existence and purification. Fed. Proc. 35:1355.

Murao, S., and Satoi, S. (1970). New pepsin inhibitors (S-PI) from streptomyces EF-44-201. Agric. Biol. Chem. 34:1265-1267.

Nasjletti, A., and Malik, K. U. (1979). Relationships between the kallikrein-kinin and prostaglandin systems. Life Sci. 25:99-110.

Nasjletti, A., and Masson, G. M. C. (1972). Studies on angiotensinogen formation in a liver perfusion system. Circ. Res. 30/31(Suppl. II):187-202.

Nasjletti, A., and Masson, G. M. C. (1973). Stimulation of angiotensinogen formation by renin and angiotensin I. Proc. Soc. Exp. Biol. Med. 142:307-310.

Nasjletti, A., Colina-Chourio, J., and McGiff, J. C. (1975). Disappearance of bradykinin in the renal circulation of dogs. Effects of kininase inhibition. Circ. Res. 37:59-65.

Needleman, P., Marshall, G. R., and Douglas, J. R., Jr. (1973). Prostaglandin release from vasculature by angiotensin II: dissociation from lipolysis. Eur. J. Pharmacol. 66:316-319.

Ng, K. K. F., and Vane, J. R. (1967). Conversion of angiotensin I to angiotensin II. Nature (Lond.) 216:762-766.

Ng, K. K. F., and Vane, J. R. (1968). Fate of angiotensin I in the circulation. Nature (Lond.) 218:144-150.

Nielsen, A. H., Lykkegaard, S., and Poulsen, K. (1979). Renin in the mouse submaxillary gland has a molecular weight of 40,000. Biochim. Biophys. Acta 576:305-313.

Obika, L. F. O. (1978). Recent development in urinary kallikrein research. Life Sci. 23:765-774.

Odya, C. E., Marinkovic, D. V., Hammond, J. J. Stewart, T. A., and Erdös, E. G. (1978). Purification and properties of prolylcarboxypeptidase (angiotensinase C) from human kidney. J. Biol. Chem. 253:5927-5931.

Oelkers, W., Schoneshofer, M., Schultze, G., Brown, J. J., Fraser, R., Morton, J. J., Lever, A. F., and Robertson, J. I. S. (1975). Effect of prolonged low-dose angiotensin II infusion on the sensitivity of adrenal cortex in man. Circ. Res. 36/37(Suppl. I):49-56.

Ondetti, M. A., Williams, N. J., Sabo, E. F., Pluscec, J., Weaver, E. R., and Kocy, O. (1971). Angiotensin-converting enzyme inhibitor from the venom of Bothrops jaracaca. Isolation, elucidation of structure and synthesis. Biochemistry 10:4033-4039.

Ondetti, M. A., Rubin, B., and Cushman, D. W. (1977). Design of specific

inhibitors of angiotensin-converting enzyme: new class of orally active antihypertensive agents. Science 196:441-444.
Oparil, S. (1976). Renin 1976. Eden Press, Montreal.
Oparil, S., and Katholi, R. (1977). Renin, Vol. 2, 1977. Eden Press, Montreal.
Oparil, S., Koerner, I. J., and Haber, E. (1974). Effects of pH and enzyme inhibitors on apparent generation of angiotensin I in human plasma. J. Clin. Endocrinol. Metab. 39:965-968.
Osborn, E. C., Hodges, N. G., Pickens, P. T., Willicombe, P. R., and Mahler, R. F. (1970). The conversion of [^{35}S]PTC-angiotensin I to PTC-angiotensin II in plasma of normotensive and hypertensive subjects. Clin. Sci. 38:217-223.
Osmond, D. H. (1972). Clinical and experimental renal weight and content of lipids and phospholipid renin "preinhibitor" in rats with renal hypertension. J. Lab. Clin. Med. 80:755-764.
Osmond, D. H., Smeby, R. R., and Bumpus, F. M. (1969a). Quantitative studies of renin preinhibitor and total phospholipids in organs and in plasma and erythrocytes of control, nephrectomized, and very old rats. J. Lab. Clin. Med. 73:795-808.
Osmond, D. H., Lewis, L. A., Smeby, R. R., and Bumpus, F. M. (1969b). Renin "preinhibitor" in blood of anephric patients in a case of hypobetalipoproteinemia, and evidence of its major association with plasma alpha lipoproteins. J. Lab. Clin. Med. 73:809-818.
Osmond, D. H., Ross, L. J., and Scaiff, K. D. (1973a). Increased renin activity after cold storage of human plasma. Can. J. Physiol. Pharmacol. 51:705-708.
Osmond, D. H., McFadzean, P. A., and Ross, L. J. (1973b). Plasma phospholipase A_2 activity in nephrectomized rats and the question of renin inhibition. Proc. Soc. Exp. Biol. Med. 144:969-973.
Osmond, D. H., Ross, L. J., and Holub, B. J. (1973c). Activity and positional specificity of a rat plasma phospholipase on phosphatidylethanolamine. Can. J. Biochem. 51:855-862.
Ostrovsky, D., Sen, S., Smeby, R. R., and Bumpus, F. M. (1967). Chemical assay of phospholipid renin preinhibitor in canine and human blood. Circ. Res. 21:497-505.
Overturf, M., Leonard, M., and Kirkendall, W. M. (1974). Purification of human renin and inhibition of its activity by pepstatin. Biochem. Pharmacol. 23:671-683.
Overturf, M., Wyatt, S., Boaz, D., and Fitz, A. (1975). Angiotensin I [Phe^8-His^9] hydrolase and bradykinase from human lung. Life Sci. 16:1669-1682.
Overturf, M., Druilhet, R., and Kirkendall, W. M. (1976). Effect of human kidney lipids on human kidney renin activity. Biochem. Pharmacol. 25:2443-2453.
Overturf, M., Druilhet, R., and Kirkendall, M. W. (1977). In vitro effects

of streptomyces protease inhibitors on human kidney renin activity. J. Biochem. 81:1579-1582.

Overturf, M. L., Druilhet, R. E., and Kirkendall, W. M. (1979a). Renin: multiple forms and prohormones. Life Sci. 24:1913-1924.

Overturf, M. L., Druilhet, R. E., and Fitz, A. E. (1979b). The effects of kallikrein, plasmin and thrombin on hog kidney renin. J. Biol. Chem. 254:12078-12083.

Page, I. H., and Bumpus, F. M. (1974). Angiotensin. Springer-Verlag, New York.

Pals, D. T., Masucci, F. D., Denning, G. S., Jr., Sipos, F., and Fessler, D. C. (1971). Role of the pressor action of angiotensin II in experimental hypertension. Circ. Res. 24:673-681.

Patak, R. V., Mookerjee, B. K., Bentzel, C. J., Hysert, P. E., and Lee, J. B. (1976). Abolition by indomethacin of the anti-hypertensive and natriuretic effects of furosemide in normal and hypertensive man. Adv. Protaglandin Thromboxane Res. 2:995-1015.

Payakkapan, W., Attallah, A., Lee, J. B., and Carr, A. A. (1975). Effect of sodium intake on prostaglandin A, renin and aldosterone in normotensive humans. Kidney Int. 8(Suppl. 5):283-290.

Peach, M. J. (1971). Adrenal medullary stimulation induced by angiotensin I, angiotensin II and analogues. Circ. Res. 28(Suppl. II):107-117.

Peach, M. J., Sarstedt, C. A., and Vaughan, E. D. (1976). Changes in cardiovascular and adrenal cortical responses to angiotensin III induced by sodium deprivation in the rat. Circ. Res. 38(Suppl. II):117-121.

Peart, W. S. (1978). Renin 1978. Johns Hopkins Med. J. 143:193-206.

Pettinger, W. A. (1976). Angiotensin antagonists as diagnostic and pharmacologic tools. Abstracts of papers in "The use of angiotensin inhibitors in clinical diagnosis," 5th Kanematsu Conf. Kidney, Satellite Symp. 4th Meet., Int. Soc. Hypertension, Sydney, Australia.

Pettinger, W. A., T. K., and Tanaka, K. (1975). Radioimmunoassay and pharmacokinetics of saralasin in the rat and hypertensive patients. Clin. Pharmacol. Ther. 17:146-158.

Pfeiffer, F. R., Hoke, S. C., Miao, C. K., Tedeschi, R. E., Pasternak, J., Hahn, R., Erickson, R. W., Levin, H. W., Burton, C. A., and Weisbach, J. A. (1971). Lysophosphatidylethanolamine and 2-desoxylysophosphatidylethanolamine derivatives: 1. Potential renin inhibitors. J. Med. Chem. 14:493-498.

Pfeiffer, F. R., Miao, C. K., Hoke, S. C., and Weisbach, J. A. (1972). Potential renin inhibitors: 2. Ethanolamine and ethylamine derivatives of phospholipids. J. Med. Chem. 15:58-60.

Pickens, P. T., Bumpus, F. M., Lloyd, A. M., Smeby, R. R., and Page, I. H. (1965). Measurement of renin activity in human plasma. Circ. Res. 17:438-448.

Piquilloud, Y., Reinharz, A., and Roth, M. (1970). Studies on the angiotensin converting enzyme with different substrates. Biochim. Biophys. Acta 206:136-142.

Pletka, P., and Hickler, R. B. (1974). Renal vein renin (RVR) and renal vein prostaglandins (PG) in renal hypertension. Kidney Int. 6:85A.
Poulsen, K., Burton, J., and Haber, E. (1973). Competitive inhibitors of renin. Biochemistry 12:3877-3882.
Poulsen, K., Burton, J., and Haber, E. (1975). Purification of hog renin by affinity chromatography using the synthetic competitive inhibitor [D-Leu^6]-Octapeptide. Biochim. Biophys. Acta 400:258-262.
Poulsen, K., Vuust, J., Lykkegaard, S., Nielsen, A. H., and Lund, T. (1979). Renin is synthesized as a 50,000 dalton single-chain polypeptide in cell-free translation systems. FEBS Lett. 98:135-138.
Priest, J. N., Ahmed, M., and Nuttall, F. Z. (1976). Pathologic hypofunction of the renin-angiotensin-aldosterone system. Postgrad. Med. 59:86-93.
Printz, M. P., and Dworschack, R. T. (1977). Evidence for the glycoprotein nature of kidney renin. Biochim. Biophys. Acta 494:162-171.
Printz, M. P., Printz, J. M., and Dworschack, R. T. (1977). Human angiotensinogen. J. Biol. Chem. 252:1654-1662.
Printz, M. P., Printz, J. M., and Gregory, T. J. (1978). Identification of angiotensin in animal brain homogenates. Circ. Res. 43(Suppl. I):21-27.
Pugsley, D. J., Beilin, L. J., and Peto, R. (1975). Renal prostaglandin synthesis in the Goldblatt hypertensive rat. Circ. Res. 36/37(Suppl. I): 81-88.
Pugsley, D., Beilin, L., and Peto, R. (1976). Renal prostaglandin synthesis in experimental renal clip hypertension in the rat. Adv. Prostaglandin Thromboxane Res. 2:595-598.
Rahkit, S., Bagli, J. F., and Deghenghi, R. (1969). Phospholipids: Part I. Synthesis of phosphatidyl ethanolamines. Can. J. Chem. 47:2906-2910.
Ramsay, D. J. (1979). The brain renin angiotensin system: a re-evaluation. Neuroscience 4:313-321.
Reid, I. A. (1979). The brain renin-angiotensin system: a critical analysis. Fed. Proc. 38:2255-2259.
Rettig, R., Speck, G., Simon, W., Schelling, P., Fahrer, A., and Ganten, D. (1978). In vivo enzyme activity of purified human brain renin. Klin. Wochenschr. 56(Suppl. I):43-45.
Rieger, D., Romero, J. C., Lazar, J., and Hoobler, S. W. (1972). Definition and use of renin reaction velocity in the study of human hypertension. J. Lab. Clin. Med. 80:342-350.
Robertson, A. L., and Khairallah, P. A. (1972). Effects of angiotensin II and some analogues on vascular permeability in the rabbit. Circ. Res. 31:923-931.
Robertson, A. L., and Khairallah, P. A. (1973). Arterial endothelial permeability and vascular disease. The "Trap Door" effect. Exp. Mol. Pathol. 18:241-260.
Robertson, A. L., and Khairallah, P. A. (1974). Effects of angiotensin II on the permeability of the vascular wall. In Angiotensin, I. H. Page and F. M. Bumpus (Eds.). Springer-Verlag, New York, pp. 500-510.

Romero, J. C., Mak, S. W., and Hoobler, S. W. (1974). Effect of blockade of angiotensin-I converting enzyme on the blood pressure of renal hypertensive rabbits. Cardiovasc. Res. 8:681-687.

Romero, J. C., Ott, C. E., Aguilo, J. J., Torres, V. E., and Strong, C. G. (1975). Role of prostaglandins in the reversal of one-kidney hypertension in the rabbit. Circ. Res. 37:683-689.

Romero, J. C., Dunlap, C. L., and Strong, C. G. (1976). The effect of indomethacin and other anti-inflammatory drugs on the renin-angiotensin system. J. Clin. Invest. 58:282-288.

Rubin, I. (1972). Purification of hog renin. Properties of purified hog renin. Scand. J. Clin. Lab. Invest. 29:51-58.

Rubin, B., Antonaccio, M. J., and Horovitz, Z. P. (1978). Captopril (SQ 14,225) (D-3-mercapto-2-methylpropanoyl-L-proline): a novel orally active inhibitor of angiotensin-converting enzyme and antihypertensive agent. Prog. Cardiovasc. Dis. 21:183-194.

Rumpf, K. W., Frenzel, S., Lowitz, H. D., and Scheler, F. (1975). The effect of indomethacin on plasma renin activity in man under normal conditions and after stimulation of the renin-angiotensin system. Prog. Int. Congr. Prostaglandins, Florence, Italy, p. 182.

Ryan, J. W. (1974). The fate of angiotensin II. In Angiotensin, I. H. Page and F. M. Bumpus (Eds.). Springer-Verlag, New York, pp. 81-110.

Ryan, J. W., Stewart, J. M., Leary, W. P., and Ledingham, J. G. (1970). Metabolism of angiotensin I in the pulmonary circulation. Biochem. J. 120:221-223.

Ryan, J. W., Ryan, U. S., Schultz, D. R., Whitabker, C., and Chung, A. (1975). Subcellular localization of pulmonary angiotensin-converting enzyme (kininase II). Biochem. J. 146:497-499.

Sambhi, M. P., and Wiedeman, C. E. (1972). Renin activation in the venous plasma from the involved kidney in the patient with renal hypertension. J. Clin. Invest. 51:22-30.

Sambhi, M. P., Eggena, P., Barrett, J. D., and Wiedeman, C. E. (1974). Renin "activation" in benign essential hypertension. In Mechanisms of Hypertension, M. P. Sambhi (Ed.). Excerpta Medica, Amsterdam, pp. 124-132.

Sambhi, M. P., Eggena, P., Barrett, J. D., Tuck, M., Wiedeman, C. E., and Thananopavarn, C. (1975). A circulating renin activator in essential hypertension. Circ. Res. 36/37(Suppl. I):28-37.

Sander, C. E., West, D. W., and Huggins, C. G. (1971). Peptide inhibitors of pulmonary angiotensin I converting enzyme. Biochim. Biophys. Acta 242:662-667.

Saruta, T., and Kaplan, N. M. (1972). Adrenocortical steroidogenesis: the effects of prostaglandins. J. Clin. Invest. 51:2246-2251.

Satoh, S., and Zimmerman, B. G. (1975). Influence of the renin-angiotensin system on the effect of prostaglandin synthesis inhibitors in the renal vasculature. Circ. Res. 36/37(Suppl. I)89-96.

Satoi, S., and Murao, S. (1973). Inhibition of acid proteases by a pepsin inhibitor (S-PI). Agric. Biol. Chem. 37:2579-2587.

Scharpe, S., Eid, M., Cooreman, W., and Lauwers, A. (1976). α-1 antitrypsin, an inhibitor of renin. Biochem. J. 153:505-507.

Scholkens, B. A., and Jung, W. (1974). Renin inhibition by pepstatin in experimental hypertension. Arch. Int. Pharmacodyn. 208:24-34.

Scholkens, B. A., and Steinbach, R. (1975). Increase of experimental hypertension following inhibition of prostaglandin biosynthesis. Arch. Int. Pharmacodyn. 124:328-334.

Sealey, J. E., and Laragh, J. H. (1975). "Prorenin" in human plasma? Methodological and physiological implications. Circ. Res. 36/37 (Suppl. I):10-16.

Sealey, J. E., Gerten, J. N., Ledingham, J. G., and Laragh, J. H. (1967). Inhibition of renin by heparin. J. Clin. Endocrinol. Metab. 27:699-705.

Sealey, J. E., Moon, C., Laragh, J. H., and Alderman, M. (1976). Plasma prorenin: cryoactivation and relationship to renin substrate in normal subjects. Am. J. Med. 61:731-738.

Sealey, J. E., Atlas, S. A., Laragh, J. H., Oza, N. B., and Ryan, J. W. (1978). Human urinary kallikrein converts inactive to active renin and is a possible physiological activator of renin. Nature (Lond.) 275:144-145.

Semple, P. F., and Morton, J. J. (1975). Angiotensin II and its heptapeptide and hexapeptide fragments in arterial and venous blood of man. Clin. Sci. Mol. Med. 48:2.

Semple, P. F., and Morton, J. J. (1976). Angiotensin II and angiotensin III in rat blood. Circ. Res. 38(Suppl. II):122-125.

Sen, S., Smeby, R. R., and Bumpus, F. M. (1967). Isolation of a phospholipid renin inhibitor from kidney. Biochemistry 6:1572-1581.

Sen, S., Smeby, R. R., and Bumpus, F. M. (1968). Antihypertensive effect of an isolated phospholipid. Am. J. Physiol. 214:337-341.

Shigezane, K., and Mizoguchi, T. (1973). Synthesis of antirenin active peptides: III. C-Terminal carbinol analogues of peptides related to the partial structure of angiotensinogen as renin inhibitor. Chem. Pharm. Bull. (Tokyo) 21:972-980.

Sibley, P. L., Keim, G. R., Keysser, C. H., Kulesza, J. S., Miller, M. M., and Zaidi, I. H. (1978). SQ 14,225, an orally active inhibitor of angiotensin-converting enzyme: acute and subacute toxicity in animals. Toxicol. Appl. Pharmacol. 45:315-316.

Silverstein, E., Friedland, J., Lyons, H., and Kitt, M. (1975). Serum angiotensin converting enzyme in sarcoidosis. Clin. Res. 22:352A.

Sirois, P., and Gagnon, D. J. (1974). Release of prostaglandins from the rabbit renal medulla. Eur. J. Pharmacol. 28:18-24.

Skeggs, L. T. (1974). Biochemical relationships of the renin-angiotensin system. Hosp. Pract. 9:145-154.

Skeggs, L. T., Marsh, W. H., Kahn, J. R., and Shumway, N. P. (1954). The existence of two forms of hypertension. J. Exp. Med. 99:275-282.

Skeggs, L. T., Kahn, J. R., Lentz, K., and Shumway, N. (1957). The preparation, purification, and amino acid sequence of a polypeptide renin substrate. J. Exp. Med. 106:439-453.

Skeggs, L. T., Lentz, K. E., Kahn, J. R., and Shumway, N. (1958). The synthesis of a tetradecapeptide renin substrate. J. Exp. Med. 108: 283-297.

Skeggs, L. T., Lentz, K. E., Hochstrasser, H., and Kahn, J. R. (1963). The purification and partial characterization of several forms of hog renin substrate. J. Exp. Med. 118:73-98.

Skeggs, L. T., Lentz, K. E., Kahn, J. R., and Hochstrasser, H. (1967). Studies on the preparation and properties of renin. Circ. Res. 20/21 (Suppl. II):91-100.

Skeggs, L. T., Lentz, K. E., Kahn, J. R., and Hochstrasser, H. (1968). Kinetics of the reaction of renin with nine synthetic peptide substrates. J. Exp. Med. 128:13-34.

Skeggs, L. T., Lentz, K. E., Kahn, J. R., Dorer, F. E., and Levine, M. (1969). Pseudorenin—a new angiotensin-forming enzyme. Circ. Res. 25:451-462.

Skeggs, L. T., Lentz, K. E., Kahn, J. R., Levine, M., and Dorer, F. E. (1972). Multiple forms of human kidney renin. In Hypertension 72, J. Genest and E. Koiw (Eds.). Springer-Verlag, New York, pp. 149-160.

Skeggs, L. T., Dorer, F. E., Kahn, J. R., Lentz, K. E., and Levine, M. (1976). The biochemistry of the renin-angiotensin system and its role in hypertension. Am. J. Med. 60:737-748.

Skinner, S. L. (1967). Improved assay methods for renin "concentration" and "activity" in human plasma. Methods using selective denaturation of renin substrate. Circ. Res. 20:391-402.

Skinner, S. L., Cran, E. J., Gibson, P., Taylor, R., Walters, W. A. W., and Catt, K. J. (1975). Angiotensin I and II, active and inactive renin, renin substrate, renin activity, and angiotensinase in human liquor amnii and plasma. Am. J. Obstet. Gynecol. 121:626-630.

Smeby, R. R., Sen, S., and Bumpus, F. M. (1967). A naturally occurring renin inhibitor. Circ. Res. 20/21(Suppl. II):129-133.

Soffer, R. L. (1976). Angiotensin-converting enzyme and the regulation of vasoactive peptides. Annu. Rev. Biochem. 45:73-94.

Soffer, R. L., Reza, R., and Caldwell, P. R. B. (1974). Angiotensin-converting enzyme from rabbit pulmonary particles. Proc. Natl. Acad. Sci. 71:1720-1724.

Solomon, T., Cavero, I., and Buckley, J. P. (1974). Inhibition of the central pressor effects of angiotensin I and II. J. Pharm. Sci. 63:511-515.

Spark, R. F. (1972). Low renin hypertension and the adrenal cortex. N. Engl. J. Med. 287:343-349.

Speckart, P., Golub, M., Zia, P., Zipser, R., and Horton, R. (1976). The effect of angiotensin II and indomethacin on immunoreactive prostaglandin "A" levels in man. Prostaglandins 11:481-488.

Steele, J. M., Neusy, A. J., and Lowenstein, J. (1976). The effects of Des-Asp[1]-angiotensin II on blood pressure, plasma aldosterone concentration, and plasma renin activity in the rabbit. Circ. Res. 38(Suppl. II): 113-116.

Stevens, R. L., Micalizzi, E. R., Fessler, D. C., and Pals, D. T. (1972). Angiotensin I converting enzyme of calf lung. Method of assay and partial purification. Biochemistry 11:2999-3007.

Stokes, G. S., Weber, M. A., and Thornell, I. R. (1974). β-blockers and plasma renin activity in hypertension. Br. Med. J. 1:60-62.

Streeten, D. H. P., Anderson, G. H., and Dalakos, T. G. (1976). Angiotensin blockade: its clinical significance. Am. J. Med. 60:817-824.

Strong, C. G., Boucher, R., Nowaczynski, W., and Genest, J. (1966). Renal vasodepressor lipid. Proc. Mayo Clin. 41:433-452.

Summy-Long, J., and Severs, W. B. (1974). Angiotensin and thirst. Studies with a converting enzyme inhibitor and a receptor antagonist. Life Sci. 15:569-582.

Symonds, E. M., Stanley, M. A., and Skinner, S. L. (1968). Production of renin by in vitro culture of human chorion and uterine muscle. Nature (Lond.) 217:1152-1153.

Taylor, A. A. (1977). Use of renin and aldosterone measurements to define pathophysiology. Pp. 599-603 in J. R. Mitchell (Moderator), "Renin-aldosterone profiling in hypertension." Ann. Intern. Med. 87:596-612.

Terragno, N. A., Malik, K. U., Nasjletti, A., Terragno, D. A., and McGiff, J. C. (1976). Renal prostaglandins. Adv. Prostaglandins Thromboxane Res. 2:561-571.

Tewksbury, D. A., Frome, W. L., and Dumas, M. L. (1977). Characterization of human angiotensinogen. J. Biol. Chem. 253:3817-3820.

Thurau, K., and Mason, J. (1974). The intrarenal function of the juxtaglomerular apparatus. In MTP International Review of Science, Physiology Series One. Vol. 6, K. Thurau (Ed.). University Park Press, Baltimore, pp. 357-389.

Thurston, H. (1976). Vascular angiotensin receptors and their role in blood pressure control. Am. J. Med. 61:768-778.

Tinker, D. O., Schwartz, J. H., Osmond, D. H., and Ross, L. J. (1973). Dog kidney phospholipids and the question of renin inhibition. Can. J. Biochem. 51:863-875.

Tobian, L., and O'Donnell, M. (1976). Renal prostaglandins in relation to sodium regulation and hypertension. Fed. Proc. 35:2388-2392.

Tobian, L., O'Donnell, M., and Smith, P. (1974). Intrarenal prostaglandin levels during normal and high sodium intake. Circ. Res. 34/35(Suppl. I): 83-86.

Tsai, B. S., Peach, M. J., Khosla, M. C., and Bumpus, F. M. (1975). Synthesis and evaluation of [Des-Asp[1]]angiotensin I as a precursor for [Des-Asp[1]]angiotensin II ("angiotensin III"). J. Med. Chem. 18:1180-1183.

Turcotte, J. G., Boyd, R. E., Quinn, J. G., and Smeby, R. R. (1973). Isolation and renin-inhibitory activity of phosphoglyceride from shark kidney. J. Med. Chem. 16:166-168.

Turker, R. K., Page, I. H., and Bumpus, F. M. (1974). Antagonists of angiotensin II. In Angiotensin, I. H. Page and F. M. Bumpus (Eds.). Springer-Verlag, New York, pp. 162-184.

Umezawa, H., Aoyagi, T., Morishima, H., Matsuzaki, M., Hamada, M., and Takeuchi, T. (1970). Pepstatin, a new pepsin inhibitor produced by actinomycetes. J. Antibiot. 23:259-262.

Vander, A. J. (1968). Direct effects of prostaglandin on renal function and renin release in anesthetized dog. Am. J. Physiol. 214:218-221.

Vapaatalo, H., and Parantainen, J. (1978). Prostaglandins: their biological and pharmacological role. Med. Biol. 56:163-183.

Varkarakis, M. J., Szolnoky, A., and Murphy, G. P. (1975). Direct effect of prostaglandins in renal function and renin release in the presence of renal ischemia in the dog. Invest. Urol. 12:302-308.

Vecsei, P., Hackenthal, E., and Ganten, D. (1978). The renin-angiotensin-aldosterone system. Klin. Wochenschr. 56(Suppl. I):5-21.

Verberckmoes, R., van Damme, B., Clement, J., Amery, A., and Michielsen, P. (1976). Bartter's syndrome with hyperplasia of renomedullary cells: successful treatment with indomethacin. Kidney Int. 9:302-307.

Vinci, J. M., Gill, J. R., Bowden, R. E., Pisano, J. J., Izzo, J. L., Radfar, N., Taylor, A. A., Zusman, R. M., Bartter, F. C., and Keiser, H. R. (1978). The kallikrein-kinin system in Bartter's syndrome and its response to prostaglandin synthetase inhibition. J. Clin. Invest. 61:1671-1682.

Weigand, K., Wernze, H., and Falge, C. (1977). Synthesis of angiotensinogen by isolated rat liver cells and its regulation in comparison to serum albumin. Biochem. Biophy. Res. Commun. 75:102-110.

Weinberger, M. H., and Rosner, D. R. (1972). Renin release by rat kidney slices in vitro. In Control of Renin Secretion, T. A. Assaykeen (Ed.). Plenum Press, New York, pp. 145-150.

Weinberger, M. H., Collins, D., Dowdy, A. J., Nokes, G. W., and Luetscher, J. A. (1969). Hypertension induced by oral contraceptives containing estrogen and gestagen. Ann. Intern. Med. 71:891-902.

Weinberger, M. H., Aoi, W., and Henry, D. P. (1975). Direct effect of beta-adrenergic stimulation on renin release by rat kidney slice in vitro. Circ. Res. 37:318-324.

Werning, C., Vetter, W., Weidmann, P., Schweikert, H. U., Stiel, D., and Siegenthaler, W. (1971). Effect of prostaglandin E_1 on renin in the dog. Am. J. Physiol. 220:852-856.

Wilson, C. M., Ward, P. E., Erdös, E. G., and Gecse, A. (1976). Studies on membrane-bound renin in the mouse and rat. Circ. Res. 38(Suppl. II): 95-98.

Winer, N., Walkenhorst, W. G., Helman, R., and Lamy, D. (1972). Effects of adrenergic antagonists in states of increased renin secretion.

In Control of Renin Secretion, T. A. Assaykeen (Ed.). Plenum Press, New York, pp. 65-81.

Woods, J. W., Pittman, A. W., Pulliam, C. C., Werk, E. E., Waider, W., and Allen, C. A. (1976). Renin profiling in hypertension and its use in treatment with propranolol and chlorthalidone. N. Engl. J. Med. 294:1137-1143.

Workman, R. J., McKown, M. M., and Gregerman, R. I. (1974). Renin: inhibition by proteins and peptides. Biochemistry 13:3029-3035.

Yamamoto, K., Iwao, H., Abe, Y., and Morimoto, S. (1974). Effect of Ca on renin release in vitro and in vivo. Jap. Circ. J. 38:1127-1131.

Yang, H. Y. T., Erdös, E. G., and Chiang, T. S. (1968). New enzymatic route for the inactivation of angiotensin. Nature (Lond.) 218:1224-1226.

Yang, H. Y. T., Erdös, E. G., and Levin, Y. (1970). A dipeptidyl carboxypeptidase that converts angiotensin I and inactivates bradykinin. Biochim. Biophys. Acta 214:374-376.

Yu, R., Anderton, J., Skinner, S. L., and Best, J. B. (1972). Renin in anephric man. Am. J. Med. 52:707-711.

Zachariah, N. Y., Smeby, R. R., Sen, S., Bumpus, F. M., and Singh, C. (1975). Phospholipase A_2 in experimental hypertension. Am. J. Physiol. 228:1782-1786.

Zakheim, R. M., Mattiolo, L., Molteni, A., Mullis, K. B., and Bartley, J. (1975). Prevention of pulmonary vascular changes of chronic alveolar hypoxia by inhibition of angiotensin I-converting enzyme in the rat. Lab. Invest. 3:57-61.

Zakheim, R. M., Molteni, A., Mattioli, L., and Mullis, K. B. (1976). Angiotensin I-converting enzyme and angiotensin II levels in women receiving an oral contraceptive. J. Clin. Endocrinol. Metab. 42:588-589.

Zanchetti, A., and Stella, A. (1975). Neural control of renin release. Clin. Sci. Mol. Med. 48:215-223.

Zanchetti, A., Stella, A., Leonetti, G., Morganti, A., and Terzoli, L. (1976). Control of renin release: a review of experimental evidence and clinical implications. Am. J. Cardiol. 37:675-691.

Zschiedrich, H., Hofbauer, K. G., Hackenthal, E., Baron, G. D., and Gross, F. (1975). Intrarenal formation of angiotensin II in the rat: interference by saralasin and SQ 20881. Clin. Sci. Mol. Med. 48:37-40.

Zusman, R. M., Spector, D., Caldwell, B. V., Speroff, L., Schneider, G., and Mulrow, P. J. (1973a). The effect of chronic sodium loading and sodium restriction on plasma prostaglandin A, E and F concentrations in normal humans. J. Clin. Invest. 52:1093-1098.

Zusman, R., Spector, D., Caldwell, B. V., Speroff, L., Forman, B., Schneider, G., and Mulrow, P. (1973b). Prostaglandin A concentrations in plasma of normal and hypertensive humans. J. Clin. Invest. 52:93.

Zusman, R. M., Snider, J. J., Cline, A., Caldwell, B. V., and Speroff, L. (1974). Antihypertensive function of a renal-cell carcinoma. N. Engl. J. Med. 290:843-845.

8 Prostaglandins and Cardiac Muscle

PHILIP B. HOLLANDER / Ohio State University College of Medicine, Columbus, Ohio

Acceptance or even postulation of a unitary mechanism justifying the vast number of actions attributed to prostaglandins on the cardiovascular system and in particular on specific elements thereof has yet to be advanced. Although many authors have substantiated the facts that the major actions of prostaglandins on vascular smooth muscle are not markedly influenced by cholinergic, adrenergic, histaminergic, or serotonergic inhibitors or antagonists, no such generalization may yet be made for the myocardial system. It is usually accepted that the pulmonary system very efficiently destroys circulating prostaglandins and essentially eliminates cardiovascular effects directly attributed to prostaglandins present in the circulatory system. Similarly, as has been reported by many investigators for tissues other than heart, prostaglandins do not appear to be stored in cardiac tissue and the main source for prostaglandin may be myocardial and/or coronary blood vessels synthesis. It can be suggested that the results and actions of prostaglandin synthesis in heart is fourfold: (1) alteration in cardiac electropharmacology, (2) modulation of local and/or coronary blood flow, (3) alteration in myocardial force and cardiac output, and (4) inhibition or precipitation of cardiac dysfunction. This chapter deals with these four prostaglandin-induced activities after briefly documenting the capacity of heart muscle to mediate prostaglandin synthesis, use, and biotransformation or metabolism.

PROSTAGLANDIN HISTORY, ASSAY, SYNTHESIS, AND METABOLISM

It was first reported by Kurzrod and Lieb (1), then Goldblatt (2), and followed by Euler (3) that fresh human semen and seminal plasma markedly modulated contractile responses of human uterus or smooth muscle. Since these simple beginnings and after isolation of the active principle called prostaglandin, which was so named since Euler implicated the prostate gland as the main source, extensive investigations attempting to define the pharmacology, physiology, and biochemistry have been voluminously reported. Prostaglandins appear to be omnipresent among all mammalian tissues investigated, usually in a concentration mean of 1 μg/g wet weight of tissue; seminal plasma is unique, with a concentration of about 100 μg/ml. An acceptable analysis and assay for prostaglandin was developed less than 15 years ago (4), which suggests that concentrations reported previous to that date may be suspect. The Vane analysis was based on a superfusion technique of a serial arranged series of isolated assay tissues, each with individual sensitivities. It was shown that both PGE_1 and PGE_2 were 60-90% metabolized or destroyed after one passage through many physiological systems. The precise mechanism for this tissue response has yet to be resolved, but data suggest that there must be enzymatic systems which specifically biotransform circulating prostaglandins to inactive forms. These systems for biotransformation may be located at surface membrane-linked systems to effect such a rapid transformation. Conclusive data are not yet at hand to indicate that prostaglandins enter permeable cell membranes to any large degree. Typically, prostaglandin assays have been standardized with three methods, yielding (1) 1 Euler unit (5) = 4.5 μg PGE_1, (2) 1 Eliasson HSF-PG unit (6) = 10 μg PGE_1, and (3) 1 Hawkins and Labrum unit (7) = 20 μg PGE_1. Two useful conversion factors for use of PGE_1 are: $\mu g/ml \times (2.82 \times 10^{-6}) = M$; $M \times (3.55 \times 10^{5}) = \mu g/ml$.

It is now generally accepted that the heart, like most other tissues, can take exogenous arachidonic acid and produce prostaglandins. Prostaglandins synthesized in heart demonstrate a dose-dependent depression of coronary resistance or increase in flow that appears to coincide with detection of a prostaglandinlike substance in coronary outflow (8). Since these effects were not produced when arachidonic acid was absent, and the heart was not traumatized prior to prostaglandin assay, it may be suggested that hearts utilize arachidonic acid (an accepted precursor to prostaglandin synthesis) to produce prostaglandin. These data would also suggest that cardiac tissue has the essential machinery to synthesize prostaglandin, a process necessary if one is to postulate the previously indicated four prostaglandin modulations of cardiac functions. That prostaglandin synthesis is indeed a basis of cardiac function modulation is substantiated by work of many laboratories as well as ours (unpublished data), since prior administration of indomethacin or aspirin, two substances known to inhibit prostaglandin synthesis (9), abolishes the cardiac effects coincident with administration of arachidonic acid. Similarly, it has been reported by many investigators that somewhat less than 50% of administered prostaglandins is recovered after one passage through cardiac systems. These data together with those indicated previously would suggest that there may be a functional prostaglandin-synthesizing metabolizing system, currently associated with prostaglandin synthetase and dehydrogenase, to regulate prostaglandin synthesized by cardiac tissues. The essential elements appear to be present in heart muscle to synthesize, use, and metabolize or biotransform prostaglandin; hence the functional aspects may now be considered.

ALTERATIONS IN CARDIAC ELECTROPHARMACOLOGY

Membrane Structure

Alteration of cardiovascular responses by prostaglandins may be elucidated by investigations of their electrophysiological and electropharmacological properties. Increasing numbers of biophysical and biomedical investigations during the last few decades have illustrated to some degree the fundamental processes basic to excitation and contraction of cardiovascular systems. Stimulation or excitation is intimately associated with ions and cellular membrane activities, whereas contraction is associated with ions and contractile proteins. Most, if not all, cellular stimulation of physiological and pharmacological origin is initially presented to the plasma membrane of cardiac muscle cells. The concept of a cell membrane was first introduced by Nageli and Cramer (10) as the boundary between the inside and outside of cells that appears to possess some distinctive properties. Each myocardial fiber is usually invested with an outer or surface plasma membrane and an inner or basement membrane; both in conjunction are designated the sarcolemma. The plasma membrane is about 90-100Å thick and is covered with a granular basement membrane about 50Å thick. The plasma membrane (1) is the site of electrical activities coincident with cellular activation, (2) appears to form the structural framework containing processes modulating semipermeable characteristics separating intracellular cytoplasm from extracellular milieu, and (3) is the region containing constituents involved in active transport of materials essential for maintenance of tissue viability. The basement membrane, with its glycoprotein fractions, may also be involved in ion regulation since it has been postulated that negatively charged constituents afford sites for calcium binding (11).

Membrane Excitation Process

Under most normal and some abnormal conditions, excitation always precedes contraction. Cellular or membrane excitation of cardiac cells is generally electrical in nature, whereas smooth muscle cells excitation is mainly chemical in nature. Selected physiological ions serve as vehicles for the variations in time/voltage waveforms registered with appropriate instrumentation. When myocardial cells are at rest, the interior of the cell has an electrical potential ranging from about -75 to -100 mV relative to the species and exterior milieu of the cell. This resting potential is primarily the result of the semipermeability of the plasma membrane, which is essentially impermeable to Na^+ when compared to K^+ (a factor of more than 100:1

favoring K^+). The semipermeable membrane may produce an electrochemical potential because of the difference in K^+ between the inside and outside of cardiac cells (12,13). When the heart cell membrane is adequately stimulated, by reduction of the resting membrane potential (-75 to -100 mV) to activation threshold (-55 to -45 mV), a regenerative process is initiated, resulting in an altered membrane potential.

The reduction in membrane potential or depolarization process from the resting potential produces a time/voltage change, action potential, with a reverse or overshoot membrane potential ranging from +20 to +35 mV. It is now usually accepted, due to the efforts of too many competent investigators to list, that the depolarization of the cardiac action potential (designated as phase 0) is produced by two distinct phenomena. The initial or fast phase of the action potential is related primarily to Na^+ influx, while the latter phase of the depolarization is related to both Na^+ and Ca^{2+} influx. The Ca^{2+} influx is much slower and of a longer duration than Na^+ influx. These results were obtained using tetrodotoxin and Mn^{2+}. Tetrodotoxin, a puffer fish poison, will selectively block only the fast Na^{2+} channel, while Mn^{2+} can selectively block only the slow or Ca^{2+} channel (14). If it is accepted that the maximum depolarization rate of the action potential is related to activity of the fast Na^+ channel, and the overshoot amplitude, or positivity of the action potential is related to both Na^+ and the slow or Ca^{2+} channel, then, as will be indicated later, prostaglandins produce a dose-related response in these channels. The tissue selected for study will also show differences.

The cellular membrane potential in Purkinje fibers of the heart does not remain in a plus voltage depolarization state as found with ventricle muscle. Purkinje fibers show an almost immediate return toward zero membrane potential, brought about primarily through an efflux of Cl^- from cells. The repolarization phase associated with Cl^- efflux is designated phase 1. Thereafter the cellular action potential of both Purkinje and ventricle fibers demonstrate a slowly changing plateau region lasting about three-fourths of the total duration of the action potential. By contrast, the duration of phase 0 or the depolarization of the Purkinje and ventricular action potential lasts less than 6 msec, whereas the duration of the action potential plateau exceeds 150 msec. The plateau, designated phase 2 of the action potential, is maintained by a slow inward current carried primarily by Ca^{2+}, which appears to be activated by the fast inward Na^+ current when the depolarization potential approximates -35 mV. The inward Na^+ current has not completely ceased during the plateau of the action potential and its contribution to the total effect cannot be ignored (15,16). Upon cessation of the slow inward Ca^{2+} current, and the residual inward Na^+ current, approximately coincident with the end of the action potential plateau, the final repolarization of the action potential or restitution to the resting potential of myocardial cells occurs. It is during the final repolarization phase of the action potential, designated phase 3, that K^+ efflux increases and carries the outward current required for repolarization. At least eight ion-associated current channels or pores in or on the surface membrane of cells have been identified (17). The small increase in intracellular Na^+ and loss of K^+ ions coincident with an action potential cycle are actively pumped and exchanged during the resting state, phase 4, to restore intracellular milieu found prior to action potential activity. The resting potential usually remains stable in nonpathological cells, modulated by the semipermeability characteristics of the membrane-active ion pumping with K^+ and Na^+ fluxes balanced.

If a cell membrane demonstrated spontaneous depolarization during phase 4, a process designated diastolic depolarization, prior to the eventual fast potential change associated with phase 0, that cell possesses the ability of myogenicity or automaticity characteristic of pacemaker cells of the heart. Myocardial cells demonstrating automaticity or pacemaker-like activity show a slow decline in the diastolic resting potential toward zero membrane potential and an associated varying membrane permeability of K^+. As in other nonautomatic cells, phase 0 is carried by Na^+ ions but not to such a high degree. The slow time/voltage-dependent changes that occur during phase 4 of the pacemaker membrane potential are found in cells located at the sinoatrial node of the atrium and atrioventricular node of the His-Purkinje system. The latter myogenic system only becomes apparent during abnormal conduction, excitation, or other pathological conditions (18).

Excitation-Contraction

The amount of Ca^{2+} entering cells during an action potential is not sufficient to produce activation of the contractile machinery. There may be some form of "trigger" or lever of an internal store to cascade Ca^{2+} release coincident with postulated activation of myocardial proteins producing contraction. Our current state of understanding precludes a complete description of the process resulting in myocardial contraction together with membrane excitation, usually referred to as excitation-contraction. Stated briefly, ventricular action potentials with their influx of Na^+ and Ca^{2+} during depolarization together with Ca^{2+} influx during the plateau establishes the condition not only to increased Ca^{2+} activity within myocardial cytoplasm essential for activation of contractile elements, but also delivers electrical activation that spreads over cell surfaces and tubules to enhance further release of Ca^{2+}. There is some general agreement that myocardial tension generated depends on the amount of ionic Ca^{2+} within cellular cytoplasm. The increased Ca^{2+} appears also to initiate ATP splitting and thereby activates cross-bridges associated with actin-myosin proteins. Ca^{2+} appears to bind to troponin elements located on or near actin filaments, which in turn causes a conformational change in tropomyosin, thereby making available the active sites for splitting adenosine triphosphate (ATP) (19, 20).

At Ca^{2+} concentrations of less than 10^{-7} M, myofibrils are apparently relaxed, whereas at Ca^{2+} concentrations approaching 10^{-5} M, myofibrils are fully contracted. It may be stated that myocardium increases tension with an increase in both extra- and intracellular Ca^{2+}. Then (ionic) Ca^{2+} must decrease for myofibril relaxation to occur. Although there appears to be some relationship between extracellular Ca^{2+} concentration (activity) and contraction, reports that completely substantiate the premise that Ca^{2+} entering cells during action potential activity directly influences myocardial tension during that membrane activity are not yet available for mammalian hearts. Relaxation may be initiated by repolarization of the myocardial cellular and tubular action potential, which reduces the amount of Ca^{2+} entering cellular interiors. The sarcoplasmic reticulum is also a promising site to sequester intracellular Ca^{2+}, thereby reducing the critical Ca^{2+} level necessary for contraction and promoting relaxation. It may be thus postulated that repolarization of the action potential, sequestration of Ca^{2+} by sarcoplasmic reticulum and mitochondria, and passive and active removal of Ca^{2+} across membranes all serve to reduce intracellular concentrations (activities) equal to or less than 10^{-7} M and thereby promote relaxation (21).

If the data obtained in vascular smooth muscle are similar to that observed in myocardium, it may be suggested that depolarization of plasma membrane with its possible release and augmented ion fluxes may underlie the mechanism for stimulation (22). It may also be suggested that the effects of prostaglandins act directly not only on membrane properties but also on excitation-contraction acting through Ca^{2+}. It has been reported that Ca^{2+} exchange appears to be stimulated by PGE_1 (23). Thus prostaglandins may produce greater contractile response in low Ca^{2+} milieu. The antithesis of this suggestion of course would be that low concentrations of prostaglandins may inactivate intracellular Ca^{2+} and produce depression or relaxation of muscles through previously indicated troponin and ATPase mechanisms. This premise may be supported since it was reported that prostaglandins decrease the threshold and alter tissue activity during electrical activation (24).

ELECTROPHARMACOLOGY OF PROSTAGLANDINS

Although there are many prostaglandins other than PGE_1 and PGE_2, these two prostaglandins have been extensively tested to establish their electropharmacology (25, 26; unpublished data). PGE_1 was without effect on the resting potential of hearts of dogs, cats, rabbits, guinea pigs, and rats in concentrations $\leq$ 30 ng/ml, whereas PGE_2 showed a statistically significant decrease ($p < 0.05$) in the resting potential in all species at concentrations $\geq$ 30 ng/ml. Higher concentrations of both PGE_1 and PGE_2 produced aberrant membrane activity and may account for the depression or alteration in the resting potential observed. PGE_1 and PGE_2 were without effect on the total action potential magnitude, but there was an increase at lower doses and a decrease at higher doses in the overshoot of the action potential beyond the zero level. These changes in overshoot were also observed in the depolarization rate of the action potential, increasing at lower doses (less than

5 ng/ml) and decreasing at higher doses (less than 30 ng/ml). Both PGE_1 and PGE_2 decreased the duration of the plateau, increased the decay slope of the plateau, made the onset of phase 3 of the action potential more negative, and increased the duration of the terminal part of the action potential. It would appear that PGE_1 and PGE_2 are qualitatively similar on the above-indicated parameters of the membrane electrical responses.

It is of some interest that the resting potential was not changed, suggesting that its basis in the electrochemical distribution of K^+ was equivalent to the control. Augmentation of the plateau effects as well as the overshoot suggest that there were changes in these parts underlying the action potential; these activities are usually associated with Na^+ and Ca^{2+} currents. It is well documented that increased Ca^{2+} flux will produce the effects recorded with PGEs on both the overshoot and plateau of action potentials. Similarly, celluline-A produced the same effects as those seen with low concentrations of PGEs on the overshoot and maximum depolarization rate of the action potential (25-28). It would appear that the decrease in the depolarization rate of the action potentials, its overshoot, and prolongation of the duration and other characteristics observed with higher doses of PGE mimic effects observed with some agents used to control or inhibit arrhythmias. It has yet to be resolved whether these effects are operant through the Na^+, Ca^{2+}, or K^+ channel or combinations thereof.

The usual influence of changes in concentration of K^+, Ca^{2+}, and Mg^{2+} in tissue media supporting tissue treated with prostaglandins may be said to mimic most other agonists; some responses can also be evoked in K^+ depolarized smooth muscles (29). Like catecholamines, prostaglandins will counteract the effect of K^+ depolarized muscles but Ca^{2+} must be present for the effects to be produced. Low Ca^{2+} and K^+ both augment the effects reported for PGE_1, while $PGE_{1\alpha}$ appears to be relatively insensitive to Ca^{2+} concentration for progression of its activities (30).

The differences in responses of the various prostaglandins on animals seems to be related to the species employed, tissue used for testing, and prostaglandin selected. Dogs subject to pentobarbital anesthesia, surgically vagotomized, or pentolinium-induced ganglionic blockade are sensitized to depressor action of prostaglandins; rats do not appear to demonstrate this effect; $PGF_{2\alpha}$ is a vasodepressor in cats and rabbits and a pressor in rats and dogs (31, 32). PGE_1 100-1000 ng/ml always produced positive inotropy, chronotropy, and some augmented coronary blood flow when Langendorff perfused guinea pig hearts were incubated with low Ca^{2+} (unpublished data). Although similar effects with PGE_1 were reported for rabbit atria (33), use of PGA_1 was without influence on guinea pig, rabbit, or toad, whereas $PGF_{2\alpha}$ depressed these tissues (34).

MODULATION OF LOCAL OR CORONARY BLOOD FLOW

There is a general depressor effect on systemic blood pressure induced by an intravenous bolus injection of PGE_1, PGE_2, PGA_1, or PGA_2. Biphasic dose/response data are produced by PGE_1, PGE_2, PGA_1, and $PGF_{1\alpha}$ when tested on peripheral resistance vessels of dogs. Coronary systems relax in doses ranging from 1 to 100 ng/ml and contract in doses up to 10,000 ng/ml (22). It was also reported that both rabbit and dog coronary vessels contracted only in doses of 0.1 ng/ml (24), while it was reported that PGE_1 decreased coronary resistance or increase coronary flow (9); these data indicate that not all blood vessels, even those in the same system, respond in a similar manner. In fact, it has been reported that $PGF_{2\alpha}$ is without any measurable effect on dog coronary flow (31), while the same prostaglandin exerts a central effect that may thus directly influence cardiovascular actions reported (35). The basal synthetic rate of prostaglandin in dogs was 18.6 ± 4.9 ng/min for normal coronary blood flow and 35.3 ± 5.8 ng/min after postocclusive hyperemia or other conditions that produced increased metabolic demands. Prostaglandin synthesis could effectively be blocked by indomethacin or meclofenamate, which in turn would prevent reactive hyperemia due to coronary occlusion (36). It is of no small interest that these latter agents could effect their action without changes in Ca^{2+}, Na^+, or K^+ flux. The initial conditions of the pathology would markedly alter these physiological concentrations of these ions. This work was corroborated and extended to show that $PGF_{1\alpha}$ and $PGF_{2\alpha}$ were ineffective using the experimental protocol employed with PGE (37). Use of PGE_1 and PGE_2 to produce hyperemia in rats was ineffective when compared to that observed in dogs and rabbits, even at doses of 10 ng/ml (38). However, even though there was no significant change in chronotropic or inotropic responses of rat heart with PGE_1 and PGE_2, the actions of these agents may be specific for coronary vessels since PGE_1, PGE_2, PGA, and $PGF_{2\alpha}$, although effective on vasculature, are without effect on cat papillary muscles (39).

The route of prostaglandin administration appears also to influence the responses elicited by prostaglandins. Close intraarterial injection to coronary arteries increased myocardial force and coronary flow by an apparent vasodilation, which in turn produced an increased cardiac output in the face of unaltered blood pressure or heart rate (40). This is in contrast to an increased cardiac output without vasodilation when prostaglandins were injected intravenously elsewhere, provided that they were not administered into the pulmonary vascular passage (41). One should recall that an increased cardiac output is usually associated with a (subsequent) decrease in blood pressure, suggesting a decrease in peripheral resistance. Coronary blood flow or vasodilation due to prostaglandins may be altered by aspirin, suggesting a negative feedback role for prostaglandins, since prostaglandins synthesis can be decreased or blocked by aspirin.

Intraaortic administration is more effective in augmenting vasodepressor effects and myocardial intrinsic activity when compared to intravenous administration. However, administration of prostaglandins intraarterially at the level of the abdomen shows no difference of activity when compared to intravenous administration. Although there is no unanimity among investigators as to the assigned role that prostaglandins play in the total cardiovascular system, the registered effective concentrations in ng/ml, synthetic, and metabolic systems established in the cardiovascular systems all strongly suggest that prostaglandins have a role as modulators and mediators of physiological activity (42,43). It may also be stated that some parts of the cardiovascular synthesis system of prostaglandins differ from that reported for other systems. A microsomal fraction prepared from canine myocardium was found to contain an active prostaglandin synthetase (average 10 nmol PGE_2/mg protein per min), which demonstrated a capability of forming PGE_2 from arachidonic acid in the presence of reduced glutathione and essential cofactors such as L-adrenaline, hydroquinone, and p-aminophenol. It was also found that aspirin or phospholipase A, which have been reported to alter prostaglandin synthesis in other tissues, alter the activities of myocardial prostaglandin synthesis (44).

ALTERATIONS IN MYOCARDIAL FORCE

PGE_1 (33) and PGE_2 (45,46) in rabbit atria, and PGE_1 and PGE_2 (47) in guinea pig atria and ventricle (unpublished data), produced positive inotropy, whereas PGE_1 is without any significant effect on dog papillary (48) or cultured chicken hearts (49). Similarly, PGE_1 is without significant effect on the contractile force or heart rate of cat or rabbit Landendorff preparations (50-52), whereas PGE_1 increases the contractile force of rat, guinea pig, frog, and chicken heart (50,52,35). $PGF_{1\alpha}$ or $PGF_{1\beta}$ enhanced contractility of rat and guinea pig hearts without altering heart rate or coronary flow (38, 53), whereas $PGF_{2\alpha}$ and PGA_2 are without effect on the chronotropic or inotropic responses of isolated chicken and rabbit hearts, respectively. Contrary to the reported lack of effect of PGE_1 (2.5×10^{-7} M) on dog papillary, 1-3 μg of PGE_1 directly into dog atrium increases myocardial force and coronary flow without alterations in heart rate (54). Similarly, an intravenous bolus injection or even continuous infusion of PGE_1 directly into dog hearts increases chronotropic and inotropic responses while decreasing systemic arterial pressure (41,55,56). The variable effects of a specific prostaglandin is modulated by the site of injection. PGA_1 produced an effect similar to that of PGE_1 (41) even when the heart rate was kept constant with propranolol, whereas $PGF_{2\alpha}$ was without significant effect when administered under identical conditions (57). Close intracoronary injection of PGE_1 increases both coronary flow and myocardial contractility without alterations in chronotropy or systemic pressure. These differential effects of coronary flow and contractility may be separate and distinct since it was shown that coronary flow could be increased without changes in contractile force. PGE_1 may thus act in two separate sites, those dealing with coronary reactivity and with contractility of myocardium (40).

It has been suggested that PGE_1 may produce its effect by interfering with the release of catecholamines at prejunctional sites (58), since it was reported that PGE_1 decreased the effects of sympathetic stimulation on inotropy and appearance of norepinephrine in the perfusate of isolated Langendorff perfused rabbit hearts. One may thus raise the question whether prostaglandins affect their activity through the sympathetic nervous system or its receptors (58, 59). This inhibition of catecholamine activity through inhibition of release may be the mechanism by which the arrhythmic effects of isoprenaline on dog hearts are abolished by the administration of prostaglandins. Many pharmacologic reports on the interaction between atropine, other antimuscarinic agents, antihistamines, serotonin antagonists, α- and β-adrenergic antagonists, and prostaglandins are in the literature. The reports seem to indicate that they are without significant effect on the actions of prostaglandins on the myocardial or vascular system. These data would suggest that prostaglandins, when effective, elicit their response through systems separate from that associated with propranolol, diphenhydramine, or reserpine since these agents do not alter the dose/responses attributed to prostaglandins (34, 50). It may be that myocardial changes induced by prostaglandins are related to calcium metabolism, essential for changes in force. The presence or absence of prostaglandin may directly/indirectly influence myocardial response. There appears to be a decrease in right ventricular hypertrophy induced by chronic hypoxic pulmonary hypertension when prostaglandin synthesis is decreased by aspirin administration (60). A decrease in cardiac contractile force was produced by prostacyclin derivatives, (6R)-PGI_1 and (6S)-PGI_1 (61).

Although the site or mechanism of prostaglandin action on inotropy still remains to be proved directly, it is generally agreed that myocardial contraction is associated with membrane activation, with calcium acting as the excitation-contraction coupling (link). The positive inotropy in dogs induced with PGE_2 and PGA_2 (62) has yet to be directly related to the postulate of Ca^{2+} metabolism. However, the positive inotropic action of PGE_1 appears to be related to Ca^{2+} metabolism as indicated by increased Ca^{2+} permeability, mobilization, intracellular activation by displacement from a poll or storage site, or simply uptake (32, 33, 52, 63) or antagonism of the effects of K^+ which may accumulate within cells under abnormal states (38). Like smooth muscle the mechanism of action does not appear to be related to a catecholamine activation since reserpine or propranolol pretreatment does not block the positive inotropic responses of guinea pig and rat hearts (52, 64). However, when positive inotropy is induced, PGE_1- and $PGF_{1\alpha}$-like catecholamines appear to be associated with an increase in adenylcyclase activity, increased cyclic AMP concentration, and phosphorylase (53, 63). Because of the similarities in subsequent intracellular responses induced by systems, one is tempted to speculate that there may be separate membrane receptor quantities for each drug class. But both types of drugs in their association with individual receptors eventually modulate a subsequent common pathway leading to changes in contractile magnitude. That the receptor quantity may be different can be extrapolated from the changes in transmembrane potential responses under the influence of different prostaglandins. It would be of no small interest to establish whether a negative inotropic response produced a decrease in cyclic AMP, phosphorylase, and other associated intracellular changes in constituents associated with contractile activity.

Inhibition of Cardiac Arrhythmias

It was indicated previously that prostaglandins and specifically PGE_1 interacted with many substances in their usual role on physiological systems. PGE_1 interfered with catecholamine-induced vasopressor (64) and lipolytic effects (42) and angiotensin-induced vasopressor effects (65). Detailed studies using these vasoactive drugs together with prostaglandins on coronary responses have yet to be delineated, including their effects on cardiac dysfunction. But the suggestion that prostaglandins are released by adrenergic nerve stimulation in rabbit hearts to influence coronary flow indicates that there are further effects on myocardial function to be investigated (66). It was further reported that indomethacin augments catecholamine release from these nerves as well as altering prostaglandin synthesis. Reports on the antiarrhythmic properties of prostaglandins acting directly on the heart soon appeared (67-70) and it was shown that PGE_1 was able to regularize the rhythm of ischemia-induced ventricular tachycardia.

Another report showed that PGE_1 sensitized hearts to arrhythmogenic effects of ouabain (33). Minimal doses of ouabain (10^{-8} M) that were just effective on cardiac inotropy became fully therapeutically effective after administration of PGE_1 (10 ng). Fully therapeutic doses (10^{-7} M) of ouabain, which was normally nontoxic in conjunction with 10 ng PGE_1, invariably produced dysrhythmia. PGE_1, like a toxic dose of ouabain, decreases the intracellular K^+ without increasing the intracellular Na^+ usually observed with ouabain. These data would add to the premise that prostaglandins act specifically at membranes. It was also of interest that PGE_2 was without effect on the fibrillation threshold even though it was effective to block arrhythmias in hypoxic hearts (68). $PGF_{2\alpha}$ was also tested for its antiarrhythmic properties (71,72), and it was subsequently shown that $PGE_{2\alpha}$ was effective on other experimentally induced dysfunctions (73,74). Although it was shown that $PGE_{2\alpha}$ was effective in the inhibition of 60-80% of arrhythmias produced by $BcCl_2$ and aconitine, further experiments suggested that PGE_2 and PGA_2 were also effective; $PGF_{2\alpha}$ was the most effective of the three prostaglandins tested. The variety of changes in intracellular electrolytes or autonomic transmitter release modulation does not allow fro a concise definition or conclusion regarding prostaglandin action on arrhythmias. What is definite, however, is that the antiarrhythmic properties of these prostaglandins do not compromise cardiac function, as is usually observed with other classical antiarrhythmic agents.

There is a paucity of human studies relating actions of prostaglandins and cardiac dysfunction. A brief infusion of PGE (0.2 to 0.7 μg/kg per min) for 4-10 min produced tachycardia, moderate hypotension, and lowered cardiac output (75). Intravenous administration of PGE_1 (0.1-0.2 μg/kg per min) for about 20 min produced an increased heart rate of about 20 beats/min (76). Generally, administration of PGE_1 to healthy subjects produced decreased peripheral resistance, increased cardiac output, increased in stroke volume, increased heart rate, and decreased end-diastolic pressure, despite increases in other characteristics.

Vane reported in 1976 a metabolite of prostaglandin endoperoxides PGG_2 and PGH_2 which had properties that differed from other prostaglandins (77). Following identification of the chemical structure, the trivial name prostacyclin (PGI_2) was assigned, and PGI_2 was synthesized by the Upjohn Company. The prostacyclin synthetase system is apparently widespread in most tissues when microsomal fractions thereof and PGH_2 is used as substrate. Even though the presence of the enzyme suggests formation of PGI_2, direct proof of in vivo formation has yet to be reported (78). PGI_2 produced a dose-related (1.0-3 μg/kg i.v. dose) decrease in mean arterial blood pressure, total peripheral resistance, and pulmonary arterial pressure and an increase in heart rate, left ventricular dp/dt, rate of pressure development with respect to time, and cardiac index. Generally, these effects qualitatively resemble PGE_2. That PGI_2 is physiologically effective may be suggested since it is the major prostaglandin released from isolated perfused rabbit and rat hearts. When PGI_2 production is curtailed, a decrease in coronary blood flow and decreased heart rate was observed (79). It was shown previously that PGAs and PGEs may inhibit a barium- or sconitine-induced arrhythmia. PGI_2 in doses of 0.25-2.0 μg/kg also produced a dose-dependent antiarrhythmic effect (80).

SUMMARY

This chapter briefly reviews current and significant effects of prostaglandins on the physiology and electropharmacology of the cardiovascular system. It is tempting to suggest that prostaglandins initiate their functional sequella by interaction(s) with (1) membrane components of cell, which (2) produce changes in membrane permeability to ions and concurrent excitability, resulting in (3) excitation-contraction coupling. These processes all satisfy the suggested four-functional activities of heart indicated in the introduction and associated with prostaglandins. That prostaglandins are effective modifiers of cardiac function and can be synthesized and/or metabolized within cardiac coronary cells may at this time be an accepted fact. What ideally remains to be resolved is the mechanism by which prostaglandins effect their actions and the reasons for the diversity of their induced responses. Although it was demonstrated that prostaglandins can perturbate electrical activity of plasma membranes, modifying Na^+, Ca^{2+}, and K^+ movements, there were observed differences in these activities, ranging from no response to plus-and-minus effects. These data would suggest that all membranes, like all prostaglandins, are not and do not respond the same, even though they occupy a similar frame of reference. That this is indeed the case can be seen from the differences in responses between hearts of different species when challenged by different prostaglandins. Yet it can be stated that Ca^{2+} and an energy source (ATP?) are prerequisites for responses elicited by prostaglandins. Differences in sensitivities, and indeed ability to induce a change in chronotropy, inotropy, automaticity, synthesis, use, or biotransformation, all relate to both Ca^{2+} and an energy source/utilization process which appears to be modulated by prostaglandins. Obviously, an understanding of these characteristics as modulated by prostaglandins would serve to define the four fundamental processes indicated at the beginning of this chapter.

REFERENCES

1. Kurzrod, R., and Lieb, C. C. Biochemical studies of human semen: II. The action of semen on the human uterus. Proc. Soc. Exp. Biol. Med. 28:268-272, 1930.
2. Goldblatt, M. W. A depressor substance in seminal fluid. J. Soc. Chem. Ind. (Lond.) 52:1056-1057, 1933.
3. Euler, U. S. von. Zur Kenntnis der pharmakologischen Wirkungen von nativsekreten und extrackten männlicher accessorischer Geschlechtsdrüsen. Arch. Exp. Pathol. Pharmakol. 175:78-84, 1934.
4. Vane, J. R. The use of isolated organs for detecting active substances in the circulating blood. Br. J. Pharmacol. Chemother. 23:360-373, 1964.
5. Bergstrom, S., Duner, H., Euler, U. S. von, Pernow, B., and Sjovall, J. Observations on the effects of infusion of prostaglandin E in man. Acta Physiol. Scand. 45:145-151, 1959.
6. Bydgeman, M., and Eliasson, R. The effect of prostaglandin from human seminal fluid on the motility of the non-pregnant human uterus in vitro. Acta Physiol. Scand. 59:43-51, 1963.
7. Hawkins, D. F., and Labrum, A. H. Semen prostaglandin levels in 50 patients attending a fertility clinic. J. Reprod. Fertil. 2:1-10, 1961.
8. Needleman, P. The synthesis and function of prostaglandins in the heart. Fed. Proc. 35(12):2376-2381, 1976.
9. Vane, J. R. Inhibition of prostaglandin synthesis as a mechanism of action of aspirin-like drugs. Nature (New Biol.) 231:232-235, 1971.
10. Nageli, K. W., and Cramer, K. Pflanzenphysioloische Untersuchungen. Schultess, Zurich, 1855.
11. Langer, G. A. Ion fluxes in cardiac excitation and contraction and their relation to myocardial contractility. Physiol. Rev. 48:708-757, 1968.
12. Hodgkin, A. L., and Keynes, R. D. Action transport of cations in giant axons from sepia and loligo. J. Physiol. (Lond.) 128:28-60, 1955.
13. Weidman, S. J. Effect of the cardiac membrane potential on the rapid availability of the sodium-carrying system. J. Physiol. (Lond.) 127:213-227, 1955.

14. Trautwein, W. Membrane currents in cardiac muscle fibers. Physiol. Rev. 53:793-835, 1973.
15. Reuter, H. J. Dependence of slow inward current in Purkinje fibers on extracellular calcium concentration. J. Physiol. (Lond.) 192:479-492, 1967.
16. Reuter, H., and Beeler, G. W. Calcium current and activation of contraction in ventricular myocardial fibers. Science 163:399-401, 1969.
17. Fozzard, H. A., and Beeler, G. W. The voltage clamp and cardiac electrophysiology. Circ. Res. 37:403-413, 1975.
18. Hollander, P. B. Pharmacological methods in membrane biophysics. T.I.T. J. Life Sci. 1:1-24, 1971.
19. Winegrad, S. J. Studies of cardiac muscle with a high permeability to calcium produced by treatment with ethylenediaminetetraacetic acid. J. Gen. Physiol. 58:71-93, 1971.
20. Katz, A. M. Physiology and Biophysics of the Heart. Raven Press, New York, Chap. 7, 1977.
21. Bassingthwaighte, J. B., and Reuter, H. Calcium movements and excitation-contraction coupling in cardiac cells. In Electrical Phenomena in the Heart, W. C. DeMello (Ed.). Academic Press, New York, pp. 353-395, 1972.
22. Strong, C. G., and Bohr, D. F. Effects of prostaglandins E_1, E_2, A_1, and $F_{1\alpha}$ on isolated vascular smooth muscle. Amer. J. Physiol. 213:725-733, 1967.
23. Klaus, W., and Piccinini, F. Uber die Wirkung von Prostaglandin E_1 auf den Ca-Hautshalt isolierter Meerschwainchenherzen. Experientia 23:556-557, 1967.
24. Khairallah, P. A., Page, I. H., and Turker, R. K. Some properties of prostaglandin E_1 action on muscle. Arch. Int. Pharmacodyn. Ther. 169:328-341, 1967.
25. Kecskemeti, V., Kelemen, K., and Knoll, J. Effect of prostaglandin E_1 on the cardiac transmembrane potentials. Eur. J. Pharmacol. 24:289-295, 1973.
26. Kecskemeti, V., Kelemen, K., and Knoll, J. Microelectrophysiological analyses of the cardiac effect of prostaglandin E_2. Pol. J. Pharmacol. Pharm. 26:171-176, 1974.
27. Knoll, J. Celluline: a tissue substance with a highly specific cardiotonic activity. 3rd Int. Pharmacol. Congr. Abstr. Short Commun., Sao Paulo, p. 196, 1966.
28. Kelemen, K., Kecskemeti, V., Scultety, L., and Friedman, T. Activity index of frog heart ventricle cells: analyses of the correlation between resting potential and activity of the sodium carrier system in the frog heart by means of celluline and adranuline. Acta Physiol. Hung. 33:269-284, 1968.
29. deBoer, J., Houtsmuller, V. M. T., and Vergroesen, A. J. Inotropic effects on prostaglandins, fatty acids and adenosene phosphates on hypodynamic frog hearts. Prostaglandins 3:805-825, 1973.

30. Bydgeman, M. The effect of different prostaglandins on the human myometrium in vitro. Acta Physiol. Scand. 63(Suppl. 242):1-78, 1964.
31. Nakano, J. Effects of prostaglandins E_1, A_1 and $F_{2\alpha}$ on the coronary and peripheral circulation. J. Proc. Soc. Exp. Biol. Med. 127:1160-1163, 1968.
32. January, C. T., and Schottelius, B. A. Electrophysiologic and inotropic actions of prostaglandins $F_{2\alpha}$ in rat myocardium. Proc. Soc. Exp. Biol. and Med. 147:403-406, 1974.
33. Tuttle, R. S., and Skelly, M. M. Interactions of prostaglandin E_1 and ouabain on contractility of isolated rabbit atria and intracellular cation concentration. In Prostaglandin Symposium of the Worcester Foundation for Experimental Biology, P. W. Ramwell and J. E. Shaw (Eds.). Interscience, New York, pp. 309-320, 1967.
34. Nutter, D. O., and Ratts, T. Direct actions of prostaglandins E_1, A_1 and $F2\alpha$ on myocardial contraction. Prostaglandins 3:323-336, 1973.
35. Horton, E. W., and Main, I. H. M. Further observations on the central nervous actions of prostaglandins $F_{2\alpha}$ and E_1. Br. J. Pharmacol. Chemother. 30:568-581, 1967.
36. Alexander, R. W., Kent, K. M., Pisano, J. J., Keiser, H. R., and Cooper, T. Regulation of postocclusive hyperemia by endogenously synthesized prostaglandins in the dog heart. J. Clin. Invest. 55:1174-1181, 1975.
37. Hollenberg, M., Walker, R. S., and McCormick, P. O. Cardiovascular responses to intracoronary infusion of prostaglandin E_1, $F_{1\alpha}$ and $F_{2\alpha}$. Arch. Int. Pharmacodyn. 174:66-73, 1968.
38. Vergroesen, A. J., deBoer, J., and Gottenbos, J. J. Effects of prostaglandins on perfused isolated rat hearts. In Prostaglandins, G. Bergstrom and B. Samuelsson (Eds.). Interscience, New York, pp. 211-218, 1967.
39. Ogletree, M. L., Beardsley, A. C., and Lefer, A. M. Myocardial actions of prostaglandins in isolated cat cardiac tissue. Life Sci. 16:1923-1930, 1975.
40. Nakano, J. Effect of changes in coronary arterial blood flow on the myocardial contractile force. Jap. Heart J. 7:78-86, 1966.
41. Nakano, J., and McCurdy, J. R. Cardiovascular effects of prostaglandin E_1. J. Pharmacol. Exp. Ther. 156:538-547, 1967.
42. Bergstrom, S., Carlson, L. A., and Oro, L. Effect of prostaglandins on catecholamine induced changes in the free fatty acids in plasma and in blood pressure in the dog. Acta Physiol. Scand. 60:170-180, 1964.
43. Weeks, J. R. Introduction to cardiovascular research on prostaglandins. Adv. Prostaglandin Thromboxane Res. 1:395-401, 1976.
44. Limas, L., Constantinos, J., and Cohn, J. N. Isolation and properties of myocardial prostaglandin synthetase. Cardiovasc. Res. 7:623-628, 1973.
45. Levy, T. V., and Killebrew, E. Inotropic effects of prostaglandin E_2 on isolated cardiac tissue. Proc. Soc. Exp. Biol. Med. 136:1227-1231, 1971.

46. Krebs, R., and Schror, K. Actions of prostaglandin E_2 on myocardial mechanics, coronary vascular resistance and oxygen consumption in the guinea pig. Isolated heart preparation. Br. J. Pharmacol. 55:403-408, 1975.
47. Sabatini-Smith, B. Action of prostaglandins E_1 and $F_{2\alpha}$ on calcium flax in the isolated guinea pig atria and fragmented cardiac sarcoplasmic reticulum. Pharmacologist 12:239-245, 1970.
48. Antonaccio, M. J., and Lucchesi, B. R. The interaction of glucogen with theophylline, PGE_1, isoproterenol, ouabain and $CaCl_2$ on dog isolated papillary muscle. Life Sci. 9:1081-1089, 1970.
49. Spereiakis, N., and Lehmkuhl, D. Insensitivity of cultured chick heart cells to autonomic agents and tetrodotoxin. Am. J. Physiol. 209:693-698, 1965.
50. Berti, F., Lentati, R., and Usardi, M. M. The species specificity of prostaglandin E_1 effects on isolated heart. Med. Pharmacol. Exp. 13: 233-240, 1965.
51. Euler, U. S. von. On the specific vasodilating and plain muscle stimulating substances from accessory genital glands in man and certain animals (prostaglandin and vesiglandin). J. Physiol. (Lond.) 88:213-234, 1936.
52. Mantegazza, P. La prostaglandina E_1 Come sostanza sensibilizzatrice per il calcio a livello del cuore isolato di cavia. Atti Accad. Med. Lomb. 20:66-79, 1965.
53. Sobel, B. E., and Robison, A. K. Activation of guinea pig myocardial adenyl cyclase by prostaglandins. Circulation 40(Suppl. III):III-189, 1969.
54. Katori, M., Takeda, K., and Imai, S. Effects of prostaglandin E_1 and $F_{2\alpha}$ on heart-lung preparation of the dog. Tohoku J. Exp. Med. 10: 67-72, 1970.
55. Nakano, J., and Cole, B. Effects of prostaglandins E_1 and $F_{2\alpha}$ on systemic, pulmonary and splenic circulation in dogs. Am. J. Physiol. 217:222-227, 1969.
56. Emerson, T. E., Jr., Kelks, G. W., Dougherty, R. M., Jr., and Hodgmen, R. E. Effects of prostaglandin E_1 and $F_{2\alpha}$ on venous return and other parameters in the dog. Am. J. Physiol. 200:243-249, 1971.
57. DuCharme, K. E., Weeks, J. R., and Montgomery, R. G. Studies on the mechanisms of hypertensive effect of prostaglandin $F_{2\alpha}$. J. Pharmacol. Exp. Ther. 160:1-10, 1968.
58. Wennmalm, A., and Hedqvist, P. Prostaglandin E_1 as inhibitor of the sympathetic neuroeffector system in rabbit heart. Life Sci. 9:931-937, 1970.
59. Schror, K. K., and Forester, W. Interactions between isoproterenol and prostaglandin E_2 in the dog heart in situ. Pol. J. Pharmacol. 26:143-149, 1974.
60. Kentera, D., Susic, D., and Zdravkovic, M. Effect of verapamil and

aspirin on experimental chronic hypoxic pulmonary hypertension and right ventricular hypertrophy in rats. Respiration 37:192-196, 1979.

61. Sehzor, K. The action of the dehydro derivatives of prostacyclin (6R)-PGI, and (6S)-PGI, on the heart and the coronary vasculature. Naunyn-Schmiedeberg's Arch. Pharmacol. 306:213-217, 1979.
62. Nakano, J. Metabolism of prostaglandin E_1 in kidney and lung. Fed. Proc. 29:746, 1970.
63. Piccinini, F., Pomarelli, P., and Chiarra, A. Further investigation on the mechanism of the inotropic action of prostaglandin E_1 in relation to the ion balance in the frog heart. Pharmacol. Res. Commun. 1:381-390, 1969.
64. Weeks, J. R., and Wingerson, F. Cardiovascular action of prostaglandin E_1 evaluated using unanesthetized relatively unrestrained rats. Fed. Proc. 23:327, 1964.
65. Holmes, S. W., Horton, E. W., and Main, I. H. M. The effect of prostaglandin E_1 on response of smooth muscle to catecholamines, angiotensin and vasopressin. Br. J. Pharmacol. 37:705-722, 1969.
66. Wennmalm, A. Studies on mechanisms controlling the secretion of neurotransmitters in the rabbit heart. Acta Physiol. Scand. 82:1-36, 1971.
67. Zijlstra, W. G., Brunsting, J. R., Ten Hoor, F., and Vergroesen, A. J. Prostaglandin E_1 and cardiac arrhythmia. Eur. J. Pharmacol. 18:392-395, 1972.
68. Mest, H. J., Schror, K., and Forester, W. Antiarrhythmic properties of PGE_2: preliminary results. Adv. Biosci. 9:385-393, 1973.
69. Mest, H. J., Blass, K. E., and Forester, W. Effect of archidonic, linoleic, enolenic and oleic acid on experimental arrhythmias in cat, rabbit and guinea pigs. Prostaglandins 14:163-172, 1977.
70. Bayer, B. L., and Forester, W. Actions of prostaglandin precursors and other unsaturated fatty acids on conduction time and refraction period in the cat heart in sites. Acta Biol. Med. Ger. 37:833-835, 1978.
71. Forester, W., Mest, H. J., and Mentz, P. The influence of $PGF_{2\alpha}$ on experimental arrhythmias. Prostaglandins 3:895-904, 1973.
72. Koss, M. C., and Nakano, T. Reflex bradycardia and hypotension produced by prostaglandin $F_{2\alpha}$ in the cat. Br. J. Pharmacol. 56:245-253, 1976.
73. Mest, H. J., Mentz, P., and Forester, W. Effect of prostaglandins on experimental arrhythmias. Pol. J. Pharmacol. Pharm. 26:151-158, 1974.
74. Mest, H. J., and Forester, W. Vergleich der antiarrhythmischen Wirkungen von PGA_1, and PGA_2, PGE_1, PGE_2, PGF_2 Am $BaCl_2$-arrhythmie Modell des wachen Kaninchens. Arch. Int. Pharmacodyn. Therap. 217:152-161, 1975.
75. Bergstrom, S., Eliasson, R., Euler, U. S. von, and Sjovall, J. Some biological effects of two crystalline prostaglandin factors. J. Acta Physiol. Scand. 45:133-144, 1959.

76. Bergstrom, S., Carlson, L. A., Ekelund, L. G., and Oro, L. Effect of prostaglandin E_1 on blood pressure, heart rate and concentration of free fatty acids of plasma in man. Proc. Soc. Exp. Biol. Med. 118: 110-112, 1965.
77. Vane, J. R. Adv. Prostaglandin Thromboxane Res. 2:791, 1976.
78. Weeks, J. R. The general pharmacology of prostacyclin PGI_2 (PGX): a new prostaglandin especially active on the cardiovascular system. Acta Biol. Med. Ger. 37:707-714, 1978.
79. TenHoor, F., deDeckere, E. A. M., Haddeman, E., Hornstra, G., and Vendelmans-Starrenburg, A. The production of prostaglandin I_2 in the heart and blood vessels and its physiological role in heart function and thromboregulation. Acta Biol. Med. Ger. 37:729-730, 1978.
80. Mest, H. J., and Forester, W. The antiarrhythmic action of prostacyclin (PGI_2) on acomtine induced arrhythmias in rats. Acta Biol. Med. Ger. 37:827-828, 1978.

9 Differential Actions of the Prostaglandins on the Pulmonary Vascular Bed

PHILIP J. KADOWITZ / ALBERT L. HYMAN / CARL A. GRUETTER* / ERNST WM. SPANNHAKE / Tulane University School of Medicine, New Orleans, Louisiana

STAN GREENBERG / University of South Alabama College of Medicine, Mobile, Alabama

In most organ systems so far studied, including the lung, the fatty acid precursor arachidonic acid, which is derived from the breakdown of phospholipids in cell membranes, is converted into the cyclic endoperoxide intermediates, PGG_2 and PGH_2, by a microsomal cyclooxygenase (7, 8, 23). The endoperoxide intermediates (PGG_2 and PGH_2) are then converted by specific terminal enzymes into primary prostaglandins (PG), thromboxane A_2 (TxA_2), or prostacyclin (PGI_2) (1, 5, 6, 8, 9, 22-24). The distribution and activity of terminal enzymes determine the pattern and relative quantities of vasoactive and bronchoactive products formed from endoperoxide intermediates in an organ system (10, 11, 24). Many reports indicate that the endoperoxide intermediate PGH_2, and the endoperoxide analogs PGE_2, $PGF_{2\alpha}$, and PGD_2, all increase pulmonary resistance in a variety of species (10, 12, 14-18, 28). In contrast, PGE_2 has dilator activity in the pulmonary circulation of fetal and neonatal animals (3). The pulmonary vascular effects of TxA_2 are uncertain, but this labile substance has potent smooth muscle-stimulating and platelet-aggregating activity and its breakdown product, TxB_2, has modest pressor activity in the pulmonary vascular bed (9, 19). In contrast to the effects of PGH_2, PGE_2, PGD_2, $PGF_{2\alpha}$, and TxB_2, the newly discovered product of arachidonic acid metabolism, PGI_2, has pulmonary vasodilator activity (9, 19). However, the effects arachidonic acid has on the pulmonary vascular bed are controversial. Arachidonic acid has been shown to increase pulmonary vascular resistance in a number of species when injected as a bolus and to contract isolated segments of rabbit intrapulmonary artery (4, 10, 12, 14, 15, 26, 27, 29). These responses were blocked by indomethacin, suggesting that in the lung, arachidonate, when administered as a bolus, is converted to vasoactive substances that have pulmonary vasoconstrictor and bronchoconstrictor activity (10, 12, 14, 15, 24, 26, 29). It has, however, recently been

*Present affiliation: Marshall University School of Medicine, Huntington, West Virginia

reported that arachidonic acid has depressor activity in the pulmonary circulation when the prostaglandin precursor is infused and that infusions of the precursor acid decreased pulmonary vascular resistance in the intact chest cat and dog (12, 14, 27). The purpose of the present chapter is to compare responses to the endoperoxide PGH_2, primary prostaglandins (PGE_2, $PGF_{2\alpha}$, and PGD_2), arachidonic acid, and prostacyclin (PGI_2) in the canine and feline pulmonary vascular bed. In addition, the effects of the prostaglandins and a PGH_2 analog on isolated intrapulmonary vessels are contrasted.

METHODS

The pulmonary vascular effects of PGH_2, primary prostaglandins, arachidonic acid, and prostacyclin were investigated in intact chest mongrel dogs unselected as to sex, weighing 14.2-26.8 kg. The dogs were anesthetized with pentobarbital sodium (30 mg/kg i.v.) and strapped to a Philips heart table in the supine position. A specially designed 20 F double-lumen balloon catheter was introduced through a jugular vein into the arterial branch of the left lower lung lobe under fluoroscopic guidance. A 1.5-mm Teflon catheter with its tip positioned about 2 cm distal to the tip of the perfusion catheter was used to monitor perfusion pressure in the lobar artery. Catheters with side holes near the tip were passed into the main pulmonary artery and femoral artery and into a small intrapulmonary vein and the left atrium transseptally. Precautions were taken to ensure that pressure measurements were made without wedging in veins 2-3 mm in diameter. Briefly, a 0.9-mm Teflon catheter with two side holes near the tip were passed through a 6-mm Teflon catheter that previously had been wedged in a small intrapulmonary vein. The 0.9-mm catheter was then withdrawn 1-3 cm from the wedge position until pressure dropped abruptly. The 0.9-mm catheter was fixed in place with a Cope adaptor after the large catheter had been withdrawn to the left atrium. These methods have been described in detail previously (12, 16). All vascular pressures were measured with Statham P23Db transducers zeroed at the level of the right atrium, and mean pressures were recorded on an oscilloscopic recorder (Model DR-12, Electronics for Medicine) or Grass Model 7 polygraph. After all catheters had been positioned and the dogs heparinized (1000 IU/kg i.v.) the balloon on the perfusion catheter was distended with 2-4 ml of 50% sodium diatrizoate (Hypaque Winthrop) until pressure in the lobar artery and small vein decreased to near left atrial pressure. The vascularly isolated left lower lobe was then perfused with a Sarns roller pump (Model 3500) with blood withdrawn from the right atrium. The pumping rate was adjusted so that mean pressure in the perfused lobar artery approximated mean pressure in the main pulmonary artery and thereafter was not changed during the experiment. The pumping rate averaged 245 ml/min. These dogs spontaneously breathed room air, or room air enriched with oxygen, through a cuffed endotracheal tube.

For studies in the feline pulmonary vascular bed of adult cats of either sex, weighing 2.3-4.1 kg, were anesthetized with pentobarbital sodium, 35 mg/kg i.v. and were strapped in the supine position to a Philips fluoroscopic table. The cats spontaneously breathed room air, or room air enriched with oxygen, through a cuffed endotracheal tube. A specially designed 5 or 6 F triple-lumen balloon perfusion catheter was passed under fluoroscopic guidance from an external jugular vein into the arterial branch to the left lower lung lobe. After the lobar artery was vascularly isolated by distension of the balloon cuff on the catheter, and the animals heparinized (1000 IU/kg i.v.), the lung was perfused with blood withdrawn from the femoral artery or vein through the catheter lumen immediately beyond the balloon cuff. Perfusion pressure in the lobar artery was measured through the third lumen, 5 mm distal to the perfusion port. The lobe was perfused with a Harvard Model 1210 peristaltic pump and the perfusion rate was adjusted so that arterial pressure in the perfused lobe approximated mean pressure in the main pulmonary artery and was not changed during an experiment. Flow rates in left lower lobe averaged 48 ± 4 ml/min. Left atrial pressure was measured with a transseptally placed 3 or 4 F Teflon catheter. Aortic pressure was measured with a 3 or 4 F catheter inserted into the aorta by way of a femoral artery. These procedures have been described recently (14). All vascular pressures were measured with Statham P23Db transducers zeroed at right atrial level, and mean pressures obtained by electronic integration were recorded on an Electronics for Medicine Model DR-12 recorder.

Bovine lungs were obtained from a local slaughterhouse. Upon removal from the animal they were placed in ice-cold physiologic saline solution (PSS) (see below) for immediate transport to the laboratory. Canine lungs were obtained via thoracotomy from adult mongrel dogs (14-23 kg) anesthetized with pentobarbital sodium (30-45 mg/kg i.v.). The dogs had received heparin (300-1000 IU/kg) and were exsanguinated via a catheter placed in the femoral artery just prior to lung removal. New Zealand white rabbits weighing 2.1-3.3 kg were sacrificed by cervical dislocation and exsanguination, and lungs were removed via thoracotomy.

Segments of intrapulmonary artery (IPA) and intrapulmonary vein (IPV) 1-5 cm in length were carefully dissected from the lung tissue. Rabbit IPA and IPV were 1.5-2.5 mm in diameter and consisted of the main lobal vessels. Bovine vessels were 4-5 mm in diameter and were probably second- to fourth-order branches of main lobar vessels. Vessel segments were removed indiscriminately from upper and lower lobes of the three species and were placed in PSS for preparation. The PSS consisted of (in millimolar): NaCl, 125; KCl, 2.7; $CaCl_2$, 1.8; glucose, 11; and Tris [tris(hydroxymethyl)-aminomethane, Sigma Trizma base buffer], 23.8. The pH was adjusted to 7.4 with a small quantity of 6 N HCl.

After removal of excess connective tissue, a helical strip (1.5-5 mm wide and 7-15 mm in length) was cut from each vascular segment. Cotton thread ties were fixed to both ends of each strip. By means of the ties, one end of each strip was anchored in the bottom of a 10-ml muscle bath and the other end was attached to a force-displacement transducer (Grass Model FT03C). Isometric force output was recorded on a Grass polygraph (Model 79D). In the muscle bath each strip was bathed by PSS maintained at 37 ± 0.5°C and bubbled continuously with 100% oxygen.

Resting loads on the vascular strips were (in grams): bovine IPA, 4; bovine IPV, 3; rabbit IPA, 1; rabbit IPV, 0.5; canine IPA, 3; and canine IPV, 2. These loads resulted in tensile stresses in IPA and IPV which approximate tangential stresses estimated to exist in the vascular wall in vivo. After a 2-hr equilibration period, each vascular strip was exposed to one of several vasoactive substances to determine a reference response. In most cases, a depolarizing potassium solution (127 mM K^+ was employed; 127 mM K^+ was similar to PSS except that the NaCl of the PSS was replaced with an equimolar concentration of KCl to increase the level of K^+ to 127 mM. Some bovine vessels were exposed to 10^{-7} M serotonin (5-HT). The magnitudes of contraction in bovine IPA and IPV elicited by this concentration of 5-HT and 127 mM K^+ were similar.

Bovine and canine vascular strips that did not respond to these vasoactive substances with an increased force output of at least 250 mg were not included in the study. Only those rabbit IPA and IPV that exhibited an increased force output of at least 100 and 50 mg, respectively, in response to 127 mM K^+ were used in the study.

Once responses to 127 mM K^+ or 10^{-7} M 5-HT reached maximum, the vascular strips were rinsed several times with PSS and, after returning to baseline, were allowed to remain in PSS for 1 hr. Strips were then exposed to one of the substances either as a single concentration or in a cumulative manner. After responses to the desired concentration reached maximum, the strips were rinsed with PSS and allowed to return to baseline. After remaining in PSS for 1 hr, some of the strips were reexposed to the same substance, whereas others were exposed to 127 mM K^+ or 10^{-7} M 5-HT. When the cyclooxygenase inhibitor indomethacin was employed, it was added to the bathing media 30 min prior to and remained present during subsequent exposure of the strips to arachidonic acid (AA) or the analog.

Arachidonic acid (NuChek) 99% pure and indomethacin (Merck) were freshly prepared as sodium salts: arachidonic acid in 10% ethanol in 100 mM sodium carbonate and indomethacin in 100 mM sodium carbonate in normal saline. Prostaglandins D_2, E_2, and $F_{2\alpha}$ and the PGH_2 analog (Upjohn) were dissolved in absolute ethanol and stored at -20°C. Working solutions were freshly prepared in saline. PGI_2 was prepared in 20 mM Tris buffer, pH 8.5, and was stored in a freezer. PGH_2 was prepared in dry acetone and diluted in chilled saline and injected rapidly.

All values are expressed as the mean ± standard error of the mean unless otherwise indicated. Tests of significance for group and paired comparisons were done according to standard statistical methods (25). A p value of less than 0.05 was considered significant.

RESULTS

The effects of bolus injections of arachidonic acid and of primary prostaglandins on the pulmonary vascular bed in the intact chest dog and cat are illustrated in Figs. 1 and 2. All of the bisenoic PGs, the PGH_2 analog, and arachidonic acid increased lobar arterial pressure in the dog and cat. In the dog under conditions of controlled flow, $PGF_{2\alpha}$ is about tenfold more active than PGE_2, which in turn is about 10-20 times more active than arachidonic acid. In the dog the stable endoperoxide analog is about tenfold more active than $PGF_{2\alpha}$ (Fig. 1). Although not shown in Fig. 1, the pressor activities of $PGF_{2\alpha}$ and PGD_2 were quite similar. Arachidonic acid, $PGF_{2\alpha}$, PGD_2, and PGH_2 analog all increased transpulmonary pressure and small vein pressures in the dog. The effects of the PGH_2 analog on transpulmonary (airway) pressure and small vein pressure are shown in Fig. 3. In addition to increasing lobar arterial pressure, arachidonic acid increased airway resistance and decreased dynamic lung compliance and in this respect is similar to, but much less potent than, $PGF_{2\alpha}$, PGD_2, and the PGH_2 analog (26). The effects of arachidonic acid on the canine and feline pulmonary vascular beds were abolished after administration of indomethacin or meclofenamate, 2.5-5 mg/kg i.v.

In the intact chest cat, $PGF_{2\alpha}$ was a very potent vasoconstrictor agent in that pulmonary vascular resistance was nearly doubled at a dose of 10 ng

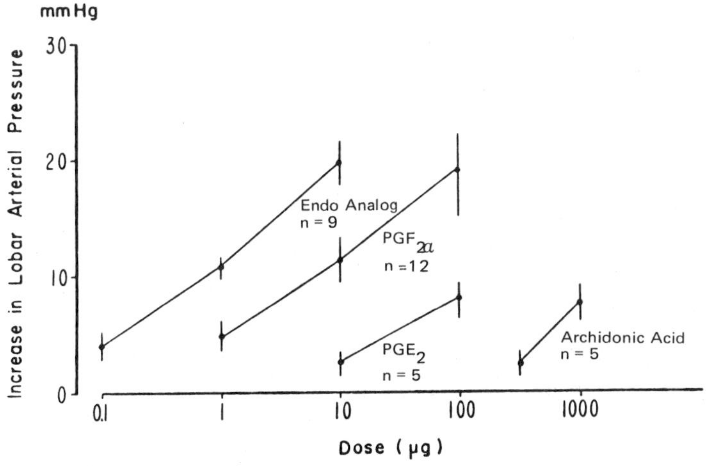

FIG. 1. Dose-response curves showing increases in lobar arterial pressure in response to graded doses of an endoperoxide (PGH_2) analog, $PGF_{2\alpha}$, PGE_2, and arachidonic acid in the intact chest dog. n indicates the number of animals studied and the blood flow to the left lower lobe was maintained constant with a pump. All substances were injected as a rapid bolus into the perfused lobar artery.

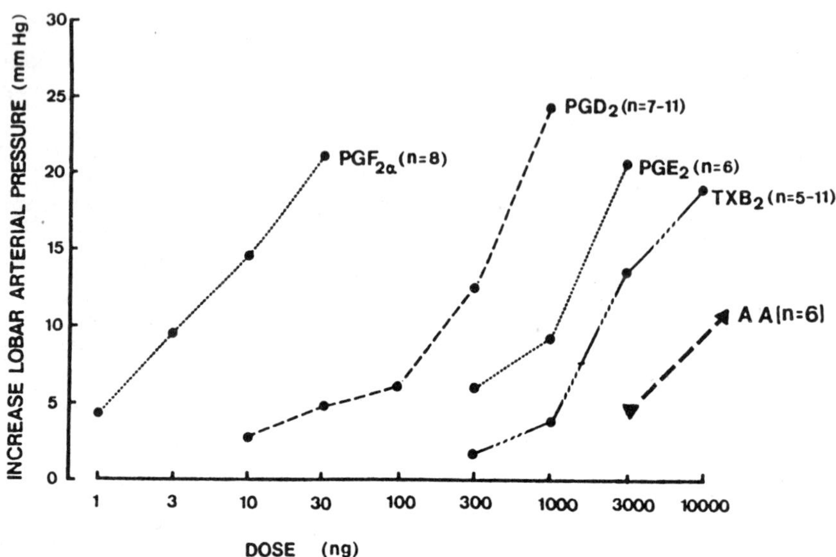

FIG. 2. Dose-response relationships comparing increased in lobar arterial pressure in response to bolus injections of graded doses of $PGF_{2\alpha}$, PGD_2, PGE_2, thromboxane (Tx) B_2, and arachidonic acid in the intact-chese cat. n indicates the number of animals studied. The blood flow to the left lower lobe was held constant with a pump.

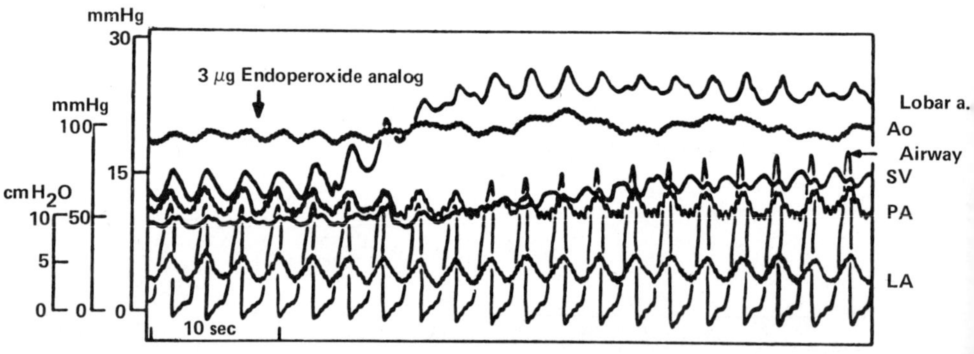

FIG. 3. Records from an experiment illustrating the effects of an endoperoxide analog on vascular pressures and translobar airway pressure in the dog. Blood flow to the left lower lobe was maintained constant with a pump and the endoperoxide analog was injected into the perfused lobar artery. Pressures in the lobar artery (lobar a), the pulmonary artery (PA), the small vein (SV), and the left atrium (LA) are on the 0-30 mmHg scale. Pressure in the aorta (Ao) is on the 0-100 mmHg scale and translobar (airway) pressure is on the 0-10 cm H_2O scale.

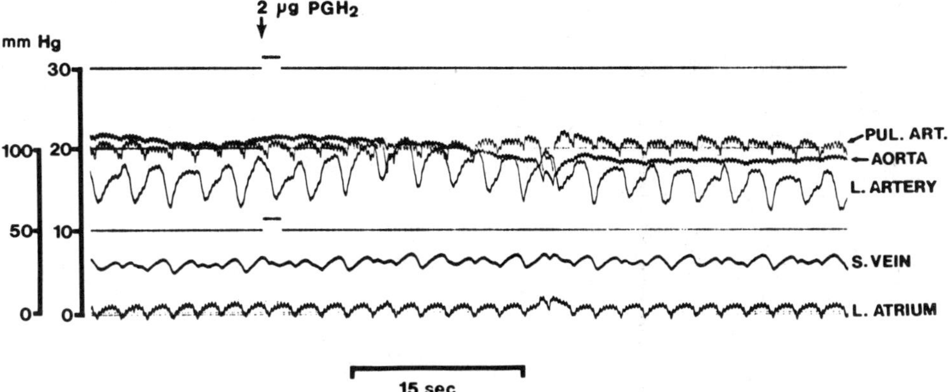

FIG. 4. Tracings from an experiment illustrating the effect of injection of a 2-μg bolus of PGH_2 on the canine pulmonary vascular bed under conditions of controlled pulmonary blood flow.

(Fig. 2). In the cat, PGD_2 was approximately 30 times less active than $PGF_{2\alpha}$, whereas PGE_2 was 100- to 300-fold less potent than $PGF_{2\alpha}$. Arachidonic acid, when administered as a rapid bolus, was threefold less active than PGE_2 (Fig. 2). Although not shown in Fig. 2, the stable PGH_2 analog was about threefold more active than $PGF_{2\alpha}$ in the intact chest cat. The effects of the endoperoxide PGH_2 on the canine pulmonary vascular bed are illustrated in Fig. 4. The endoperoxide itself, when injected as a 2-μg bolus into the perfused lobar artery, produced a modest increase in lobar arterial and

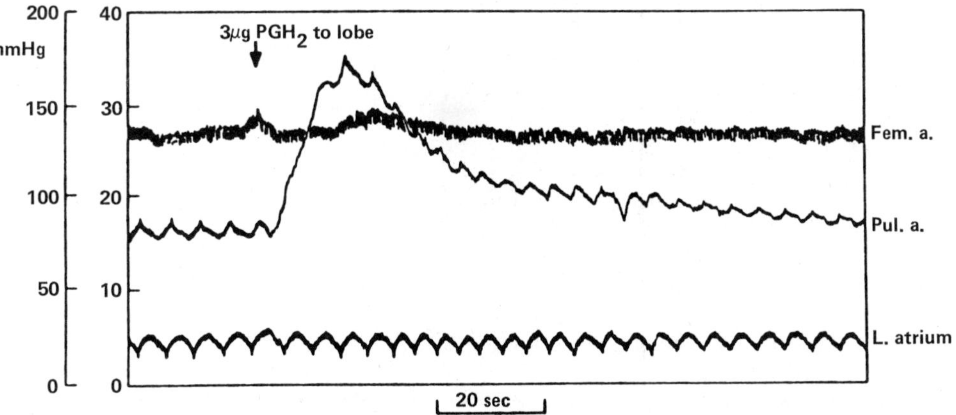

FIG. 5. Record from an experiment illustrating the effect of a bolus injection of 3 μg of PGH_2 into the feline pulmonary vascular bed when blood flow was maintained constant with a pump.

TABLE 1 Pulmonary Vasodilator Effects on PGI_2 Under Resting Conditions and When Pulmonary Vascular Resistance Is Enhanced by Infusion of an Enderoxide Analog[a]

	Pressure (mmHg SE)			
	Lobar artery	Small vein	Left atrium	Aorta
Control	15.9 ± 0.8	10.5 ± 0.6	1.8 ± 0.4	120 ± 5
PGI_2, 1-10 g	14.0 ± 1.0[b]	9.2 ± 0.6[b]	1.8 ± 0.4	99 ± 8[b]
	Infusion of 11α,9α-PGH_2 analog (1-5 μg/min)			
Control	31.5 ± 1.3	21.4 ± 1.0	1.7 ± 0.2	125 ± 1.5
PGI_2, 1-10 μg	25.1 ± 2.6[b]	17.1 ± 1.3[b]	1.6 ± 0.2	106 ± 5.2[b]

[a] n = 6.
[b] $p < 0.05$ when compared to corresponding control (paired comparison).

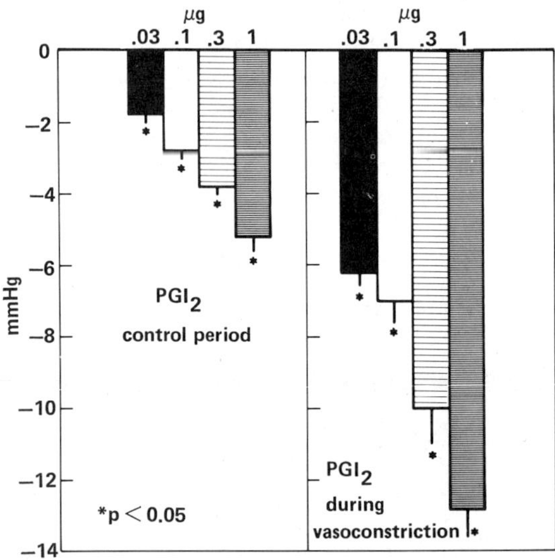

FIG. 6. Dose-response relationship showing decreases in lobar arterial pressure in response to bolus injections of PGI_2 under resting conditions and when lobar vascular resistance was increased by infusion of a PGH_2 analog. Blood flow to the lobe was held constant with a pump in the intact chest cat.

TABLE 2 Effects of Arachidonic Acid Infusion on the Pulmonary Vascular Bed When Tone Is Elevated[a]

	Lobar arterial pressure (mmHg)	
	Dog	Cat
Control	13.4 ± 0.5	14.5 ± 2.0
Tone enhanced	26.0 ± 1.5[b,c]	34.3 ± 2.7[b,d]
Arachidonate infusion	20.4 ± 0.8[b] (200 μg/min)	20.5 ± 0.8[b] (60–150 μg/min)

[a] n = 5 (dog), 4 (cat).
[b] $p < 0.05$ when compared to control, paired comparison.
[c] Tone enhanced by infusion of 15-methyl-$PGF_{2\alpha}$.
[d] Tone enhanced by infusion of an endoperoxide analog.

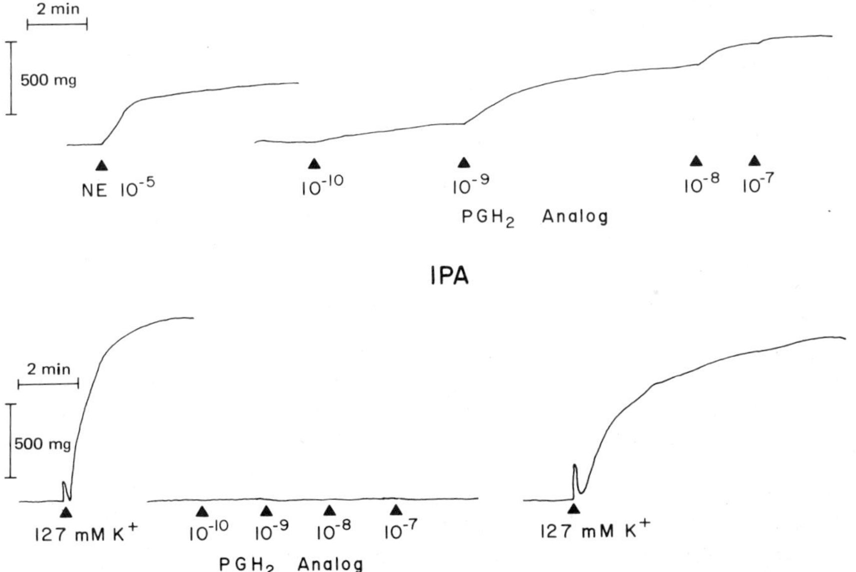

FIG. 7. Tracings from an experiment illustrating the effect of a PGH_2 analog on isometric force output in canine intrapulmonary artery (IPA) and canine intrapulmonary vein (IPV). Reference responses to norepinephrine (NE) 10^{-5} M in the vein and 127 mM K^+ in the artery are shown in the figure.

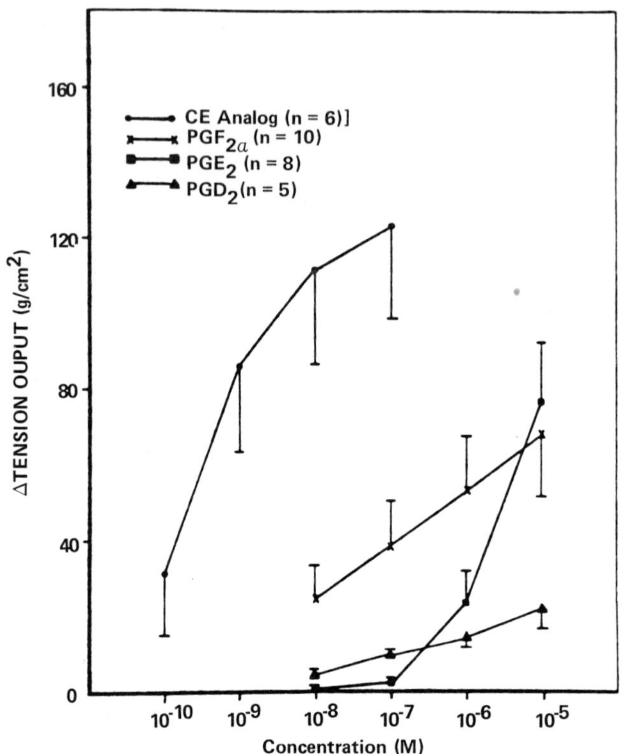

FIG. 8. Dose-response relationships for a PGH_2 (CE) analog, $PGF_{2\alpha}$, PGE_2, and PGD_2 on isometric tension in canine intrapulmonary vein (IPV). The vasoactive substances were added to the bath in a cumulative manner. n indicates the number of strips.

small vein pressures and decreased aortic pressure in the dog. The endoperoxide PGH_2 was far less active than its stable analogs in increasing pulmonary vascular resistance in the dog. The endoperoxide PGH_2 also had modest pressor activity in the feline pulmonary vascular bed, where it was approximately 100-fold less active than its stable analogs (Fig. 5).

In contrast to the effects of primary prostaglandins, PGH_2, and stable PGH_2 analogs, the newly discovered prostaglandin PGI_2 had vasodilator activity in the pulmonary vascular bed. The vasodilator actions of PGI_2 in the canine pulmonary vascular bed are summarized in Table 1. PGI_2 produced small but significant reductions in lobar arterial and small vein pressures without affecting left atrial pressure. Although the effects of PGI_2 were quite modest under resting conditions when tone was low, they were greatly enhanced when pulmonary vascular resistance was increased by infusion of a stable PGH_2 analog (Table 1). In the feline pulmonary vascular bed,

PGI_2 caused small dose-related decreases in lobar arterial pressure without affecting left atrial pressure (Fig. 6). The pulmonary vasodilator effects of PGI_2 were also greatly enhanced in the cat when pulmonary vascular resistance was increased by infusion of a PGH_2 analog (Fig. 6).

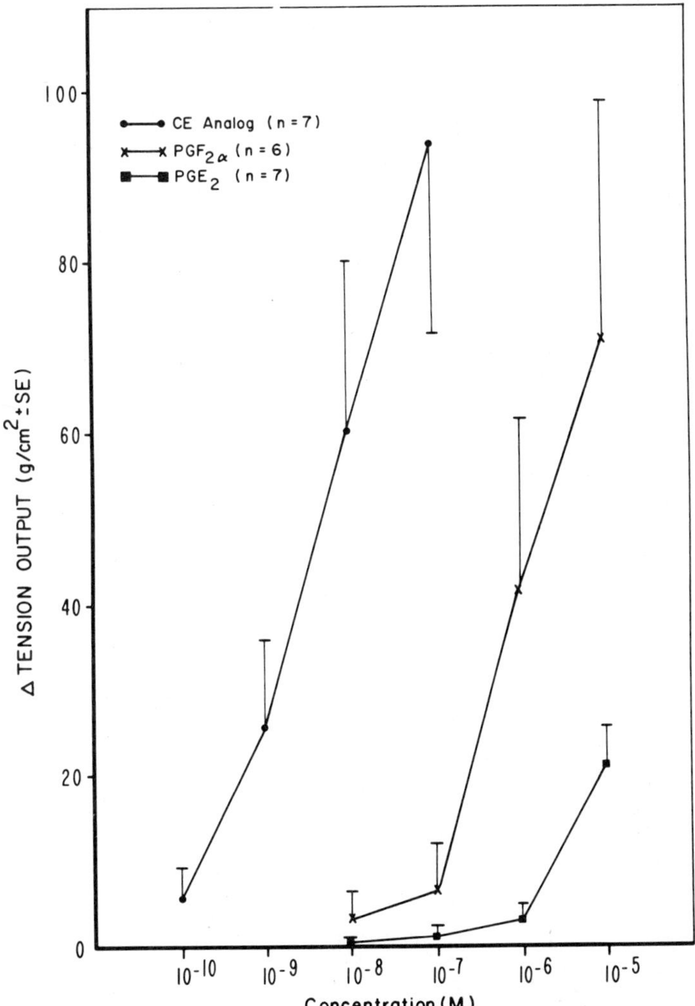

FIG. 9. Dose-response curves for a PGH_2 (CE) analog, $PGF_{2\alpha}$ and PGE_2 on isometric tension output in isolated bovine intrapulmonary vein (IPV). Dose-response curves were determined in a cumulative manner. n indicates the number of strips.

TABLE 3 Dose-Response Relationships for PGH_2 Analogs (I and II) in Isolated Canine Saphenous Vein[a]

	Concentration endoperoxide analog (M)				
	10^{-12}	10^{-11}	10^{-10}	10^{-9}	10^{-8}
Analog I (11α, 9α)	72[b]	76	81	87	95
Analog II (9α, 11α)	9	14	27	51	68

[a] n = 8.
[b] Percent reference response to norepinephrine (10^{-5} M).

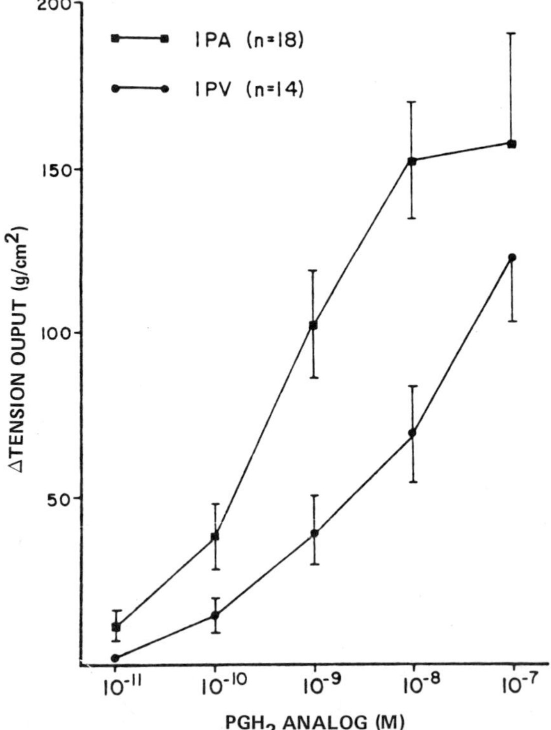

FIG. 10. Dose-response curves comparing the effects of a PGH_2 analog on isometric tension development in rabbit intrapulmonary artery (IPA) and vein (IPV). Dose-response curves were determined in a cumulative manner. n indicates the number of strips.

It has been reported that PGI_2 is the major product of arachidonic acid metabolism in isolated vascular tissue (22). However, when administered as a rapid bolus, arachidonic acid had pressor activity. It has also been reported that arachidonic acid decreases pulmonary vascular resistance in the cat and dog when administered by infusion (14, 27). The effects of infusions of arachidonic acid on the feline and canine pulmonary vascular beds are summarized in Table 2. In both species arachidonic acid had no significant dilator activity when pulmonary vascular resistance was at resting levels. However, when pulmonary vascular resistance was increased by infusion of a PGH_2 analog or 15-methyl-$PGF_{2\alpha}$, arachidonic acid infusions decreased lobar arterial pressure in the dog and in the cat (Table 2).

The effects of the PGH_2 analog, norepinephrine, and 127 mM K^+ on contractile activity in isolated intrapulmonary artery and vein from the dog are illustrated in Fig. 7. The PGH_2 analogs have marked smooth muscle-stimulating activity in canine intrapulmonary vein but had no activity in arterial segments of approximately the same size (Fig. 7). The contractile activities of the PGH_2 analog, $PGF_{2\alpha}$, PGE_2, and PGD_2 on canine intrapulmonary vein are compared in Fig. 8. The PGH_2 analog was much more potent than the bisenoic prostaglandins. The PGH_2 analogs also had marked contractile activity in isolated canine saphenous vein (Fig. 9 and Table 3) and in bovine intrapulmonary vessels. The effects of the bisenoic prostaglandins and a PGH_2 analog on bovine intrapulmonary vein are illustrated in Fig. 10. The PGH_2 analog has marked stimulating activity in the bovine vein, whereas PGD_2, $PGF_{2\alpha}$, and PGE_2 were less active (Fig. 9). All of these substances also had stimulatory activity in bovine intrapulmonary arterial segments. In rabbit intrapulmonary vessels the PGH_2 analogs had significant stimulatory activity in both intrapulmonary artery and vein (Fig. 10). The analog had greater activity in the artery than in the vein (Fig. 10), and PGE_2, $PGF_{2\alpha}$, and PGD_2 had significant contractile activity in both rabbit artery and vein. The activities of PGD_2 and the PGH_2 analogs were equal in rabbit intrapulmonary vein.

DISCUSSION

Results of the studies described above show that when injected as a rapid bolus, the prostaglandin precursor arachidonic acid increases lobar arterial pressure in the intact dog and cat. Inasmuch as pulmonary blood flow was held constant and left atrial pressure was unchanged, the rise in lobar arterial pressure reflects an increase in pulmonary vascular resistance in both species. The primary prostaglandins (PGE_2, PGD_2, and $PGF_{2\alpha}$), as well as PGH_2 and a stable PGH_2 analog, all increase pulmonary vascular resistance in the dog and cat (10, 12, 15-18, 26, 28, 29). In the dog, in addition to increasing lobar arterial pressure, arachidonic acid, the bisenoic prostaglandins, and the PGH_2 analogs all increase small intrapulmonary vein pressure (12, 16-18). The increases in lobar arterial and small vein pressures suggest that these substances increase pulmonary vascular resistance by constricting intrapulmonary veins and upstream segments believed to be small arteries. The PGH_2 analog had marked contractile activity on isolated segments of intrapulmonary vein from the dog, cow, and rabbit, suggesting that in these species, increases in venous pressure would be expected to increase capillary hydrostatic pressure. This would increase the amount of fluid leaving the capillary bed and may interfere with gas exchange and lead to pulmonary edema. The bisenoic prostaglandins were less effective than the PGH_2 analogs but still had a significant effect on contractile activity of intrapulmonary veins. The PGH_2 analogs and bisenoic prostaglandins also had contractile activity on canine saphenous vein, suggesting that substances could have effects on venous pressures in the peripheral vascular bed.

Arachidonic acid also increased transpulmonary pressure when the lung was ventilated at constant volume with a positive pressure ventilator (12). In experiments in which the effects of archidonic acid on lung function were investigated further, the increase in transpulmonary pressure was associated with a transient rise in lung resistance and a sustained fall in dynamic compliance (26). The endoperoxide analog, $PGF_{2\alpha}$, and PGD_2 all increased lung resistance and decreased dynamic compliance and in this regard were similar to, but much more potent than, arachidonic acid (26, 28). The effects of PGE_2 on the pulmonary vascular bed and on the airways were modest when this substance was injected in the same doses as PGD_2 or $PGF_{2\alpha}$ (12, 15, 18, 26). Pulmonary vasoconstrictor, bronchoconstrictor, and systemic vasodepressor responses to arachidonic acid were blocked after administration of indomethacin, a cyclooxygenase inhibitor (10-12, 15, 26). These data suggest that the effects of arachidonic acid on the airways, pulmonary, and peripheral vascular beds are due to the conversion of the substrate into vasoactive and bronchoactive metabolites in the cyclooxygenase pathway. The pulmonary vasoconstrictor response to arachidonic acid is associated with increased synthesis of E- and F-like prostaglandins; however, it is not known if PGD_2 or TxB_2 are produced by the lung in the intact dog (12). The effects of arachidonic acid on the pulmonary vascular bed were not dependent on the presence of platelets or other formed elements, in that the response to arachidonic acid was not diminished when the lung was perfused with a dextran solution (12). These findings suggest that the substrate is converted to vasoactive substances by the lung itself and that platelet aggregation or release of vasoactive products from the platelets plays little or no role in this response (12).

In contrast to the pressor effects of $PGF_{2\alpha}$, PGD_2, and PGE_2, or the PGH_2 analog, which may mimic the effects of TxA_2 on the pulmonary vascular bed, the newly discovered bicyclic prostaglandin PGI_2 had vasodilator activity in the canine and feline pulmonary vascular beds (13, 20). The pulmonary vasodilator effects of PGI_2 were modest under resting conditions but were greatly enhanced when pulmonary vascular resistance was increased actively by infusion of a vasoconstrictor substance (13). Although PGI_2 had vasodilator activity, arachidonic acid, when administered as a bolus, consistently increased pulmonary vascular resistance in the intact dog and cat and in the isolated dog lung (10,12,15,26,29). These results suggest that under physiologic conditions in the intact state, the predominant products formed in the lung when arachidonate is injected as a bolus are vasoconstrictor in nature. Alternatively, it is possible that both vasoconstrictor and vasodilator metabolites are formed but that the activity of the vasoconstrictors overshadows the action of any simultaneously formed PGI_2-like substances. It has been reported that PGI_2 is the predominant metabolite formed from arachidonic acid and endoperoxide intermediates in vascular tissue (2,5,22). Indeed, we have observed that slow infusions of arachidonic acid decrease lobar vascular resistance in the intact dog and cat. However, this vasodilator effect is observed only when pulmonary vascular tone is enhanced. The explanation for the divergent responses to rapidly injected arachidonic acid and slowly infused arachidonic acid are uncertain at the present time. It is, however, possible that when excessive amounts of substrate are converted to PGH_2, the endothelial prostacyclin synthetase may be overwhelmed and the endoperoxide may isomerize to PGD_2 and PGE_2 or be reduced to $PGF_{2\alpha}$.

We have reported that administration of cyclooxygenase inhibitors such as indomethacin and meclofenamate results in a slow gradual increase in pulmonary vascular resistance in the intact dog (21). It has been shown that a PGI_2-like substance is continually released by the lung (6). We have, therefore, suggested that under resting conditions, the pulmonary vascular bed is maintained in a dilated state by production of a vasodilator product in the cyclooxygenase pathway (10,21). Recent evidence suggests that this vasodilator product in the cyclooxygenase pathway is a PGI_2-like substance (6, 13,20).

REFERENCES

1. Anggard, E., and Samuelsson, B. Prosynthesis of prostaglandins from arachidonic acid in guinea pig lung. J. Biol. Chem. 240:3518-3521, 1965.
2. Bunting, S., Gryglewski, R., Moncada, S., and Vane, J. R. Arterial walls generate from prostaglandin endoperoxides a substance (prostaglandin X) which relaxes strips of mesenteric and coeliac arteries and inhibits platelet aggregation. Prostaglandins 12:897-913, 1976.
3. Cassin, S., Tyler, T., Leffler, C., and Wallis, R. Pulmonary and systemic vascular responses of perinatal goats to prostaglandins E_1 and E_2. Am. J. Physiol. 236:H828-H832, 1979.
4. Gruetter, C. A., McNamara, D. B., Hyman, A. L., and Kadowitz, P. J. Contractile responses of intrapulmonary vessels from three species to arachidonic acid and an epoxymethano analog of PGH_2. Can. J. Physiol. Pharmacol. 56:206-215, 1978.

5. Gryglewski, R. J., Bunting, S., Moncada, S., Flower, R. J., and Vane, J. R. Arterial walls are protected against deposition of platelet thrombi by a substance (prostaglandin X) which they make from prostaglandin endoperoxides. Prostaglandins 12:685-713, 1976.
6. Gryglewski, R. J., Korbut, R., Ocetkiewicz, A., Spawinski, J., Wojtaszek, B., and Swies, J. Lungs as a generator of prostacyclin—Hypothesis on physiological significance. Naunyn-Schmiedebergs Arch. Pharmacol. 304:45-50, 1978.
7. Hamberg, M., Svensson, J., Wakabayshi, T., and Samuelsson, B. Isolation and structure of two prostaglandin endoperoxides that cause platelet aggregation. Proc. Natl. Acad. Sci. USA 71:345-349, 1974.
8. Hamberg, M., and Samuelsson, B. Prostaglandins endoperoxides: VII. Novel transformations of arachidonic acid in guinea pig lung. Biochem. Biophys. Res. Commun. 61:942-949, 1974.
9. Hamberg, M., Svensson, J., and Samuelsson, B. Thromboxanes: a new group of biologically active compounds derived from prostaglandin endoperoxides. Proc. Natl. Acad. Sci. USA 72:2994-2998, 1975.
10. Hyman, A. L., Chapnick, B. M., Kadowitz, P. J., Lands, W. E. M., Crawford, C. G., Fried, J., and Barton, J. Unusual pulmonary vasodilator activity of a novel prostacyclin analog: comparison with endoperoxides and other prostanoids. Proc. Natl. Acad. Sci. USA 12:5711-5715, 1977.
11. Hyman, A. L., Kadowitz, P. J., Lands, W. E. M., Crawford, C. G., Fried, J., and Barton, J. Coronary vasodilator activity of 13,14-dehydroprostacyclin methyl ester: comparison with PGI_2 and other prostanoids. Proc. Natl. Acad. Sci. USA 75:3522-3526, 1978.
12. Hyman, A. L., Mathe, A. A., Matthews, C. C., Bennett, J. T., Spannhake, E. W., and Kadowitz, P. J. Modification of pulmonary vascular responses to arachidonic acid by alterations in physiologic state. J. Pharmacol. Exp. Ther. 207:388-401, 1978.
13. Hyman, A. L., and Kadowitz, P. J. Pulmonary vasodilator activity of prostacyclin (PGI_2) in the intact cat. Circ. Res. 45:404-409, 1979.
14. Hyman, A. L., Spannhake, E. W., and Kadowitz, P. J. Divergent actions of archidonic acid on the feline pulmonary vascular bed. Am. J. Physiol. 239:H40-H46, 1980.
15. Kadowitz, P. J., Spannhake, E. W., Feigen, L. P., Greenberg, S., and Hyman, A. L. Comparative effects of arachidonic acid, bisenoic prostaglandins and an endoperoxide analog on the canine pulmonary vascular bed. Can. J. Physiol. Pharmacol. 55:1369-1377, 1977.
16. Kadowitz, P. J., and Hyman, A. L. Influences of a prostaglandin endoperoxide analog on the canine pulmonary vascular bed. Circ. Res. 40:282-287, 1977.
17. Kadowitz, P. J., Gruetter, C. A., McNamara, D. B., Gorman, R. R., Spannhake, E. W., and Hyman, A. L. Comparative effects of the endoperoxide PGH_2 and an analog on the pulmonary vascular bed. J. Appl. Physiol. 42:953-958, 1977.

18. Kadowitz, P. J., Joiner, P. D., and Hyman, A. L. Effects of prostaglandins E_2 on pulmonary vascular resistance in intact dog, swine and lamb. Eur. J. Pharmacol. 31:72-80, 1975.
19. Kadowitz, P. J., and Hyman, A. L. Comparative effects of thromboxane B_2 on the canine and feline pulmonary vascular bed. J. Pharmacol. Exp. Ther. 213:300-305, 1980.
20. Kadowitz, P. J., Chapnick, B. M., Feigen, L. P., Hyman, A. L., Nelson, P. K., and Spannhake, E. W. Pulmonary and systemic vasodilator effects of the newly-discovered prostaglandin PGI_2. J. Appl. Physiol. 45:408-413, 1978.
21. Kadowitz, P. J., Chapnick, B. M., Joiner, P. D., and Hyman, A. L. Influences of inhibitors of prostaglandin synthesis on the canine pulmonary vascular bed. Am. J. Physiol. 299:941-946, 1975.
22. Moncada, R., Gryglewski, R., Bunting, S., and Vane, J. R. An enzyme isolated from arteries transforms prostaglandin endoperoxides to an unstable substance that inhibits platelet aggregation. Nature (Lond.) 263:663-665, 1976.
23. Nugteren, D. H., and Hazelhof, E. Isolation and properties of intermediates in prostaglandin biosynthesis. Biochim. Biophys. Acta 326: 448-461, 1973.
24. Pace-Asciak, C. R. Oxidative biotransformations of arachidonic acid. Prostaglandins 13:811-817, 1977.
25. Snedecor, G. W., and Cochran, W. G. Statistical Methods (6th Ed.), Iowa State University Press, Ames, Iowa, pp. 91-119, 1967.
26. Spannhake, E. W., Lemen, P. J., Wegmann, M. J., Hyman, A. L., and Kadowitz, P. J. Effects of arachidonic acid and prostaglandins on lung function in the intact dog. J. Appl. Physiol. 44:397-495, 1978.
27. Spannhake, E. W., Hyman, A. L., and Kadowitz, P. J. Dependence of the airway and pulmonary vascular effects of arachidonic acid upon route and rate of administration. J. Pharmacol. Exp. Ther. 212:584-590, 1980.
28. Wasserman, M. A., DuCharme, E. W., Griffin, R. L., DeGraaf, G. L. and Robinson, F. G. Bronchopulmonary and cardiovascular effects of prostaglandins D_2 in the dog. Prostaglandins 13:255-269, 1977.
29. Wicks, T. C., Rose, J. C., Johnson, M., Ramwell, P. W., and Kot, P. A. Vascular response to arachidonic acid in the perfused canine lung. Circ. Res. 38:167-171, 1976.

10 Prostaglandins and the Platelet Prostanoid Compounds

GESINA L. LONGENECKER / University of South Alabama College of Medicine, Mobile, Alabama

Platelets, which are circulating pieces of megakaryocyte cytoplasm (Harker, 1974), are excitable. The most familiar excitable responses are adhesion, which generally refers to the sticking of platelets to anything but other platelets (e.g., glass, blood vessel subendothelium, or surfaces of prosthetic valves), and aggregation, which usually refers to the sticking of platelets to each other. Both adhesion and aggregation are involved in the formation of platelet plugs or white thrombi at sites of vascular injury, and account in part for the role of platelets in a tremendous range of activities, from primary hemostasis to maintenance of blood vessel integrity, and even to atherogenesis and the initiation of transient ischemic attack.

Although the processes of adhesion and aggregation occur in vivo, they are simplest to quantitate in vitro. Aggregation is presently more frequently studied than adhesion. The most commonly used method for studying the aggregation process is based on the turbidometric (light transmission) method first described by Born (1962), and subsequently reviewed by O'Brien (1971), Attar et al. (1973), and others. Much of the discussion in the rest of this chapter of the effects of various compounds on the aggregation process is based on results obtained using this methodology.

Some stimuli which can elicit platelet aggregation in vivo and in vitro include adenosine diphosphate (ADP), epinephrine, collagen, and thrombin, although a number of other agents also cause aggregation (e.g., ristocetin, some sepharoses, and mechanical stimuli). If the stimulus is mild, aggregation may persist for only a short while and then regress. The process is reversible aggregation. However, if the stimulus is sufficiently strong, a reaction is triggered within the platelets, accompanied by tight coalescence of the platelets, so-called irreversible aggregation. The reaction that is triggered is the release reaction, appropriately named because during it a host of compounds are released, or are formed and released, into the surrounding medium. Among the compounds that may be released are ADP and serotonin (from dense bodies), lysosomal enzymes, platelet coagulation factors, and mitogenic substance (from α granules). Several excellent reviews and monographs describe the phenomenology of aggregation, effects of various stimulators, release of the compounds above, the involvement of platelets in the initiation and complications of disease, and the pharmacology of platelet function. A few of them are: Weiss (1972, 1976, 1978); Mustard and Packham (1970, 1975); Mustard et al. (1977); Packham and Mustard (1977); Mannuci and Gorini (1972); Caprino and Rossi (1974); de Gaetano and Garattini (1978); and Gordon (1976). Details of platelet structures may be found in White (1979).

Other compounds that may be released are not in storage but rather are synthesized de novo; these include the prostaglandins, the thromboxanes, and their precursor endoperoxides. These compounds as a group will be referred to as the prostanoid compounds. There are also several review articles which deal at least in part with this latter with respect to platelets: Smith et al. (1976a); Samuelsson et al. (1975, 1976, 1978); Gorman (1978); Harris et al. (1979); and Malmsten (1979). It is the purpose of this chapter to examine the prostanoid synthetic capabilities of platelets and also the consequences of these capabilities with respect to platelets themselves.

ASPECTS OF NOMENCLATURE IN BRIEF

The alphabetic designation of the prostaglandins (PG) is a function of the substitutions occurring on the cyclopentane ring of the basic structure (see Fig. 1), especially at positions 9 and 11 [e.g., A = 9-keto, 10-11 unsaturation; D = 9-hydroxy, 11-keto; E = 9-keto, 11-hydroxy; F_a = 9,11-keto; G and H = 9,11-dioxygen bridge (9,11-epoxy), or endoperoxide]. The numerical designation is primarily a function of the degree of unsaturation of the side chains. An exception occurs with the endoperoxides, where the alphabetic designation changes for side chain differences (PGG_2 = 15-OOH; PGH_2 = 15-hydroxy). Prostaglandins and thromboxanes may originate from more than one substrate: those with one double bond in the side chain (e.g., PGE_1) are formed from dihomo-γ-linolenic acid (8,11,14-eicosatrienoic acid), and those with two double bonds from arachidonic acid (5,8,11,14-eicosatetraenoic acid). Compounds with three double bonds are not found in significant quantities because of the extremely low occurrence of the precursor 5,8,11,14,17-eicosapentaenoic acid, although the formation of thromboxane A_3 by human platelet microsomes supplied with this substrate has been noted (Needleman, 1976a). Figure 1 has been numbered for reference to the nomenclature. The nomenclature and structure have recently been reviewed in detail by Gorman (1978).

FORMATION OF PROSTAGLANDINS AND RELATED COMPOUNDS BY PLATELETS

The ability of many tissues to convert fatty acids into prostaglandins has been known for nearly 20 years. The observation that prostaglandins of the E series were able to alter platelet responses to aggregating agents (Kloeze, 1967; Emmons et al., 1967) led Clausen and Srivastava (1972) to examine whether there was production of PGs from labeled acetate and other precursors by platelet suspensions. They found that platelets provided with precursor materials were capable of forming PGs, with those identified being PGEs (PGE_1 and PGE_2). The amount of label incorporated into PGs approximated 10%. Platelets possess a cytoplasmic system for de novo fatty acid synthesis (malonyl CoA, fatty acid synthetase, etc.), unlike other formed elements of blood (Karpatkin, 1977), which probably accounts for at least some of the label incorporation, while some incorporation probably occurs as a result of chain lengthening of fatty acids already present. The PGs are short-lived in the circulation because of rapid clearance by the lung (Flower, 1977). Thus Clausen and Srivastava concluded that the production of PG by platelets in the circulation could be of importance.

Subsequent to the observation that platelets could produce PG from acetate, Silver et al. (1973) demonstrated that exposure of platelets to arachidonic acid resulted in both PG production and aggregation. (It should be noted that PG alone, i.e., added exogenously, never resulted in aggregation; PG simply modified the response to aggregating agents such as ADP.) Smith et al. (1973) demonstrated the formation of PGE_2 and $PGF_{2\alpha}$ by platelets responding to ADP, epinephrine, or collagen. A number of other prostaglandins have subsequently been found to be released from platelets under varying conditions, including $F_{1\alpha}$ and $F_{2\alpha}$ (Patrono et al., 1975), D_1 (Falardeau et al., 1976), and D_2 (Smith et al., 1976b).

Shortly after the capability of PG production was identified, another compound of interest was identified and shown to be produced by platelets from arachidonic acid. This was labile aggregation-stimulating substance (LASS) (Willis, 1973, 1974; Willis and Kuhn, 1973). LASS was subsequently shown to be an endoperoxide precursor of the PGs (Willis et al., 1974b). The halflife of LASS was about 2 min at pH 7.6 and room temperature. Unlike the PGs, LASS alone could directly induce aggregation. PGE_1 could lessen LASS aggregation, and PGE_2 could increase it. Willis et al. therefore concluded that LASS and PGE_2 acting in concert might be responsible for aggregation, with release induced by such already described agents as ADP or collagen. Willis did not exclude the possibility that the endoperoxide was contaminated with some other, also active, compound(s), since the techniques for identification were not direct chemical ones. Vargaftig and Zirinis (1973) also identified the existence of a compound(s) distinct from the PG formed during arachidonic acid-induced aggregation. Hamberg et al. (1974) succeeded in isolating two compounds, characterized as endoperoxides, and given the designation PGG_2 and PGH_2. The existence of these intermediates had actually been suspected by Samuelsson (1965) for nearly 10 years on the basis of oxygen labeling experiments.

Further elaboration of the pathways in arachidonic acid conversion occurred subsequently. Hamberg and Samuelsson (1974) showed that arachidonic acid undergoes conversion via two parallel pathways: one by way of a lipoxygenase, with conversion to hydroxyeicosatetraenoic acid (HETE), the other by way of cyclooxygenase, with conversion to endoperoxides, and eventually several end products, some of which were novel. These previously unidentified conversions proved to be of great interest.

An end product of the cyclooxygenase pathway, in fact the major metabolite of PGG_2, was shown to be thromboxane B_2 (TxB_2) (Hamberg and Samuelsson, 1974). Hamberg et al. (1975) then demonstrated the existence of an intermediate step in the conversion of PGG_2 to TxB_2. The complete conversion sequence was from PGG_2 to thromboxane A_2 (TxA_2), a highly unstable intermediate, and then to TxB_2. TxA_2, like the endoperoxides, proved to be a potent aggregator of platelets (and a potent vasoconstrictor), whereas TxB_2 was inactive in this respect. Indeed, because of the rapid (about 30 sec) conversion of endoperoxides to TxA_2, and also because of dose-response/time-action data for aggregation of indomethacin (a cyclooxygenase inhibitor)-treated platelets by small quantities of untreated platelets in the process of aggregating after addition of arachidonic acid, Hamberg et al. (1975) and Svensson et al. (1976) concluded that it is TxA_2 that is predominantly responsible for platelet aggregation. The role of TxA_2 in aggregation has since been questioned, subsequent to the development of some specific inhibitors of various steps in the pathways, as is discussed in a later section. A scheme for the conversion of arachidonic acid to some of its various end products is given in Fig. 1. Inhibitors, which are discussed in the next section, are indicated in the figure.

Although it is not formed by the platelets themselves, one other compound needs to be mentioned at least—prostacyclin. The prostaglandin endoperoxides are converted by blood vessel microsomes into a unique, unstable, prostanoid compound called prostacyclin (originally PGX, now PGI_2) (Moncada et al., 1976a,b; Gryglewski et al., 1976). PGI_2, in addition to its unique structure, also has unique properties: it is a potent inhibitor of platelet aggregation induced by various agents,

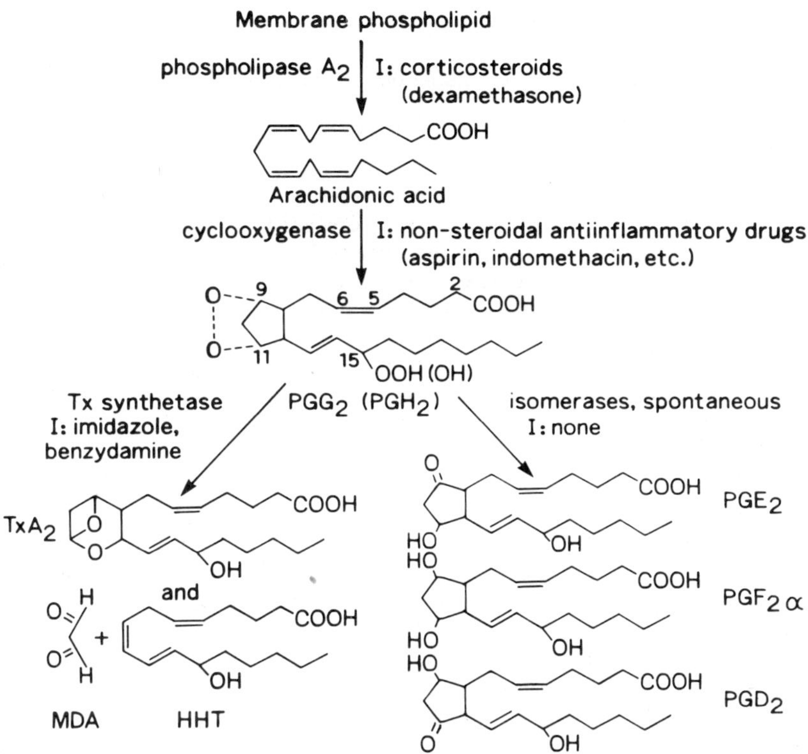

FIG. 1. Some steps in the conversion of arachidonic acid to active products by platelets. PGG_2 and PGH_2, endoperoxides; PG, prostaglandins; TxA_2, thromboxane A_2; MDA, malondialdehyde; HHT, 12L-hydroxy-5, 8, 10-heptadecanoic acid; I, inhibitor(s). (Data from Moncada and Vane, 1978, 1979; Diczfalusy et al., 1977; Hammarstrom and Falardeau, 1977; Gorman, 1978.)

and is also a vasodepressor. It has been demonstrated that vascular endothelium synthesizes the major portion of PGI_2, although other layers also synthesize some PGI_2 (decreases from endothelium toward adventitia) (Moncada et al., 1977b). The synthesis of PGI_2 can proceed from endogenously derived substrate (e.g., Bunting et al., 1976a; Dembinska-Kiec et al., 1977; Silberbauer et al., 1978), from added arachidonate or endoperoxides (e.g., Bunting et al., 1976a; Weksler et al., 1977), or perhaps even from endoperoxides being formed and released by platelets (Moncada et al., 1976a,b; Gryglewski et al., 1976; summary, Moncada and Vane, 1978, 1979). There is evidence, however, to indicate that platelet endoperoxides may only be available for conversion to PGI_2 when their conversion to TxA_2 by the platelets is inhibited (Needleman et al., 1979a). The effects of PGI_2 on platelets are discussed in greater detail in a subsequent section.

ENZYME SYSTEMS

Platelets possess "prostaglandin synthetase" activity, which was resolved by Miyamoto et al. (1974) for bovine seminal vesicles into a system that converts arachidonate to unstable endoperoxides (the cyclooxygenase) and a second system, which converts endoperoxides to PGE_2 (an isomerase). The cyclooxygenase of platelets is similar to that of other systems; hence further discussion will be confined primarily to conversions of the endoperoxides, i.e., to thromboxane synthetase (synthase), and to isomerase(s).

Cyclooxygenase

The cyclooxygenase of platelets has been reported to be microsomal and has been separated from thromboxane synthetase activity by solubilization (Triton X-100) and DEAE Sephadex chromatography (Hammarstrom and Falardeau, 1977). White and Glassman (1976), however, have reported a major portion of this activity in fractions sedimenting at less than 10,000g, which may represent an outcome of technique differences. White and Glassman found arachidonate and dihomo-γ-linolenate (DHgL) to be competitive substrates for the cyclooxygenase. This is of interest because of the reports of Willis et al. (1974a) and Farrow and Willis (1975) that DHgL can suppress platelet aggregation when given either in vivo or in vitro. These findings suggest that the endoperoxides formed from DHgL are incapable (or less capable) of inducing aggregation (although the possibility of effect from PGE_1 should not be overlooked): this point is discussed further later.

Thromboxane Synthetase

Needleman et al. (1976b) have shown that an enzyme that is capable of converting endoperoxides to a TxA_2-like substance is microsomal, in both human and horse platelets. While examining the existence and properties of the enzyme, Needleman et al. also established a superfusion bioassay method using two tissues, rat stomach and rabbit aorta: both tissues respond to endoperoxides, whereas only the aorta responds to TxA_2. Similar assays have been based on the description by Bunting et al. (1976b) of the responses of rabbit mesenteric and coeliac arteries, which relax to endoperoxides but contract to TxA_2. The action of the endoperoxides and Txs on platelets is discussed in detail later. Hammarstrom and Falardeau (1977) also demonstrated that thromboxane synthetase is microsomal, and that it is separable from cyclooxygenase as described above.

Sun (1977) has devised a radiometric TLC (thin layer chromatography) assay for thromboxane synthetase obtained from platelet microsomes. Using it, he has defined some additional factors affecting the activity of Tx synthetase:

1. There is little pH dependence between 5 and 8.5, but pH $\geq$ 9 gives depression.
2. The enzyme distributes with membranes, with the highest activity in the microsomal fraction.
3. The specific activity of the enzyme was 5.7 nmol/min per mg protein. "Short" incubation times showed no conversion of PGH_2, whereas "long" ones resulted in production of PGs.
4. The enzyme is strongly inhibited by substrate analogs (e.g., 9,11-epoxymethanoprostanoic acid).
5. The enzyme is not inhibited by NSAID (nonsteroidal anti-inflammatory drugs), nor is it affected by azide, glutathione, the PGs, HETE, or TxB_2.

Sun also points out that aggregation of platelets by endoperoxides in platelet-rich plasma does not result in the formation of significant amounts of TxA_2, whereas aggregation of washed platelets by most agents, including endoperoxides, does. The role of plasma itself in regulating the availability (formation) of the Txs therefore remains unclear. Indeed, Smith et al. (1976c) have demonstrated a stabilizing effect of plasma on TxA_2 activity.

Needleman et al. (1976a) have shown that whereas arachidonate and DHgL, as well as some additional fatty acids, cause substrate-catalyzed destruction of cyclooxygenase, they have no effect on Tx synthetase. Ho et al. (1976) isolated in human platelet microsomes an enzyme system capable of generating an unstable aggregation factor and TxB_2 from arachidonic acid. They have shown TxB_2 (the stable breakdown product of TxA_2) synthesis to be dependent on methemoglobin (hemin, hematin) and tryptophan (catecholamines, 3-indoleacetic acid) as cofactors, although they were examining the enzyme system rather than an isolated thromboxane synthetase activity.

There is controversy as to whether Tx synthetase can form thromboxanes from endoperoxides other than PGG_2-H_2: Needleman et al. (1976a) find no TxA_1 formed from PGG_1-H_1, while Falardeau et al. (1976) have demonstrated TxB_1 formation in platelets given DHgL as substrate. Needleman et al. have shown TxA_3 formation from eicosapentaenoate. Moncada (1977) feels that either a lack of TxA_1 formation or a lack of TxA_1 pro-aggregation effect would explain the in vivo effects of DHgL administration on platelet aggregation. The latter seems more likely in light of the data of Mathias et al. (1978), demonstrating increased platelet thromboxane synthesis with increased linoleate (a precursor of γ-linolenate and homo-γ-linolenate) in the diet.

Activities other than the conversion of endoperoxides to thromboxanes have been attributed to thromboxane synthetase. For example, Diczfalusy et al. (1977) have presented data supporting the conversion of endoperoxides to HHT (12L-hydroxy-5,8,10-heptadecanoic acid) and malonaldehyde by isolated thromboxane synthetase. McMillan et al. (1978) have shown that selective inhibition of thromboxane B_2 synthesis in intact human platelets is paralleled by decreased malonaldehyde formation: they conclude that thromboxane synthetase is indeed responsible for the formation of both. Anderson et al. (1978) have presented kinetic data showing that TxA_2 and HHT formation are not sequential, i.e., that the formation of each probably occurs from a separate molecule of PGH_2. They also suggest a mechanism for thromboxane synthetase more similar to a dismutase than to an isomerase.

Isomerases

The conversion of the endoperoxides to prostaglandins may proceed enzymatically or nonenzymatically. The conversion to PGE_2 is probably enzymatic: Raz and Aharony (1978) have demonstrated PGH_2 to PGE_2 isomerase activity in platelets treated with imidazole to remove thromboxane synthetase activity. This brings out a point made by Sun et al. (1977), that substrate availability is an important factor in determining the spectrum of products that occur when more than one conversion is possible. Stated somewhat differently, it would appear that there is competition for substrate for various conversions. Ordinarily only a very small percentage of conversion occurs via prostaglandins, indicating a greater success at obtaining substrate by the thromboxane synthetase pathway.

The only prostaglandin that appears to be synthesized and released in sufficient quantity to affect platelet function is PGD_2 (Oelz et al., 1977). The conversion to PGD_2 from endoperoxide may occur via the same isomerase as PGE_2, since Raz and Aharony (1978) noted its formation (although in quantities insufficient for inhibition of platelet function) along with PGE_2. Perhaps more important, however, is the finding that serum albumin has PGH_2-to-PGD_2 isomerase activity (Hamberg and Fredholm, 1976). Sun (1977; see above) had noted that suspensions of washed platelets produced primarily TxA_2, whereas platelets in plasma produced little TxA_2 and substantial PGD_2, although the differences may also occur because of protein binding of TxA_2 in plasma samples, with subsequent loss (see Fitzpatrick and Gorman, 1977). Samuelsson et al. (1978) have postulated a protective role for serum albumin against platelet aggregation (in species sensitive to PGD_2), similar to the role proposed for PGI_2.

Whether conversion to $PGF_{2\alpha}$ occurs via an isomerase (reductase) or simply via isomerization is unclear in general (Gorman, 1978), and also for platelets. A $PGF_{2\alpha}$ reductase activity has been identified in other tissues (e.g., guinea pig uterus) (Wlodawer et al., 1976), but the activity has only minimal characteristics of enzymatic conversion. The lack of specific inhibitors for any of the endoperoxide-to-prostaglandin conversions is a difficulty yet to be overcome: inhibitors have proved extremely valuable in studying other steps in arachidonate conversion, however, as discussed in the next section.

INHIBITORS OF PLATELET ENZYMES INVOLVED IN ARACHIDONATE CONVERSIONS

Cyclooxygenase Inhibitors

The nonsteroidal anti-inflammatory drugs (NSAIDs; e.g., aspirin, indomethacin, phenylbutazone) are inhibitors of platelet aggregation (see the reviews cited earlier). This action was known before the mechanism of even the anti-inflammatory effect became apparent (e.g., Zucker, 1971; Weiss, 1971), i.e., the inhibition of prostaglandin formation (Vane, 1971). Even after this latter was realized, how this had anything to do with inhibition of platelet aggregation remained temporarily uncertain, because, as mentioned earlier, the prostaglandins, which were the only known end products, were clearly not involved directly as effectors of aggregation. That NSAIDs did inhibit prostaglandin release by stimulated platelets was known, however (Smith and Willis, 1974). With the discovery of the endoperoxide intermediates and the subsequent conversion of these to thromboxane (see previous sections), and with the elucidation of the involvement of these in aggregation, the story finally began to make sense: it was not the lack of prostaglandin synthesis that was important, but the lack of synthesis of endoperoxide intermediates, the first step in arachidonate conversion. Since the endoperoxides represent a common point for subsequent divergence, no end products are formed from arachidonate. Because the inhibition occurs at such an early step, the NSAIDs are useful primarily in the study of specific steps past the cyclooxygenase, or as they have been used in "coupled" systems (e.g., Needleman et al., 1976b). White and Glassman (1976) have presented a comparison of the I_{50} values and inhibitory concentrations of several NSAIDs (and additional cyclooxygenase inhibitors).

One point that should be made about aspirin versus other NSAIDs concerns duration of inhibition: it was noted by Kocsis et al. (1973) (and by many other subsequently) that in vivo exposure of platelets to aspirin results in inhibition of cyclooxygenase activity lasting from several days to over a week, whereas the duration of inhibition by other NSAIDs generally approximates the effective life of the drug in plasma (e.g., indomethacin; Rane et al., 1978). The long duration of effect for aspirin apparently results from acetylation of the membrane-cyclooxygenase complex, an irreversible reaction (Roth et al., 1975). The NSAIDs generally have no effect on thromboxane synthetase or on the conversion of endoperoxides to prostaglandins.

Thromboxane Synthetase Inhibitors

Moncada et al. (1976c) described the use of benzydamine to inhibit Tx synthetase: inhibition was obtained only at concentrations which had some effect on the cyclooxygenase as well, however (I_{50} = 100 μg/ml, and 250 μg/ml, respectively). Subsequently, Moncada et al. (1977a) have described the use of imidazole as a thromboxane synthetase inhibitor. It apparently has a better separation of dose-response curves and does not affect cyclooxygenase at doses that inhibit Tx synthetase. 1-Methyl imidazole is actually a somewhat better inhibitor than the parent compound. David and Phillips (1971) had previously reported an inhibitory effect of imidazole buffer solution on platelet aggregation.

Gryglewski (1977) has reported that the nonacidic NSAID designated L-8027 is apparently an inhibitor of Tx synthetase, but has no effect on cyclooxygenase. An interesting point here is that L-8027 is also a very effective inhibitor of platelet aggregation, thus implicating TxA_2 in causing aggregation physiologically. The effect of L-8027 on endoperoxide-induced aggregation per se was not reported.

Polyphloretin phosphate (N-0164) was reported by Kulkarni and Eakins (1976) to inhibit Tx synthetase. However, the reported PG antagonistic behavior of the compound (Juan and Lembeck, 1976; Fredholm, 1976; Eakins et al., 1976) and its effects on exogenous endoperoxide aggregation (MacIntyre and Gordon, 1977) clouds definition of its effects.

Burimamide, an H_2-receptor histamine antagonist, and also an analog of imidazole, has been reported by Allan and Eakins (1978) to be an inhibitor of thromboxane synthetase of platelet microsomes at concentrations not affecting cyclooxygenase activity. Vincent and Zylstra (1978) find that nicotinic acid inhibits formation of TxA_2 after exposure of platelets to phospholipase A_2, with simultaneous increases in PGE_2 and $PGF_{2\alpha}$ (indicating no inhibition prior to thromboxane synthetase). The prostaglandin analog 9,11-azoprosta-5,13-dienoic acid (Gorman et al., 1977a) is an effective inhibitor of thromboxane synthesis (and second-phase platelet aggregation), also shifting synthesis toward PGE_2. (Sun, 1977, previous section, also reported inhibition by substrate analogs.) Grodzinska and Marcinkiewicz (1979) have found nictindole to inhibit TxA_2 formation by platelets exposed to several aggregating agents and also to inhibit aggregation (second phase).

Furosemide inhibits PGG_2-induced platelet aggregation (Malmsten et al., 1975). Ingerman et al. (1976) subsequently demonstrated that furosemide inhibits malonaldehyde formation by platelets exposed to arachidonate or thrombin. Inhibition of PGG_2 aggregation, together with the previously presented data that malonaldehyde formation may be catalyzed by thromboxane synthetase, may indicate some effect of furosemide on thromboxane synthetase, perhaps in addition to the proposed antagonism of ADP effect on platelets. Needleman et al. (1977) reviewed some of the problems associated with lack of selectivity, choice of assay methods, and so on, for thromboxane synthetase inhibitors.

Other

No step-specific inhibitors of the conversion of endoperoxides to PGs are currently available.

Thus, in summary, it is possible to inhibit two important sequences in the enzyme pathways of platelets. It appears that inhibition of either results in inhibition of aggregation, pointing to TxA_2 as perhaps the sole initiator of irreversible aggregation. Although this would seem the case, there are some conflicting data. The role of the various compounds produced by platelets in platelet function is discussed in some detail in the next section.

EFFECTS OF PROSTAGLANDINS, ENDOPEROXIDES, AND THROMBOXANES ON PLATELETS

The Prostaglandins

Although the prostaglandins have been known to be formed by platelets during aggregation, the role of the prostaglandins in this process has never been clear. The reader is referred to the reviews cited earlier for detailed information on the effects of prostaglandins on platelets. In examining prostaglandins for effect on platelets, it has become clear that the most reasonable role is that of modifier. Prostaglandins of the E series will modify the response of platelets to the usual stimuli: E_1 is a very effective inhibitor, whereas E_2 is a stimulator [at lower concentrations—at higher ones it acts more like E_1, perhaps because of contamination by E_1 (Kloeze, 1969)]. $PGF_{2\alpha}$ reportedly has little effect on aggregation of either human (Vargaftig and Chignard, 1975) or canine (Bridenbaugh and Lefer, 1976) platelets. However, by using submaximal ADP stimulation we have been able to demonstrate a facilitatory effect of $PGF_{2\alpha}$ on canine platelet aggregation (Longenecker, 1978, 1980). Smith et al. (1974) have demonstrated an inhibitory effect of PGD_2 on aggregation of human platelets, and indeed report it to be about twice as effective on a concentration basis as PGE_1. Because the prostaglandins are metabolized rapidly in the lung when they are released into the circulation (Flower, 1977), and because they have only modifying effects on platelet function, it is unlikely that the prostaglandins are the prime movers in platelet function (i.e., in aggregation).

Derivatives of the naturally occurring prostaglandins, however, have been shown to cause aggregation: e.g., Corey et al. (1977) have shown that 11-deoxy-15(RS)-15-methyl-$PGF_{2\alpha}$ (WY-17,186), 16-16-dimethyl-PGE_2, and a 9,11-azo derivative of PGH_2 can cause both primary aggregation and a second-phase aggregation which is both indomethacin sensitive and insensitive (i.e., they act in part like native endoperoxides). The latter is an interesting point, since it is possible that some of these compounds could also act as analogs of TxA_2, although the azo compound is not converted. The effects as endoperoxide analogs might be distinguishable from those as TxA_2 analogs by the use of thromboxane synthetase inhibitors, as above.

Other prostaglandin analogs have similar types of activity as the parent prostaglandin, but are more or less potent (e.g., Bicking et al., 1978). In some cases the metabolites of the native prostaglandins are active, or are even more active, than the parent, although this is not generally the case (e.g., Westwick, 1978).

Endoperoxides and Thromboxanes

It was pointed out earlier that the endoperoxides, unlike the prostaglandins, can cause platelet aggregation without the necessity of other stimuli (Willis et al., 1974b; Hamberg et al., 1974). The aggregation thus induced may be reversible or irreversible, and accompanied by release of ADP, serotonin, and prostanoids, but not of lysosomal enzymes (MacIntyre et al., 1978). The data cited previously (Grylewski, 1977), in which an inhibitor of Tx synthetase prevented aggregation, may present a reason to at least consider modification of the role of endoperoxides with respect to platelets. If the endoperoxides need to be converted to TxA_2 to cause aggregation, inhibition of Tx synthetase alone may prove a realistic approach to control of platelet function, bypassing the necessity of cyclooxygenase inhibition. This could have an additional benefit in that the endoperoxides would still be available for conversion to theoretically useful compounds, such as prostacyclin (PGI_2), by other tissues, such as blood vessels. Certainly, the other effects of TxA_2 (e.g., vascular spasm) might be lessened, since the endoperoxides frequently are less effective (ineffective) in causing spasm or may even cause an opposite effect (e.g., Needleman et al., 1976a; Bunting et al., 1976b). [The opposite effect (i.e., relaxation) may be due to vessel utilization of endoperoxides to form prostacyclin.]

Support for the argument that the endoperoxides themselves can cause aggregation has been advanced by Needleman et al. (1976a) on the basis of some structure-activity data for the endoperoxides. Essentially, Needleman's group used the endoperoxides PGG_1-H_1, PGG_2-H_2, and PGG_3-H_3, and looked for conversion of these to the corresponding Txs by platelet microsomes: no TxA_1 was detected, while TxA_2 and TxA_3* were formed. The interesting comparison is between effect of the endoperoxides which are converted and the corresponding Tx: both endoperoxides cause contraction of vascular strips and also cause platelet aggregation, both Txs contract vascular strips, but TxA_3 has no effect on platelet aggregation. This lends credence to the argument that the endoperoxides by themselves can cause aggregation. Support is also lent by the spectacular effects of the stable endoperoxide analogs, e.g., (15S)-hydroxy-9α, 11α (U44069)- and 11α, 9α (U46619)-(epoxymethano)-prosta-5-cis, 13-trans-dienoic acids (MacIntyre and Gordon, 1977), although whether these are converted, act as Txs per se, or differ in effect because of their (relative) stability remains to be clarified. Fitzpatrick and Gorman (1977) have pointed out that apparent lack of Tx formation can result from inappropriate timing of samples taken for Tx assay, since TxA_2 is formed early in aggregation and has mainly disappeared by the time maximum response occurs, a point that should be kept in mind.

The lack of effectiveness of TxA_3 in causing aggregation has been proposed as protective against atherosclerosis and ischemic heart disease in situations where the diet is high in eicosapentaenoic acid with respect to arachidonic acid (Dyerberg et al., 1978). This diet rearrangement apparently happens as a natural occurrence among Eskimos, and may account for their lower incidence of both atherosclerosis and heart disease, and for a "bleeding tendency." Needleman et al. (1979a) report that although eicosapentoaenoic acid is a poor cyclooxygenase substrate, it binds avidly, thereby lowering arachidonate conversion as well. They further report that both PGH_3 and TxA_3 increase platelet levels of cyclic AMP (see the next section), acting more like other classical inhibitors of aggregation, such as PGE_1 or PGI_2. In addition, PGH_3 is apparently transformed into a triene prostacyclin, PGI_3, which acts very similarly to PGI_2 with respect to platelets. Thus the antiplatelet effects of eicosapentaenoate probably result from several simultaneous effects, none of which serve to resolve completely the issue of the necessity or lack of necessity of conversion of the endoperoxides for effecting platelet aggregation.

Prostacyclin

As mentioned previously, prostacyclin (PGI_2) is a unique prostanoid compound produced by blood vessel endothelium. Actually, the original observations were for aortic microsomes (Moncada et al., 1976a,b;

---

*TxA_3 may also be accompanied by or replaced by PGD_3, an analog of PGD_2, a potent inhibitor of aggregation, which can form in the presence of albumin, as previously pointed out (p. 262).

Gryglewski et al., 1976), and were made later for intact vessel (Bunting et al., 1976a). Prostacyclin has been noted to be a very effective inhibitor of platelet aggregation: it is approximately 30 times more effective than PGE_1 against in vitro arachidonate-induced aggregation (Gryglewski et al., 1976). PGI_2 is also effective against in vitro aggregation induced by ADP, collagen, PGG_2-H_2, epinephrine, and serotonin (Moncada et al., 1976b), and may even reverse aggregation already in progress. PGI_2 has been shown to cause disaggregation of preformed platelet thrombi in vivo (Gryglewski et al., 1978), and to inhibit in vitro aggregation subsequent to its in vivo administration (Szczeklik et al., 1978). Bayer et al. (1979) have recently demonstrated a reduced mortality in rabbits given PGI_2 and subsequently arachidonate in vivo, presumably because the PGI_2 prevented vascular occlusion in the lung by arachidonate-caused platelet emboli. Because no other platelet-inhibitory prostanoid compound is clearly produced by platelets themselves in sufficient quantities to act as a feedback inhibitor, this role has been postulated for PGI_2 (see the articles cited above; also Moncada and Vane, 1978, 1979).

PLATELET RECEPTORS FOR PROSTANOID COMPOUNDS

There appear to be two basic "categories" or types of receptor sites for the prostanoid compounds on platelets: stimulatory and inhibitory, stated perhaps overly simply. The history, description, and requirements in the following discussion are by no means exhaustive, and are meant only to present an overview.

Subsequent to the observation mentioned earlier that PGE_1 and PGE_2 could modify platelet behavior (Kloeze, 1967; Emmons et al., 1967), the existence of PGE receptors on platelets was demonstrated (McDonald and Stuart, 1974; Gorman, 1974). From competitive binding data and effect of combinations of PGE_1 and E_2 on cyclic AMP content as compared to PGE_1 alone, it appeared that E_1 and E_2 shared a common receptor site (remember that the effect of E_2 is biphasic). Gorman (1974) cites the existence of high- and low-affinity prostaglandin binding sites.

Moncada et al. (1977c) have shown that N-0164 (polyphloretin phosphate) antagonized the effect of PGI_2; N-0164 was reported (see below) to antagonize the effects of PGE_1, but not PGD_2, which was also confirmed by Moncada. These findings were taken as evidence that PGI_2 and PGE_1 act on the same receptors. More recently, Siegl et al. (1979) have demonstrated both high- and low-affinity selective binding sites for PGI_2 on platelets. PGI_2 could be displaced (from the high-affinity sites) by several prostaglandins, but PGE_1 was much more effective at displacement than PGE_2 or the PGI_2 metabolite 6-keto-$PGF_{1\alpha}$. PGD_2, also an inhibitor, did not displace PGI_2. They conclude that these high-affinity sites for PGI_2 are the ones through which the inhibitory effect of PGI_2 on platelets is exerted. Nugteren (1978) has concluded that prostaglandin E_1, more or less accidentally, has some activity due to a certain similarity in structure (to PGI_2) which seems to align with current evidence. The comment could also be extended to PGE_2, especially when it acts like PGE_1, although it is obviously a less efficacious inhibitor than PGE_1.

That PGE_2 also may act at other receptor sites is supported by the fact that N-0164 antagonizes the effects of E_2 and D_2, but not E_1, on aggregation (MacIntyre and Gordon, 1977). N-0164 did not affect arachidonate-induced aggregation or aggregation induced by PGG_2/platelet microsomes (TxA_2), but did antagonize U46619 or PGG_2 alone. They conclude (1) that all stimulatory bisenoic prostaglandins, i.e., those which can alone cause aggregation, act on a single receptor site; and (2) that endogenous endoperoxides must be rapidly converted to TxA_2, which is not antagonized by N-0164. The latter would seem to distinguish exogenously added endoperoxide from that endogenously generated.

MacIntyre et al. (1978) have further refined the requirements for bisenoic prostaglandins to act on the endogenous endoperoxide receptor: (1) The configuration of the molecule should be such that the side chains are out of plane with the ring, as they are in the native compounds. The chains of E_2, $F_{2\alpha}$, and A_2 are in plane and thus they cannot affect the receptor in such a way as to produce aggregation. (2) Certain changes in C-11, C-15, and C-16 will achieve the required configuration and will probably favorably alter lipid solubility characteristics and so on. The latter conclusion is supported by the effect of modified PGE_2 analogs (e.g., 16,16-dimethyl PGE_2), which act like endoperoxides. (3) The existence of two rings (bicyclic compounds) appears to be a strong and perhaps sufficient (although not sole) stimulus for affecting the site.

From the data given above, the receptor for PGD_2 on platelets appears to be separate from that of the inhibitory PGI_2 and PGE_1. Cooper and Ahern (1979) have developed a binding assay for prostaglandins/platelets, and have used it to examine PGD_2 binding. They find the binding to be both saturable and rapid, and to be competed for by PGI_2 and PGE_1, with concentrations approximately one and two orders of magnitude higher, respectively, required for displacement. This would support separate sites for PGD_2 binding. That they may not be entirely unrelated is possible, since both PGI_2/PGE_1 and PGD_2 cause activation of adenyl cyclase (subsequent section), and thus may indeed represent only different sites on the adenyl cyclase as suggested by Moncada et al. (1977c) and by Mills and MacFarlane (1974).

A somewhat different approach to considering the PGD_2 receptor has been offered by Harris et al. (1979), who propose that PGI_2 and PGE_2 share the high-affinity PGI_2 sites described above, while PGI_2 and PGD_2 share the low-affinity PGI_2 sites. This would account for the inhibitory activity of all the compounds and also for the greater effects of PGI_2, for which a larger number of receptors would be available.

In conclusion, there appear to be inhibitory sites shared by PGI_2 and PGE_1, while a separate, but perhaps related group exists for PGD_2. There are stimulatory receptor sites for the native endoperoxides which may be shared by bisenoic prostaglandins with certain characteristics and stable synthetic bicyclic bisenoic endoperoxide analogs. These sites, however, may not be shared by TxA_2, since N-0164 interferes with exogenous endoperoxides but not with TxA_2. This also leaves open the question of the modulatory prostaglandins, especially those which are stimulatory: they may be simply partial agonists of another receptor category.

MECHANISM OF EFFECT OF PROSTAGLANDINS, ENDOPEROXIDES, AND THROMBOXANE: THE CYCLIC NUCLEOTIDES AND CALCIUM

Because of the vastness of the cyclic nucleotide-platelet function literature, only some salient features will be presented, with references sufficient for the reader to initiate an independent and more complete search. A recent review by Harris et al. (1979) on the mechanisms of effect of the prostaglandins (and related compounds) includes a discussion of platelets, the effects on platelets of the various prostanoids, and a consideration of the role of intracellular mediators such as the cyclic nucleotides.

Cyclic Nucleotides

In general, it has been found that prostaglandins which inhibit aggregation stimulate adenyl cyclase (Wolfe and Shulman, 1969; Mills and MacFarlane, 1974; Zieve and Greenough, 1969; review, Salzman et al., 1972) and result in increased levels of cyclic adenosine 3',5'-monophosphate (cAMP; Vargaftig and Chignard, 1975; Michel et al., 1976; McDonald and Stuart, 1973; Shio et al., 1971). However, there is some evidence that PGE_1 may also inhibit aggregation by a cAMP-independent mechanism (Sinha and Colman, 1978).

Most of the prostaglandins (PGE_1, PGE_2, $PGF_{2\alpha}$) are capable of stimulating adenyl cyclase activity to some extent, despite the fact that the direction of effects on aggregation differ (Longenecker et al., 1977, 1980; Longenecker, 1978, 1980). Prostacyclin, also an inhibitor of aggregation, has effects similar to PGE_1 or PGD_2; i.e., it increases cAMP, but to a much greater degree (Gorman et al., 1977b; Tateson et al., 1977). Prostaglandin stimulators of cAMP levels may not affect cyclic guanosine monophosphate (cGMP) levels (e.g., PGE_1; Miller and Gorman, 1976).

The cyclic nucleotides and their derivatives (e.g., dibutyryl cAMP) also affect platelet function when used directly, and their effects support a role for cAMP in platelet function (Salzman and Levine, 1971; Wang et al., 1977). Recent data suggest that cAMP may actually limit the availability of arachidonate to the cyclooxygenase (Minkes et al., 1977) and/or inhibit cyclooxygenase (Malmsten et al., 1976), thus accounting for its inhibitory effect. Lapetina et al. (1977) have also shown that both dibutyryl cAMP and PGI_2 inhibit phospholipase A_2 activity in washed horse platelets.

Since the ratio of cAMP to cGMP seems important in many systems, it would be "convenient" if the aggregation stimulators had different effects on either cAMP or cGMP levels in platelets. The prostanoid stimulators of aggregation may increase the concentration of cGMP and stimulate guanyl cyclase (Chiang and Kang, 1975). cGMP has been reported to be pro-aggregatory as well (Chiang et al., 1976). However, others report that PGE_2 and and $PGF_{2\alpha}$ have no effect on platelet guanyl cyclase (Asano and Hidaka, 1977). In fact, Weiss et al. (1978) have shown no effect at all of increased cGMP on either secretion or thrombin aggregation. Other aggregating agents, such as ADP, epinephrine, and collagen, depress cAMP levels rather than increase cGMP (Harris et al., 1979). Miller and Gorman (1976) demonstrated that PGG_2 has an indirect effect on cyclic nucleotide levels, i.e., no effect alone on either cAMP or cGMP, but an antagonism of PGE_1-induced increases in cAMP. Similar data have been obtained for PGH_2 and TxA_2 (Miller et al., 1977). A reciprocal relationship has been proposed between PGI_2 and TxA_2 as regulators of platelet cAMP levels (Gorman et al., 1977b, 1978; Gorman, 1979), and of platelet function.

Thus it would seem that a link between cAMP and platelet function is fairly well established. A link between cGMP and function has been suggested, but the evidence is not as convincing at present. The subsequent intracellular changes effected by altered cAMP levels are discussed in the next section.

Calcium

Intracellular changes in cAMP seem to require yet another intracellular change to achieve stimulation or inhibition of aggregation: modification of intracellular (free) calcium levels. The sequence generally held to occur for pro-aggregatory stimulation of platelets (based in part on the descriptions by Gorman, 1979; White, 1979; Harris et al., 1979; Gorman et al., 1978) includes combination of the agent with the platelet membrane, causing movement of small amounts of calcium into the platelet (or mobilization from bound sites to the free state within the platelet). This calcium can then activate phospholipase A_2, perhaps via calmodulin (calcium-dependent regulatory protein) (Wong and Cheung, 1979), resulting in liberation of arachidonate. The arachidonate is then rapidly converted to endoperoxides and TxA_2, with additional calcium mobilized from (probably) the dense tubular system by an ionophoric action of TxA_2.

Gerrard et al. (1978) have demonstrated an ability of arachidonate and the endoperoxides (PGG_2, PGH_2) to release calcium from a platelet membrane fraction, which would support the scheme presented above. Imidazole, however, had little effect on endoperoxide-induced calcium release, while aspirin inhibited arachidonate, but not endoperoxide release. Thus it is possible that calcium-releasing capacity exists for other prostanoids as well as TxA_2. The prostaglandins had no releasing ability in this system.

Calcium thus made available in the platelet is available not only for microtubule assembly, secretion, and contractile element activity, but also for inhibition of adenyl cyclase. Gorman (1979) has also proposed that released ADP, and subaggregatory amounts of other aggregation stimulators such as collagen, can also participate in calcium mobilization and thus amplify responses to other agents.

The sequence that would be necessary for an inhibition is more straightforward. The inhibitor would combine with the platelet, stimulate adenyl cyclase, and elevate cAMP. Calcium mobilization would be inhibited by the elevated cAMP and would antagonize the effect of compounds tending to increase mobilization.

Kaser-Glanzmann et al. (1977) have shown removal of calcium into membranes caused by cAMP, which is also supported by the work of Gerrard et al. (1977). Recent data by Haslam et al. (1979) suggest that increases in cAMP (e.g., caused by PGE_1) may initiate phosphorylation of certain polypeptides, which in turn lower calcium, and so on. Harris et al. (1979) state: "If increased cytoplasmic calcium is associated with platelet activation, then its removal would be expected to inhibit aggregation." The data are certainly suggestive that the case is so, but the data are far from sufficient at this point.

SUMMARY

Platelets are capable of undergoing a number of excitable reactions, one of which, the release reaction, accompanies, or is integral to, the aggregation reaction. During the release reaction a number of products formed from arachidonic acid are produced and released into the surrounding medium. These compounds include several very active ones (e.g., the endoperoxides and a thromboxane). The activity of these particular compounds can be observed in many systems, including the platelets themselves. Current data suggest that the prostaglandins act as modulators of platelet function (i.e., they enhance or inhibit aggregation due to other agents), while the endoperoxides and thromboxane A_2 may be more directly involved. There are platelet receptors for prostaglandins, particularly PGE_1 and PGD_2, for the bisenoic endoperoxides (and analogs), and for prostacyclin. Prostacyclin and PGE_1 may share common receptors. There is some controversy concerning whether both the endoperoxides and thromboxanes can induce aggregation. The mechanisms by which aggregation is affected involve the cyclic nucleotide levels/nucleotide cyclase activities of the platelets, in particular cAMP. Inhibitors of aggregation generally increase cAMP levels, while stimulators antagonize the increased cAMP levels seen with inhibitors, or may increase cGMP levels. Increased cAMP may inhibit phospholipase, thus limiting substrate to cyclooxygenase, and may also directly inhibit cyclooxygenase, accounting in part for the inhibition of aggregation and the release reaction. The final common pathway for affecting platelet function seems to involve calcium, with stimulators increasing intracellular calcium levels, and inhibitors decreasing calcium, the latter via increases in cAMP. Increased calcium stimulates phospholipase A_2 activity (via calmodulin?), leading to synthesis of stimulatory endoperoxides and TxA_2.

REFERENCES

Allan, J., and Eakins, K. E. (1978). Burimamide is a selective inhibitor of thromboxane A biosynthesis in human platelet microsomes. Prostaglandins 15:659-661.

Anderson, M. W., Crutchly, D. J., Tainer, B. E., and Eling, T. E. (1978). Kinetic studies on the conversion of prostaglandin endoperoxide PGH_2 by thromboxane synthase. Prostaglandins 16:563-570.

Asano, T., and Hidaka, H. (1977). Purification of guanylate cyclase from human platelets and effect of arachidonic acid peroxide. Biochem. Biophys. Res. Commun. 78:910-918.

Attar, S., McLaughlin, J. S., and Masaitis, C. (1973). Clinical application of platelet aggregation. South. Med. J. 66:481-485.

Bayer, B. L., Blass, K. E., and Forster, W. (1979). Anti-aggregatory effect of prostacyclin (PGI_2) in vivo. Br. J. Pharmacol. 66:10-12.

Bicking, J. B., Jones, J. H., Holtz, W. J., Robb, C. M., Kuehl, F. A., Jr., Minsker, D. H., and Cragoe, E. J., Jr. (1978). 11,12-Secoprostaglandins, 5,8-acetyl- or 8-(1-hydroxyethyl)-12-hydroxy-13-aryloxytridecanoic acids and sulfonamide isosteres as inhibitors of platelet aggregation. J. Med. Chem. 21:1011-1018.

Born, G. V. R. (1962). Aggregation of blood platelets by adenosine diphosphate and its reversal. Nature (Lond.) 184:927-929.

Bridenbaugh, G. A., and Lefer, A. M. (1976). Influence of humoral shock factors on in vitro aggregation of dog platelets. Thromb. Res. 8:599-606.

Bunting, S., Gryglewski, R. J., Moncada, S., and Vane, J. R. (1976a). Arterial walls generate from prostaglandin endoperoxides a substance (prostaglandin X) which relaxes strips of mesenteric and coeliac arteries and inhibits platelet aggregation. Prostaglandins 12:897-913.

Bunting, S., Moncada, S., and Vane, J. R. (1976b). The effects of prostaglandin endoperoxides and thromboxane A_2 on strips of rabbit coeliac artery and other smooth muscle preparations. Br. J. Pharmacol. 57:462P-463P.

Caprino, L., and Rossi, E. C. (Eds.) (1974). Platelet Aggregation and Drugs. Academic Press, New York.

Chiang, T. M. H., and Kang, A. H. (1975). The role of cyclic 3',5'-guanosine monophosphate in human platelet aggregation. Fed. Proc. 34:695.

Chiang, T. M., Dixit, S. N., and Kang, H. (1976). Effect of cyclic 3',5'-guanosine monophosphate on human platelet function. J. Lab. Clin. Med. 88:215-221.

Chignard, M., and Vargaftig, B. B. (1976). Dog platelets fail to aggregate when they form aggregating substances upon stimulation with arachadonic acid. Eur. J. Pharmacol. 38:7-18.

Clausen, J., and Srivastava, K. C. (1972). The synthesis of prostaglandins in human platelets. Lipids 7:246-250.

Cooper, B., and Ahern, D. (1979). Characterization of the platelet prostaglandin D_2 receptor. Loss of prostaglandin D_2 receptors in platelets of patients with myeloproliferative disorders. J. Clin. Invest. 64:586-590.

Corey, E. J., Gordon, J. L., MacIntyre, D. E., and Salzman, E. W. (1977). Effects of synthetic prostaglandin analogues on platelet aggregation and secretion. Br. J. Pharmacol. 59:446P-447P.

Davis, J. W., and Phillips, P. E. (1971). The effect of imidazole on human platelet aggregation. Blood 38:417-421.

de Gaetano, G., and Garattini, S. (Eds.) (1978). Platelets: A Multidisciplinary Approach. Raven Press, New York.

Dembinska-Kiec, A., Gryglewska, T., Zmuda, A., and Gryglewski, R. J. (1977). The generation of prostacyclin by arteries and by the coronary vascular bed is reduced in experimental atherosclerosis in rabbits. Prostaglandins 14:1025-1034.

Diczfalusy, V., Falardeau, P., and Hammarstrom, S. (1977). Conversion of prostaglandin endoperoxides to C_{17}-hydroxy acids catalyzed by human platelet thromboxane synthase. FEBS Lett. 84:271-274.

Dyerberg, J., Bang, H. O., Stofferson, E., Moncada, S., and Vane, J. R. (1978). Eicosapentaenoic acid and prevention of thrombosis and atherosclerosis. Lancet 2(July 15):117-119.

Eakins, K. E., Rajadhyaksha, V., and Schroer, R. (1976). Prostaglandin antagonism by sodium p-benzyl-4-(1-oxo-2-(4-chlorobenzyl)-3 phenylpropyl)phenyl phosphonate (N-0164). Br. J. Pharmacol. 58:333-339.

Emmons, P. R., Hampton, J. R., Harrison, M. J. G., Honor, A. J., and Mitchell, J. R. A. (1967). Effect of prostaglandin E_1 on platelet behavior in vitro and in vivo. Br. Med. J. 2:468-472.

Falardeau, P., Hamberg, M., and Samuelsson, B. (1976). Metabolism of 8,11,14-eicosatrienoic acid in human platelets. Biochim. Biophys. Acta 441:193-200.

Farrow, J. W., and Willis, A. L. (1975). Thrombolytic and anti-thrombotic properties of dihomo-gamma-linolenate in vitro. Br. J. Pharmacol. 55:316P-317P.

Fitzpatrick, F. A., and Gorman, R. R. (1977). Platelet rich plasma transforms exogenous prostaglandin endoperoxide H_2 into thromboxane A_2. Prostaglandins 14:881-889.

Flower, R. J. (1977). Prostaglandin metabolism in the lung. In Metabolic Functions of the Lung, Y. S. Bakhle and J. R. Vane (Eds.). Marcel Dekker, New York.

Fredholm, B. (1976). Prostaglandin inhibitory effects of polyphloretin phosphate. Acta Biol. Med. Ger. 35:1233-1239.

Gerrard, J. M., Townsend, D., Stoddard, S., Witkop, C. J., and White, J. G. (1977). The influence of prostaglandin G_2 on platelet ultrastructure and platelet secretion. Am. J. Pathol. 86:99-115.

Gerrard, J. M., Butler, A. M., Graff, G., Stoddard, S. F., and White, J. G. (1978). Prostaglandin endoperoxides promote calcium release from a platelet membrane fraction in vitro. Prostaglandins Med. 1:373-385.

Gordon, J. L. (Ed.) (1976). Platelets in Biology and Pathology. North-Holland, Amsterdam.

Gorman, R. R. (1974). Specific PGE_1 and PGE_2 binding sites in platelet membranes. Prostaglandins 6:542.

Gorman, R. R. (1978). Prostaglandins, thromboxanes, and prostacyclin. In Biochemistry and Mode of Action of Hormones II, Vol. 20, Rickenberg, H. V. (Ed.). University Park Press, Baltimore, pp. 81-107.

Gorman, R. R. (1979). Modulation of human platelet function by prostacyclin and thromboxane A_2. Fed. Proc. 38:83-88.

Gorman, R. R., Bundy, G. L., Peterson, D. C., Sun, F. F., Miller, O. V., and Fitzpatrick, F. A. (1977a). Inhibition of human platelet thromboxane synthetase by 9,11-azoprosta-5,13-dienoic acid. Proc. Natl. Acad. Sci. USA 74:4007-4011.

Gorman, R. R., Bunting, S., and Miller, O. V. (1977b). Modulation of human platelet adenylate cyclase by prostacyclin (PGX). Prostaglandins 13:377-388.

Gorman, R. R., Fitzpatrick, F. A., and Miller, O. V. (1978). Reciprocal regulation of human platelet cAMP levels by thromboxane A_2 and prostacyclin. Adv. Cyclic Nucleotide Res. 9:597-609.

Grodzinska, L., and Marcinkiewicz, E. (1979). The generation of TxA_2 in human platelet rich plasma and its inhibition by nictindole and prostacyclin. Pharmacol. Res. Commun. 11:133-146.

Gryglewski, R. J. (1977). Prostaglandin and thromboxane biosynthesis inhibitors. Naunyn-Schmiedeberg's Arch. Pharmacol. 297:585-588.

Gryglewski, R. J., Bunting, S., Moncada, S., Flower, R. J., and Vane, J. R. (1976). Arterial walls are protected against deposition of platelet thrombi by a substance (prostaglandin X) which they make from prostaglandin endoperoxides. Prostaglandins 12:685-713.

Gryglewski, R. J., Korbut, R., and Ocetkiewicz, A. (1978). Reversal of platelet aggregation. Pharmacol. Res. Commun. 10:185-189.

Hamberg, M., and Fredholm, B. B. (1976). Isomerization of prostaglandin H_2 into prostaglandin D_2 in the presence of serum albumin. Biochim. Biophys. Acta 431:189-193.

Hamberg, M., and Samuelsson, B. (1974). Prostaglandin endoperoxides. Novel transformations of arachidonic acid in human platelets. Proc. Natl. Acad. Sci. USA 71:3400-3404.

Hamberg, M., Svensson, J., Wakabayashi, T., and Samuelsson, B. (1974). Isolation and structure of two prostaglandin endoperoxides that cause platelet aggregation. Proc. Natl. Acad. Sci. USA 71:345-349.

Hamberg, M., Svensson, J., and Samuelsson, B. (1975). Thromboxanes: a new group of biologically active compounds derived from prostaglandin endoperoxides. Proc. Natl. Acad. Sci. USA 72:2994-2998.

Hammarstrom, S., and Falardeau, P. (1977). Resolution of prostaglandin endoperoxide synthetase and thromboxane synthase of human platelets. Proc. Natl. Acad. Sci. USA 74:3691-3695.

Harker, L. A. (1974). Control of platelet production. Annu. Rev. Med. 25: 383-400.

Harris, R. H., Ramwell, P. W., and Gilmer, P. J. (1979). Cellular mechanisms of prostaglandin action. Annu. Rev. Physiol. 41:653-668.

Haslam, R. J., Lynham, J. A., and Fox, J. E. B. (1979). Effects of collagen, ionophore A23187 and prostaglandin E_1 on the phosphorylation of specific proteins in blood platelets. Biochem. J. 178:397-406.

Ho, P. P. K., Walters, P., and Sullivan, H. R. (1976). Biosynthesis of thromboxane B_2: assay, isolation and properties of the enzyme system in human platelets. Prostaglandins 12:951-970.

Ingerman, C. M., Smith, J. B., and Silver, M. J. (1976). Inhibition of the platelet release reaction and platelet prostaglandin synthesis by furosemide. Thromb. Res. 8:417-419.

Juan, H., and Lembeck, F. (1976). Polyphloretin phosphate reduces the algesic action of bradykinin by interfering with E-type prostaglandins. Agents Actions 615:646-650.

Karpatkin, S. (1977). Metabolism of platelets. In Hematology, W. J. Williams, E. Beutler, A. J. Ersleo, and B. Wayne Rundles (Eds.). McGraw-Hill, New York, pp. 1187-1200.

Kaser-Glanzmann, R., Jakabova, M., George, J., and Luscher, E. (1977). Stimulation of calcium uptake in platelet membrane vesicles by adenosine 3',5'-cyclic monophosphate and protein kinase. Biochim. Biophys. Acta 466:429-440.

Kloeze, J. (1967). Influence of prostaglandins on platelet adhesiveness and platelet aggregation. In Prostaglandins: Proceedings of the Second Nobel Symposium, S. Bergstrom and B. Samuelsson (Eds.). Interscience, London, pp. 241-252.

Kloeze, J. (1969). Relationship between chemical structure and platelet aggregation activity of prostaglandins. Biochim. Biophys. Acta 187: 285-292.

Kocsis, J. J., Hernandovich, J., Silver, M. J., Smith, J. B., and Ingerman, C. (1973). Duration of inhibition of platelet prostaglandin formation and aggregation by ingested aspirin or indomethacin. Prostaglandins 3:141-144.

Kulkarni, P. S., and Eakins, K. E. (1976). N-0164 inhibits generation of thromboxane-A_2-like activity from prostaglandin endoperoxides by human platelet microsomes. Prostaglandins 12:465-469.

Lapetina, E. G., Schmitges, C. J., Chandrabose, K., and Cuatrecasas, P. (1977). Cyclic adenosine 3',5'-monophosphate and prostacyclin inhibit membrane phospholipase activity in platelets. Biochem. Biophys. Res. Commun. 76:828-835.

Longenecker, G. L. (1978). Prostaglandin $F_{2\alpha}$ stimulation of submaximal ADP-induced platelet aggregation. Fed. Proc. 37:253.

Longenecker, G. L. (1980). Effects of prostaglandin $F_{2\alpha}$ on aggregation of canine platelets. Thromb. Res. 18:369-374.

Longenecker, G. L., Kopaciewicz, L. J., Palmer, S. J., and Palmer, G. C. (1977). Activation of adenylate cyclase by prostaglandins E_1, E_2 and $F_{2\alpha}$ in homogenates of canine platelets. Adv. Cyclic Nucleotide Res. 9:738.

Longenecker, G. L., Kopaciewicz, L. J., Palmer, S. J., and Palmer, G. C. (1980). Prostaglandin stimulation of canine platelet adenylate cyclase. Thromb. Res. 19:119-124.

MacIntyre, D. E., and Gordon, J. L. (1977). Discrimination between platelet prostaglandin receptors with a specific antagonist of bisenoic prostaglandins. Thromb. Res. 11:705-713.

MacIntyre, D. E., Salzman, E. W., and Gordon, J. L. (1978). Prostaglandin receptors on human platelets. Structure-activity relationships of stimulatory prostaglandins. Biochem. J. 174:921-929.

Malmsten, C. (1979). Annotation: Prostaglandins, thromboxanes and platelets. Br. J. Haematol. 41:453-458.

Malmsten, C., Hamberg, M., Svensson, J., and Samuelsson, B. (1975). Physiological role of an endoperoxide in human platelets: hemostatic defect due to platelet cyclooxygenase deficiency. Proc. Natl. Acad. Sci. USA 72:1446-1450.

Malmsten, C., Granstrom, E., and Samuelsson, B. (1976). Cyclic AMP inhibits formation of prostaglandin endoperoxide (PGG_2) in human platelets. Biochem. Biophys. Res. Commun. 68:569-576.

Mannuci, P. M., and Gorini, S. (Eds.) (1972). Platelet Function and Thrombosis: A Review of Methods. Plenum Press, New York.

Mathias, M. M., Fine, K., Lipinski, B., and Dupont, J. (1978). Dietary linoleate effect upon prostaglandin and thromboxane synthesis. Prostaglandins 15:706.

McDonald, J. W. D., and Stuart, R. K. (1973). Regulation of cyclic AMP levels and aggregation in human platelets by prostaglandin E_1. J. Lab. Clin. Med. 81:838-849.

McDonald, J. W. D., and Stuart, R. K. (1974). Interaction of prostaglandins E_1 and E_2 in regulation of cyclic AMP and aggregation in human platelets: evidence for a common prostaglandin receptor. J. Lab. Clin. Med. 84:111-121.

McMillan, R. M., MacIntyre, D. E., Booth, A., and Gordon, J. L. (1978). Malonaldehyde formation in intact platelets is catalysed by thromboxane synthase. Biochem. J. 176:595-598.

Michel, H., Caen, J. P., Born, G. V. R., Miller, R., D'Auriac, G. A., and Meyer, P. (1976). Relation between the inhibition of aggregation and the concentration of cAMP in human and rat platelets. Br. J. Haematol. 33:27-38.

Miller, O. V., and Gorman, R. R. (1976). Modulation of platelet cyclic nucleotide content by PGE_1 and the prostaglandin endoperoxide PGG_2. J. Cyclic Nucleotide Res. 2:79-87.

Miller, O. V., Johnson, R. A., and Gorman, R. R. (1977). Inhibition of PGE_1-stimulated cAMP accumulation in human platelets by thromboxane A_2. Prostaglandins 13:599-609.

Mills, D. C. B., and MacFarlane, D. E. (1974). Stimulation of human platelet adenylate cyclase by prostaglandin D_2. Thromb. Res. 5:401-412.

Minkes, M., Stanford, N., Chi, M. M. Y., Roth, G. J., Raz, A., Needleman, P., and Majerus, P. W. (1977). Cyclic adenosine 3',5'-monophosphate inhibits the availability of arachidonate to prostaglandin synthetase in human platelet suspensions. J. Clin. Invest. 59:449-454.

Miyamoto, T., Yamamoto, S., and Hayaishi, O. (1974). Prostaglandin synthetase system—resolution into oxygenase and isomerase components. Proc. Natl. Acad. Sci. USA 71:3645-3648.

Moncada, S. (1977). Prostaglandin endoperoxides and thromboxanes: formation and effects. Naunyn-Schmiederberg's Arch. Pharmacol. 297:581-584.

Moncada, S., and Vane, J. R. (1978). Unstable metabolites of arachidonic acid and their role in haemostasis and thrombosis. Br. Med. Bull. 34:129-135.

Moncada, S., and Vane, J. R. (1979). Arachidonic acid metabolites and the interactions between platelets and blood vessel walls. N. Engl. J. Med. 300:1142-1147.

Moncada, S., Gryglewski, R., Bunting, S., and Vane, J. R. (1976a). An enzyme isolated from arteries transforms prostaglandin endoperoxides to an unstable substance that inhibits platelet aggregation. Nature (Lond.) 263:663-665.

Moncada, S., Gryglewski, R., Bunting, S., and Vane, J. R. (1976b). A lipid peroxide inhibits the enzyme in blood vessel microsomes that generates from prostaglandin endoperoxides the substance (prostaglandin X) which prevents platelet aggregation. Prostaglandins 12:715-737.

Moncada, S., Needleman, P., Bunting, S., and Vane, J. R. (1976c). Prostaglandin endoperoxide and thromboxane generating systems and their selective inhibition. Prostaglandins 12:323-336.

Moncada, S., Bunting, S., Mullane, K., Thorogood, P., Vane, J. R., Raz, A., and Needleman, P. (1977a). Imidazole: a selective inhibitor of thromboxane synthetase. Prostaglandins 13:611-618.

Moncada, S., Herman, A. G., Higgs, E. A., and Vane, J. R. (1977b). Differential formation of prostacyclin (PGX or PGI_2) by layers of the arterial wall. An explanation for the antithrombotic properties of vascular endothelium. Thromb. Res. 11:323-344.

Moncada, S., Vane, J. R., and Whittle, B. J. R. (1977c). Relative potency of prostacyclin, prostaglandin E_1 and D_2 as inhibitors of platelet aggregation in several species. J. Physiol. (Lond.), 273:2P-4P.

Mustard, J. F., and Packham, M. A. (1970). Factors influencing platelet function: adhesion, release and aggregation. Pharmacol. Rev. 22:97-187.

Mustard, J. F., and Packham, M. A. (1975). Platelets, thrombosis and drugs. Drugs 9:19-76.

Mustard, J. F., Packham, M. A., and Kinlough-Rathbone, R. L. (1977). Effects of drugs on platelets and complications of vascular disease. Adv. Exp. Biol. Med. 82:94-105.

Needleman, P., Minkes, M., and Raz, R. (1976a). Thromboxanes: selective biosynthesis and distinct biological properties. Science 193:163-165.

Needleman, P., Moncada, S., Bunting, S., Vane, J. R., Hamberg, M., and Samuelsson, B. (1976b). Identification of an enzyme in platelet microsomes which generates thromboxane A_2 from prostaglandin endoperoxides. Nature (Lond.) 261:558-560.

Needleman, P., Bryan, B., Wyche, A., Bronson, S. D., Eakins, K., Ferrendelli, J. A., and Minkes, M. (1977). Thromboxane synthetase inhibitors as pharmacological tools: differential biochemical and biological effects on platelets. Prostaglandins 14:897-907.

Needleman, P., Wyche, A., and Raz, A. (1979a). Platelet and blood vessel arachidonate metabolism and interactions. J. Clin. Invest. 63:345-349.

Needleman, P., Raz, A., Minkes, M. S., Ferrendelli, J. A., and Sprecher, H. (1979b). Triene prostaglandins: prostacyclin and thromboxane biosynthesis and unique biological properties. Proc. Natl. Acad. Sci. USA 76:944-948.

Nugteren, D. H. (1978). Platelets and prostaglandins. Agents Actions 8:296-298.

O'Brien, J. R. (1971). Platelet count techniques, platelet adhesiveness and aggregation tests. In Thrombosis and Bleeding Disorders, N. U. Bang, F. K. Beller, E. Deutsch, and E. F. Mammen (Eds.). Georg Thieme Verlag, Stuttgart/Academic Press, New York, pp. 430-436.

Oelz, O., Oelz, R., Knapp, H. R., Sweetman, B. J., and Oates, J. A. (1977). Biosynthesis of prostaglandin D_2. Formation of prostaglandin D_2 by human platelets. Prostaglandins 13:225-234.

Packham, M. A., and Mustard, J. F. (1977). Clinical pharmacology of platelets. Blood 50:555-573.

Patrono, C., Ciabattoni, G., and Grossi-Belloni, D. (1975). Release of prostaglandin $F_{1\alpha}$ and $F_{2\alpha}$ from superfused platelets: quantitative evaluation of the inhibitory effects of some aspirin-like drugs. Prostaglandins 9:557-568.

Rane, M. D., Oelz, O., Frolich, J. C., Seyberth, H. J., Sweetman, B. J., Watson, J. T., Wilkinson, G. R., and Oates, J. A. (1978). Relation between plasma concentration of indomethacin and its effect on prostaglandin synthesis and platelet aggregation in man. Clin. Pharm. Ther. 23:658-668.

Raz, A., and Aharony, D. (1978). Prostaglandin synthesis in platelets:

demonstration and role of prostaglandin H_2—E_2 isomerase. Res. Commun. Chem. Pathol. Pharmacol. 21:507-515.

Robison, G., Arnold, A., Cole, B., and Hartmann, R. (1971). Effects of prostaglandins on function and cyclic AMP levels of human blood platelets. Ann. N.Y. Acad. Sci. 180:324-331.

Roth, G. J., Stanford, N., and Majerus, P. W. (1975). Acetylation of prostaglandin synthase by aspirin. Proc. Natl. Acad. Sci. USA 72: 3073-3076.

Salzman, E. W., and Levine, L. (1971). Cyclic 3',5'-adenosine monophosphate in human blood platelets. J. Clin. Invest. 50:131-141.

Salzman, E. W., Kensler, P. C., and Levine, L. (1972). Cyclic 3',5'-adenosine monophosphate in human blood platelets: IV. Regulatory role of cyclic AMP in platelet function. Ann. N.Y. Acad. Sci. 201:61-71.

Samuelsson, B. (1965). On the incorporation of oxygen in the conversion of 8,11,14-eicosatrienoic acid to prostaglandin E_1. J. Am. Chem. Soc. 87:3011-3013.

Samuelsson, B., Granstrom, E., Green, K., Hamberg, M., and Hammarstrom, S. (1975). Prostaglandins. Annu. Rev. Biochem. 44:669-695.

Samuelsson, B., Hamberg, C., Malmsten, C., and Svensson, J. (1976). The role of prostaglandin endoperoxides and the thromboxanes in platelet aggregation. Adv. Prostaglandin Thromboxane Res. 2:737-746.

Samuelsson, B., Goldyne, M., Granstrom, E., Hamberg, M., Hammarstrom, S., and Malmsten, C. (1978). Prostaglandins and thromboxanes. Annu. Rev. Biochem. 47:997-1029.

Shio, H., Ramwell, P. W., and Jessup, S. J. (1972). Prostaglandin E_2: effects on aggregation, shape change and cyclic AMP of rat platelets. Prostaglandins 1:29-36.

Siegl, A., Smith, J. B., Silver, M. J., Nicolaou, K. C., and Ahern, D. (1979). Selective binding site for [^{3}H]prostacyclin on platelets. J. Clin. Invest. 63:215-220.

Silberbauer, K., Sinzinger, H., and Winter, M. (1978). Prostacyclin production by vascular smooth-muscle cells. Lancet 1 (June 24):1356-1357.

Silver, M. J., Smith, J. B., Ingerman, C., and Kocsis, J. J. (1973). Arachidonic acid-induced human platelet aggregation and prostaglandin formation. Prostaglandins 4:863-875.

Sinha, A. K., and Colman, R. W. (1978). Prostaglandin E_1 inhibits platelet aggregation by a pathway independent of adenosin 3',5'-monophosphate. Science 200:202-203.

Smith, J. B., and Willis, A. L. (1974). Aspirin selectively inhibits prostaglandin production in human platelets. Nature (New Biol.) 231:235-237.

Smith, J. B., Ingerman, C., Kocsis, J. J., and Silver, M. J. (1973). Formation of prostaglandins during the aggregation of human blood platelets. J. Clin. Invest. 52:965-969.

Smith, J. B., Silver, M. J., Ingerman, C. M., and Kocsis, J. J. (1974). Prostaglandin D_2 inhibits the aggregation of human platelets. Thromb. Res. 5:291-299.

Smith, J. B., Ingerman, C. M., and Silver, M. J. (1976a). Platelet prostaglandin production and its implications. Adv. Prostaglandin Thromboxane Res. 2:747-753.

Smith, J. B., Ingerman, C. M., and Silver, M. J. (1976b). Persistence of thromboxane A_2-like material and platelet release-inducing activity in plasma. J. Clin. Invest. 58:1119-1122.

Smith, J. B., Ingerman, C. M., and Silver, M. J. (1976c). Formation of prostaglandin D_2 during endoperoxide-induced platelet aggregation. Thromb. Res. 9:413-418.

Sun, F. F. (1977). Biosynthesis of thromboxanes in human platelets. I. Characterization and assay of thromboxane synthetase. Biochem. Biophys. Res. Commun. 74:1432-1440.

Sun, F. F., Chapman, J. P., and McGuire, J. C. (1977). Metabolism of prostaglandin endoperoxide in animal tissue. Prostaglandins 14:1055-1074.

Svensson, J., Hamberg, M., and Samuelsson, B. (1976). On the formation and effects of thromboxane A_2 in human platelets. Acta Physiol. Scand. 98:285-294.

Szczeklik, A., Gryglewski, R. J., Nizankowski, R., Musial, J., Pieton, R., and Mruk, J. (1978). Circulatory and anti-platelet effects of intravenous prostacyclin in healthy men. Pharmacol. Res. Commun. 10:545-556.

Tateson, J. E., Moncada, S., and Vane, J. R. (1977). Effects of prostacyclin (PGX) on cyclic AMP concentrations in human platelets. Prostaglandins 13:389-397.

Vane, J. R. (1971). Inhibition of prostaglandin synthesis as a mechanism of action for aspirin-like drugs. Nature (New Biol.) 231:232-235.

Vargaftig, B. B., and Chignard, M. (1975). Substances that increase the cyclic AMP content prevent platelet aggregation and the concurrent release of pharmacologically active substances evoked by arachidonic acid. Agents Actions 5:137-114.

Vargaftig, B. B., and Zirinis, P. (1973). Platelet aggregation induced by arachidonic acid is accompanied by release of potential inflammatory mediators distinct from PGE_2 and $PGF_{2\alpha}$. Nature (New Biol.) 214:114-116.

Vincent, J. E., and Zijlstra, F. J. (1978). Nicotinic acid inhibits thromboxane synthesis in platelets. Prostaglandins 15:629-636.

Wang, T. Y., Hussey, C. U., and Garancis, J. C. (1977). Effects of dibutyryl cyclic adenosine-monophosphate and prostaglandin E_1 on platelet aggregation and shape changes. Am. J. Clin. Pathol. 67:362-367.

Weiss, A., Baenziger, N. L., and Atkinson, J. P. (1978). Platelet release reaction and intracellular cGMP. Blood 52:524-531.

Weiss, H. J. (1971). The effects of aspirin on platelets and thrombosis. An historical review and experimental studies. In Aspirin, Platelets and Stroke, W. S. Fields and W. K. Hass (Eds.). Warren H. Green, St. Louis, Mo., pp. 51-58.

Weiss, H. J. (1972). The pharmacology of platelet inhibition. Prog. Hemostasis Thromb. 1:199-231.

Weiss, H. J. (1976). Antiplatelet drugs—a new pharmacologic approach to the prevention of thrombosis. Am. Heart J. 92:86-102.

Weiss, H. J. (1978). Antiplatelet therapy (two parts). N. Engl. J. Med. 298:1344-1347; 1403-1406.

Weksler, B. B., Marcus, A. J., and Jaffe, E. A. (1977). Synthesis of prostaglandin I_2 (prostacyclin) by cultured human and bovine endothelial cells. Proc. Natl. Acad. Sci. USA 74:3922-3926.

Westwick, J. (1978). The effect of pulmonary metabolites of prostaglandins E_1, E_2 and $F_{2\alpha}$ on ADP-induced aggregation of human and rabbit platelets. Br. J. Pharmacol. 58:297P-298P.

White, H. L., and Glasman, A. T. (1976). Biochemical properties of the prostaglandin/thromboxane synthetase of human blood platelets and comparison with the synthetase of bovine seminal vesicles. Prostaglandins 12:811-828.

White, J. G. (1979). Current concepts of platelet structure. Am. J. Clin. Pathol. 71:363-377.

Willis, A. L. (1973). Platelet synthesis of pro-aggregating material from arachidonate and its blockade by aspirin. Circulation 48(Suppl):55.

Willis, A. L. (1974). Isolation of a chemical trigger for thrombosis. Prostaglandins 5:1-25.

Willis, A. L., and Kuhn, D. C. (1973). A new potential mediator of arterial thrombosis whose biosynthesis is inhibited by aspirin. Prostaglandins 4:127-130.

Willis, A. L., Comai, K., Kuhn, D. C., and Paulsrud, J. (1974a). Dihomogamma-linolenate suppresses platelet aggregation when administered in vitro or in vivo. Prostaglandins 8:509-519.

Willis, A. L., Vane, F. M., Kuhn, D. C., Scott, C. G., and Petrin, M. (1974b). An endoperoxide aggregator (LASS) formed in platelets in response to thrombotic stimuli. Prostaglandins 8:453-507.

Wlodawer, P., Kindahl, H., and Hamberg, M. (1976). Biosynthesis of prostaglandin $F_{2\alpha}$ from arachidonic acid and prostaglandin endoperoxides in the uterus. Biochim. Biophys. Acta 431:603-614.

Wolfe, S. M., and Shulman, N. R. (1969). Adenyl cyclase activity in human platelets. Biochem. Biophys. Res. Commun. 35:265-272.

Wong, P. Y.-K., and Cheung, W. Y. (1979). Calmodulin stimulates human platelet phospholipase A_2. Biochem. Biophys. Res. Commun. 90:473-480.

Zieve, P. D., and Greenough, W. B., III (1969). Adenyl cyclase in human platelets: activity and responsiveness. Biochem. Biophys. Res. Commun. 35:462-466.

Zucker, M. B. (1971). Effects of aspirin and other anti-inflammatory agents on platelets. In Aspirin, Platelets and Stroke, W. S. Fields and W. K. Hass (Eds.). Warren H. Green, St. Louis, Mo., pp. 74-83.

11 Effects of Prostaglandins on Erythropoiesis

PETER P. DUKES / Childrens Hospital of Los Angeles and University of Southern California School of Medicine, Los Angeles, California

Erythropoiesis is the sequence of events that starts in pluripotent hematopoietic stem cells and leads ultimately, after a number of differentiation steps and cell divisions, to the appearance of mature red cells in the circulation of an organism. The initial steps occur under the influence of an erythroid-specific hematopoietic-inducive microenvironment (1) and bring into existence progenitor cells which can follow the pathway of erythroid differentiation. The number of early erythroid progenitor cells (erythroid burst-forming units BFU-E) seems to be modulated by factors termed burst-promoting activities (BPA) (2-5). Once past the earliest stages, the hormone erythropoietin appears to be the decisive factor controlling successive steps in this process. Krantz and Graber have prepared an extensive review on erythropoietin (6) to which the reader is directed for background information on this subject.

Prostaglandins have been found to play an important role in the mechanism of the elaboration of erythropoietin; they have also been reported to have direct effects on the pluripotent hematopoietic stem cells and on erythroid precursor cells. These two topics are taken up separately.

ROLE OF PROSTAGLANDINS IN THE REGULATION OF THE ELABORATION OF ERYTHROPOIETIN

Kidney, Extrarenal Sites

Schooley and Mahlmann first observed a stimulation of erythropoiesis by prostaglandins (7). They reported that PGE_1 and PGE_2 but not $PGF_{2\alpha}$ increased the erythropoiesis of polycythemic mice which are otherwise almost totally devoid of new red cell formation. They further found that the erythropoietic response of polycythemic mice, induced by an exposure to hypoxia, could be significantly potentiated if the mice were first injected with the stimulatory prostaglandins. They demonstrated that these effects were erythropoietin dependent by showing that an antiserum directed against that hormone prevented their occurrence. They suggested that the prostaglandins caused a redistribution of blood flow in the kidney of mice and implied that since that organ is the major site of erythropoietin production, this may have led to increased erythropoietin output.

Investigations performed in our laboratory (8) showed that among the primary prostaglandins PGA_2 was most effective in stimulating erythropoiesis in the exhypoxic polycythemic mouse followed by PGE_2, PGE_1, and PGA_1, whereas $PGF_{2\alpha}$ and $PGF_{2\beta}$ exhibited no effect. A dose dependence of prostaglandin effects on the production of red cells was demonstrated. Subsequently (9) two PGE_2 derivatives with protected 15-hydroxy groups: 15(S)-methyl and 16,16-dimethyl-PGE_2-methyl ester (15M-PGE_2-M and 16diM-PGE_2-M) were found to be 100 times more potent than the parent compound in the polycythemic mouse assay. Their effects were also found to be dose dependent. Comparing the dose-response curves of prostaglandins and of erythropoietin, it was found that their slopes differed and that the maximum stimulation obtainable with prostaglandins was below that obtainable with erythropoietin. The last finding suggested that the limitation of the prostaglandin effect was not caused by a lack of target cells.

The effects of the simultaneous administration of prostaglandin and of erythropoietin to the polycythemic mouse were systematically investigated (8,9). It was found that prostaglandins further increased erythropoiesis when administered with small doses of erythropoietin but had no effect when the mice received larger, but still submaximally stimulatory doses of the hormone. It also became apparent that the dose of the prostaglandin coadministered with erythropoietin determined at what dose level of the hormone the potentiating effect of the prostaglandin disappeared. Prostaglandin doses which by themselves were suboptimally stimulatory were effective in further increasing erythropoiesis in the presence of higher doses of erythropoietin than the erythropoietin dose, which represented the cutoff point for the effect with larger prostaglandin doses. The central region of the log dose-response curve of erythropoietin appeared to be parallel displaced to the left when an appropriate amount of prostaglandin was coadministered. This type of displacement suggested a more than simply additive effect which could not have resulted from the generation or release in the mice of a fixed amount of erythropoietin due to the prostaglandin administered. It was concluded that prostaglandins enhance erythropoiesis in the polycythemic mouse, not only by the stimulation of erythropoietin production, but also by a direct effect on erythroid precursor cells (8).

Evidence for a role of prostaglandins in the production of erythropoietin by the kidney was presented in several papers by Fisher and his coworkers. Paulo et al. (10) and Nelson and Fisher (11) confirmed that PGE_1 increases the erythropoiesis of the exhypoxic polycythemic mouse and that the dehydrogenase resistant analogs 15M-PGE_2 and 16diM-PGE_2 have a much higher activity in that system than does the parent compound. Nelson and Fisher (12) further reported that PGI_2, but not 6-keto-$PGF_{1\alpha}$ (its primary metabolite), also stimulates erythropoiesis in the exhypoxic polycythemic mouse. Paulo et al. (10) perfused isolated dog kidneys with a PGE_1 solution and showed that this stimulated erythropoietin release from that organ. The dogs, whose kidneys were utilized in this study, were exposed to 4 hr of hypoxia before the perfusion experiment was started. This was found to be necessary to preprogram the kidneys for erythropoietin production. Employing the same isolated dog kidney perfusion system, Gross et al. (13) demonstrated that perfusion with PGE_2, the principal renal prostaglandin, similarly increased erythropoietin release. In both sets of experiments, perfusion of the preprogrammed kidneys with saline did not lead to erythropoietin release. Mujovic and Fisher (14) and Gross et al. (15) found that renal artery constriction in the dog led to increased erythropoietin production and increased PGE levels in the renal venous effluent. Both the increased erythropoietin production and the increased prostaglandin levels in the dogs could be prevented by the administration of indomethacin, a known inhibitor of prostaglandin synthesis, suggesting an involvement of prostaglandin in erythropoietin production. Hypoxic hypoxia causes increased erythropoietin levels in dogs. Mujovic and Fisher (16) showed that this stimulus of erythropoietin production was also ineffective when the dogs were pretreated with indomethacin. Foley et al. (17) recently showed that the prostaglandin precursor arachidonic acid stimulated erythropoiesis in the exhypoxic polycythemic mouse and that it caused erythropoietin production (blocked by indomethacin pretreatment) in the preprogrammed, isolated perfused canine kidney.

Humoral, Nervous, and Local Effects of Hypoxia Leading to Prostaglandin Release and Erythropoietin Production

The findings so far presented make a role of prostaglandins in erythropoietin production or activation highly plausible. Even more impressive is the fact that hypoxia, the condition that causes erythropoietin elaboration in the organism, also causes the release of systemic humoral stimuli, specific nerve activity, and changes in affected cells which lead to the release of prostaglandins. These relationships will now be reviewed.

Hypoxia causes catecholamine release from the adrenal medulla, extramedullary chromaffin tissues, and the sympathetic nerves (18,19). Fink et al. (20,21) have shown that there are actually two separate mechanisms involving catecholamines related to the production of erythropoietin by the hypoxic rabbit. They observed that during a 5-hr hypoxic stress, renal denervation but not β-adrenergic blockade reduced erythropoietin production. Conversely, if hypoxia continued for an 18-hr period, it was β-adrenergic blockade and not renal denervation that reduced erythropoietin output. Fink and Fisher (22, 23) found that the nonselective β-adrenergic agonist isoproterenol and the β_2-specific agonist salbutamol, but not the β_1-specific agonist dobutamine, increased the rate of erythropoiesis in the polycythemic mouse and that this could be blocked by propranolol (adrenergic antagonist) pretreatment. Salbutamol infusion was shown to increase the plasma erythropoietin levels of rabbits unless they had been nephrectomized. Albuterol, another β_2-specific adrenergic agonist, has recently been reported by Przala et al. (24) to have the same effect in rabbits. All this suggested that β_2-adrenergic receptor stimulation modulated the rate of new hormone synthesis, whereas renal sympathetic nerve activity had an additional effect on release or activation of a storage form of erythropoietin.

It is possible that the increase in circulating catecholamines produced by hypoxia brings about increased renin levels. Alternatively, it may be that prostaglandin endoperoxides generated from arachidonic acid, which is released by cells under hypoxic conditions by a mechanism described below, stimulate renin release. This was suggested by Weber et al. (25), who found that rabbit renal cortex slices would release renin when incubated with arachidonic acid, PGG_2, or stable endoperoxide analogs in approximately 10^{-6} M concentration; PGE_2 (10^{-12}-10^{-6} M) had no effect. One has to assume that the renin-angiotensinogen system is in some fashion involved in the concurrently observed increase in plasma erythropoietin since Gould et al. (26) were able to demonstrate an in vivo effect of renin on erythropoietin formation in rats. They found increases of renin, angiotensinogen, and erythropoietin in the plasma of rats exposed to hypoxia; if renin (2.5 GU/100 g) was injected into these rats, the plasma concentration of angiotensinogen and of erythropoietin rose. However, renin had no such effect on rats kept at ambient pressure. Of great interest is their additional observation that anephric rats kept at ambient pressure did respond to the same dose of renin with a measurable increase in erythropoietin, suggesting a common mechanism involving angiotensins I and II in both renal and extrarenal erythropoietin formation.

At this point, one should compare the stimuli that promote prostaglandin synthesis in the kidney [reviewed by Zins (27)] with the stimuli that lead to increased erythropoietin output by that organ. Zins listed the following: ischemia (stenosis or reduced perfusion pressure), renal nerve stimulation, norepinephrine, epinephrine, angiotensin II, angiotensin I, vasopressin, and bradykinin. The first six stimuli have already been shown to be related to hypoxia and erythropoietin production. Increased catecholamine levels can bring about a rise in angiotensin II, which in turn stimulates adenylate cyclase activity in the rabbit renal papilla (28). This leads to activation of phospholipase A, and this enzyme releases arachidonate, which the prostaglandin synthetase complex converts into prostaglandins E or F via the endoperoxide intermediates. The angiotensin II mechanism is not restricted to the kidney; vascular smooth muscle cells in culture can similarly respond to angiotensin II (29); catecholamines may, however, in some instances, stimulate prostaglandin synthesis by a more direct route. Vasopressin is well known to be released by the pituitary in various stressful situations; it has been shown to cause prostaglandin synthesis and the activation of a renal adenylate cyclase (27). Bradykinin is formed by the action of kallikrein on the appropriate circulating kininogen. Kallikreins are elaborated in response to an ischemic, hypoxic condition in various organs, including the kidney (27) and the heart (30). Smooth muscle cells in culture respond to bradykinin as well as to angiotensin II by prostaglandin formation (29), possibly by a similar mechanism of action.

Finally, as referred to earlier, an intracellular process seems to operate which may explain why cells deprived of oxygen release prostaglandins into the local environment. Markelonis and Garbus (31) reported that mitochondria kept under anoxic conditions elaborate increasing amounts of free fatty acids similar to what is obtained with mitochondria "aged" in vitro or isolated from ischemic tissues. They found that the free fatty acids elaborated included the polyunsaturated precursors of prostaglandins such as arachidonic acid and postulated that these are converted into prostaglandins to be released from the ischemic tissues.

Involvement of Cyclic Nucleotides

Although it seems certain that prostaglandins (PGE_2 and/or PGA_2 and/or PGI_2) are involved in the elaboration of erythropoietin, their role in this process is not yet completely established. In the kidney they are very likely to activate a cortical adenylate cyclase. An elevated renal cyclic AMP level has been shown to precede increased plasma erythropoietin levels in rats (32), and it was possible to stimulate erythropoiesis of polycythemic mice by administration of cyclic AMP (33). Rodgers et al. (32) and Martelo et al. (34) demonstrated that a cyclic AMP-dependent protein kinase activates (phosphorylates) a renal erythropoietic factor (REF). Interaction of this factor with another protein leads to the generation of biologically active erythropoietin (35, 36). REF is of lysosomal origin (37). It is interesting to note that Rodgers et al. (38) have demonstrated a rise in renal cyclic GMP and an associated release of renal lysosomal enzymes into plasma preceding a cobalt-induced rise in circulating erythropoietin levels. Both cobalt and hypoxia-induced increases in erythropoietin output could be reduced by atropine. They therefore suggested that renal cyclic GMP participates in a cholinergic mechanism mediating lysosomal REF release, whereas renal cyclic AMP has a role in the subsequent activation of REF, leading to erythropoietin production.

EFFECTS OF PROSTAGLANDINS ON ERYTHROID CELLS AND THEIR PROGENITORS

Effects on DNA Synthetic Activity of Pluripotent Hematopoietic Stem Cells

Fehér and Gidáli (39) studied the effect of PGE_2 on the proliferative state of the pluripotent hematopoietic stem cells of mice. These cells are quantitated utilizing their ability to form spleen colonies when injected into lethally irradiated recipient mice. Their proliferative state can be characterized by their in vitro sensitivity to $[^3H]$thymidine of high specific activity. It was found that 2.5-hr preincubation of donor marrow cells with PGE_2 at concentrations from 10^{-11} to 10^{-3} M increased the fraction of spleen colony-forming cells (CFU-S) killed by the exposure to $[^3H]$thymidine to 30% from a control value of 5%. This suggested that the CFU-S, most of which are normally in the resting (G_0) phase of the cell cycle, may be triggered by PGE_2 to commence DNA synthesis indicating replication. Fehér and Gidáli (39) suggested that this prostaglandin effect was not mediated by cyclic AMP through activation of an adenylate cyclase since they found that the addition of imidazole, a potentiator of phosphodiesterase, to the incubation mixture containing PGE_2 did not reduce the fraction of CFU-S killed in the experiment. However, Byron (40) criticized this conclusion as premature since the imidazole effect was only tested at a 10^{-6} M PGE_2 concentration. More recently, Gidáli and Fehér (41) also investigated the effect on CFU-S of PGE_1 and PGE_2 administration in vivo. They found that injection of as little as 10^{-4} μg/g body weight caused a significant increase of the proportion of CFU-S in the S-phase, without affecting their total number per animal.

Effects on Erythroid Precursor Cells and Their Response to Erythropoietin

Work from our laboratory (9,42,43) suggests that erythroid-committed hematopoietic cells from the bone marrow of rats are also sensitive to prostaglandins. Such cells characteristically respond to erythropoietin with increased heme synthesis. Heme synthesis of rat marrow cells in suspension culture was found to be stimulated by various prostaglandins, most effectively by 3.3×10^{-7} M PGE_2. This effect occurred both in the presence and absence of added erythropoietin.

Another effect of the addition of erythropoietin to rat marrow cells in culture is an increase in the rate of incorporation of glucosamine into cellular material. This effect is not erythropoietin specific, but it is nevertheless of interest that glucosamine incorporation was stimulated by the same prostaglandins which were found to stimulate heme synthesis and with roughly the same order of potency.

Friend virus-transformed mouse erythroleukemia cells (FL cells) (44) in culture respond to certain inducers (e.g., dimethylsulfoxide and related compounds), but not to erythropoietin, by undergoing erythroid differentiation as manifested by the synthesis of markers such as heme and the erythrocyte membrane-specific antigen spectrin. Tabuse et al. (45) reported that 10^{-4} M PGE_1 caused similar erythroid differentiation of FL cells, based on the appearance of heme and spectrin-positive cells after 5 days of incubation. Interestingly, a dimethylsulfoxide-resistant FL cell line also was stimulated by PGE_1, but its response was confined to spectrin synthesis.

Djaldetti et al. (46) investigated the effect of PGA_2 on RNA synthesis by 12-day embryonic mouse liver erythroid cells in culture. This system responds to the addition of erythropoietin with an increase in RNA synthesis; PGA_2 (10 μg/ml) caused a 53% augmentation of RNA synthesis. The effects of PGE_2 on nucleic acid synthesis in rat marrow cell cultures were investigated in our laboratory (M. C. Datta and P. P. Dukes, unpublished observations, 1978). No major change in RNA synthesis could be detected. However, DNA synthesis was reduced by PGE_2 in a reversible fashion. PGE_2 was added either at the beginning of culture or at the end of 45 hr of preincubation. At the end of 24 hr of incubation, 3.3×10^{-7} M PGE_2 depressed DNA synthesis 31%, whereas 2.4×10^{-5} M PGE_2 depressed it 48%. The same doses of PGE_2, added to preincubated cells, depressed 26% and 96% of DNA synthesis, respectively. A detailed kinetic analysis of DNA synthesis in cultures treated with the lower dose showed no increase in synthesis at any time, but a maximum depression after 24 hr. Starting with 24 hr of incubation, an increment in surviving cells due to 3.3×10^{-7} M PGE_2 was observed which reached a maximum after 45-48 hr. In cultures washed free of PGE_2 after 45 hr of incubation, DNA synthesis increased, hour by hour, over that of controls in spite of a simultaneous decrease in nucleated cell numbers. These results indicate that whereas PGE_2 initiates DNA synthesis in CFU-S (39,41), which constitute a small fraction (< 1%) of the total cells in the bone marrow, it causes a reversible arrest of a large number of marrow cells in a non-DNA synthetic state.

Chan et al. (47,48) reported that nine different prostaglandins added to normal human marrow cells cultured in a methylcellulose-based medium enhanced the stimulatory effect of erythropoietin on the appearance of colonies derived from late erythroid progenitor cells (CFU-E) and from the early progenitor cells (BFU-E). This stimulation could be shown only if the fetal calf serum component of the medium was heat inactivated. In the presence of 1 IU/ml of erythropoietin, the maximum stimulatory effect on CFU-E (197%) was seen with PGE_1 (1.5×10^{-7} M); BFU-E were maximally stimulated by 2.0×10^{-6} M $PGF_{2\alpha}$-THAM (333%). Studies conducted in our laboratory (W. Powell and P. P. Dukes, unpublished observations, 1979) compared the effects of PGE_2 and PGI_2 on human circulating blood BFU-E incubated in a similar methylcellulose system. It was found that both prostaglandins caused a large increase in burst colonies over the number generated by 1.3 IU/ml erythropoietin by itself. This was not dependent on heat inactivation of the fetal calf serum. Whereas PGE_2 was maximally stimulatory at 10^{-7} M (300-400%) and totally inhibitory at 10^{-4} M, PGI_2 was most stimulatory at 10^{-5} M (50-150%) and still stimulatory at 10^{-4} M. The lesser effect of PGI_2 probably reflects a lesser stability in solution rather than a lower potency than that of PGE_2. These findings further support the hypothesis, alluded to in the preceding section, that certain prostaglandins can increase the number of newly formed red cells in an organism, not only by causing erythropoietin production, but also by an effect on marrow cells. Erythroid progenitor cells may be affected directly by prostaglandins or other cells, which in turn positively or negatively regulate progenitor cells, may be acted on by prostaglandins. Positive effector cells involved may be the producers of BPA (2-5); negative effector cells which may play a role are the suppressor cells described by Hoffman et al. (49). It should be noted that a report by Kurland and Moore (50) describes a suppressing effect of PGE_1 on granulocyte-macrophage progenitor cells; the same publication also reviews the modulation of other hematopoietic cells by prostaglandins.

Effects on Red Cell Deformability

Finally, it has been reported that prostaglandins affect the deformability of red cells and their resistance to hypotonic hemolysis. Allen and Rasmussen (51) and Rasmussen et al. (52) examined the effects of PGE_2 and PGE_1 on human and rat red cells. Filterability through standardized paper filters was used as a measure of their deformability. They found that PGE_2 from 10^{-12} to 10^{-10} M caused a decreased rate of filtration and increased hypotonic hemolysis, whereas PGE_1 at the same concentrations had exactly the opposite effects. At higher concentrations, both prostaglandins caused a slight decrease in hypotonic hemolysis. In the human cells, the prostaglandin-receptor interaction did not lead to an increase in intracellular cyclic AMP levels, although this did occur in the rat cells. This suggested to the authors that at least in the human red cells the prostaglandins caused a generalized change in membrane structure by a mechanism quite independent of adenylate cyclase activation. Kury et al. (53), employing spin-labeled human red cells and measuring paramagnetic resonance spectra of the spin labels, also concluded that PGE_2 at very low concentrations made the cells less deformable and PGE_1 at the same concentrations made them more deformable than untreated controls. It should be mentioned here, however, that Jay et al. (54) were unable to detect any change in deformability of human red cells in the presence of either PGE_2 or PGE_1 (10^{-13}-10^{-5} M) when they measured deformability by examining the pressures required to draw single red cells into glass micropipettes of various diameters. If further experimentation bears out the findings indicating that red cell membrane changes can be caused by prostaglandins, that would suggest that red cells can actively respond to these vasoactive substances and may therefore play a role themselves in blood pressure and flow regulation.

SUMMARY

Prostaglandins have been shown to be involved in several ways in the regulation of red cell formation and function. The elaboration of the hormone erythropoietin, which governs the replication and differentiation of erythroid precursor cells, is obligatorily linked to the synthesis of PGE_2 in the kidney in response to stimuli due to hypoxia. The replication of hematopoietic stem cells has been demonstrated to be triggered by PGE_2. This may make possible a fast replacement of those erythroid-committed progenitor cells which have been withdrawn from the earliest erythropoietin-sensitive cellular compartment by the action of erythropoietin. Certain prostaglandins, particularly of the E type, were found to stimulate in cell culture systems erythroid colony formation from progenitor cells and also heme synthesis in erythroid precursor cells, indicating that prostaglandins also stimulate erythropoiesis at the marrow cell level. Finally, the deformability of erythrocytes was shown to be decreased by a direct action of PGE_2 on their cell membranes, whereas PGE_1 had an opposite effect. This suggests that the rate of passage of red cells through the microvasculature may be modulated by their response to local prostaglandin levels.

REFERENCES

1. Curry, J. L., and Trentin, J. J. Hemopoietic spleen colony studies: I. Growth and differentiation. Dev. Biol. 15:395–413, 1967.
2. Iscove, N. N. Erythropoietin-independent stimulation of early erythropoiesis in adult marrow cultures by conditioned media from lectin-stimulated mouse spleen cells. In Hematopoietic Cell Differentiation (ICN-UCLA Symposia on Molecular and Cellular Biology, Vol. 10), D. W. Golde, M. J. Cline, D. Metcalf, and C. F. Fox (Eds.). Academic Press, New York, pp. 37-52, 1978.
3. Wagemaker, G. Induction of erythropoietin responsiveness in vitro. In Hematopoietic Cell Differentiation (ICN-UCLA Symposia on Molecular and Cellular Biology, Vol. 10), D. W. Golde, M. J. Cline, D. Metcalf, and C. F. Fox (Eds.). Academic Press, New York, pp. 109-118, 1978.
4. Aye, M. T. Erythroid colony formation in cultures of human marrow: effects of leukocyte conditioned medium. J. Cell. Physiol. 91:68-78, 1977.
5. Meytes, D., Ma, A., Ortega, J. A., Shore, N. A., and Dukes, P. P. Human erythroid burst-promoting activity produced by phytohemagglutinin-stimulated radioresistant peripheral blood mononuclear cells. Blood 54:1050-1057, 1979.
6. Krantz, S. B., and Graber, S. E. Erythropoietin. In Physiological Pharmacology, Vol. 5, W. S. Root and N. I. Berlin (Eds.). Academic Press, New York, pp. 509-554, 1974.

7. Schooley, J. C., and Mahlmann, L. J. Stimulation of erythropoiesis in plethoric mice by prostaglandins and its inhibition by antierythropoietin. Proc. Soc. Exp. Biol. Med. 138:52 3-524, 1971.
8. Dukes, P. P., Shore, N. A., Hammond, D., Ortega, J. A., and Datta, M. C. Enhancement of erythropoiesis by prostaglandins. J. Lab. Clin. Med. 82:704-712, 1973.
9. Dukes, P. P., Shore, N. A., Hammond, D., and Ortega, J. A. Prostaglandins and erythropoietin action. In Erythropoiesis, K. Nakao, J. W. Fisher, and F. Takaku (Eds.). University of Tokyo Press, Tokyo, pp. 3-14, 1975.
10. Paulo, L. G., Wilkerson, R. D., Roh, B. L., George, W. J., and Fisher, J. W. The effects of prostaglandin E_1 on erythropoietin production. Proc. Soc. Exp. Biol. Med. 142:771-775, 1973.
11. Nelson, P. K., and Fisher, J. W. Erythroid progenitor cell activation by prostaglandins E (PGE). Blood 52(Suppl. 1):212, 1978.
12. Nelson, P. K., and Fisher, J. W. Erythropoietic effects of PGI_2 and 6-keto-$PGF_{1\alpha}$. Fed. Proc. 37:607, 1978.
13. Gross, D. M., Brookins, J., Fink, G. D., and Fisher, J. W. Effects of prostaglandins A_2, E_2 and $F_{2\alpha}$ on erythropoietin production. J. Pharmacol. Exp. Ther. 198:489-496, 1976.
14. Mujovic, V. M., and Fisher, J. W. The effects of indomethacin on erythropoietin production in dogs following renal artery constriction: I. The possible role of prostaglandins in the generation of erythropoietin by the kidney. J. Pharmacol. Exp. Ther. 191:575-580, 1974.
15. Gross, D. M., Mujovic, V. M., Jubiz, W., and Fisher, J. W. Enhanced erythropoietin and prostaglandin E production in the dog following renal artery constriction. Proc. Soc. Exp. Biol. Med. 15:498-500, 1976.
16. Mujovic, V. M., and Fisher, J. W. The role of prostaglandins in the production of erythropoietin (ESF) by the kidney: II. Effects of indomethacin on erythropoietin production following hypoxia in dogs. Life Sci. 16:463-473, 1975.
17. Foley, J. E., Gross, D. M., Nelson, P. K., and Fisher, J. W. The effects of arachidonic acid on erythropoietin production in exhypoxic polycythemic mice and the isolated perfused canine kidney. J. Pharmacol. Exp. Ther. 207:402–409, 1978.
18. Fowler, N. O., Shabetai, R., and Holmes, J. C. Adrenal medullary secretion during hypoxia, bleeding and rapid intravenous infusion. Circ. Res. 9:427-435, 1961.
19. Kotchen, T. A., Hogan, R. P., Boyd, A. E., Li, T.-K., Sing, H. C., and Mason, J. W. Renin, noradrenaline and adrenaline responses to simulated altitude. Clin. Sci. 44:243-251, 1973.
20. Fink, G. D., Paulo, L. G., and Fisher, J. W. Effects of beta adrenergic blocking agents on erythropoietin production in rabbits exposed to hypoxia. J. Pharmacol. Exp. Ther. 193:176-181, 1975.

21. Fink, G. D., and Fisher, J. W. Erythropoietin production after renal denervation or beta-adrenergic blockade. Am. J. Physiol. 230:508-513, 1976.
22. Fink, G. D., and Fisher, J. W. Stimulation of erythropoiesis by beta adrenergic agonists: I. Characterization of activity in polycythemic mice. J. Pharmacol. Exp. Ther. 202:192-198, 1977.
23. Fink, G. D., and Fisher, J. W. Stimulation of erythropoiesis by beta adrenergic agonists: II. Mechanisms of action. J. Pharmacol. Exp. Ther. 202:199-208, 1977.
24. Przala, F., Gross, D. M., Beckman, B., and Fisher, J. W. Influence of albuterol on erythropoietin production and erythroid progenitor cell activation. Am. J. Physiol. 236:H422-H426, 1979.
25. Weber, P. C., Larsson, C., Anggard, E., Hamberg, M., Corey, E. J., Nicolaou, K. C., and Samuelsson, B. Stimulation of renin release from rabbit renal cortex by arachidonic acid and prostaglandin endoperoxides. Circ. Res. 39:868-874, 1976.
26. Gould, A. B., Goodman, S. A., and Green, D. An in vivo effect of renin on erythropoietin formation. Lab. Invest. 28:719-722, 1973.
27. Zins, G. R. Renal prostaglandins. Am. J. Med. 58:14-24, 1975.
28. Danon, A., Chang, L., Sweetman, B., Nies, A., and Oates, J. Synthesis of prostaglandins by the rat renal papilla in vitro: mechanism of stimulation by angiotensin II. Biochim. Biophys. Acta 388:71-83, 1974.
29. Alexander, R. W., and Gimbrone, M. A. Stimulation of prostaglandin E synthesis in cultured human umbilical vein smooth muscle cells. Proc. Natl. Acad. Sci. USA 73:1617-1620, 1976.
30. Needleman, P. The synthesis and function of prostaglandins in the heart. Fed. Proc. 35:2376-2381, 1976.
31. Markelonis, G., and Garbus, J. Elaboration of medium chain free fatty acids and long chain fatty acid prostaglandin precursors by isolated anoxic rat liver mitochondria. FEBS Lett. 51:7-10, 1975.
32. Rodgers, G. M., Fisher, J. W., and George, W. J. The role of renal adenosine 3',5'-monophosphate in the control of erythropoietin production. Am. J. Med. 58:31-38, 1975.
33. Gidari, A. S., Zanjani, E. D., and Gordon, A. S. Stimulation of erythropoiesis by cyclic adenosine monophosphate. Life Sci. 10:895-900, 1971.
34. Martelo, O. J., Toro, E. F., and Hirsch, J. Activation of renal erythropoietic factor by phosphorylation. J. Lab. Clin. Med. 87:83-88, 1976.
35. Gordon, A. S., Zanjani, E. D., and McLaurin, W. D. The renal erythropoietic factor (REF or erythrogenin. In Renal Pharmacology, J. W. Fisher and E. J. Cafruny (Eds.). Appleton-Century-Crofts, New York, pp. 141-165, 1971.
36. Peschle, C., and Condorelli, M. Biogenesis of erythropoietin: evidence for proerythropoietin in a subcellular fraction of kidney. Science 190: 910-912, 1975.

37. Libbin, R. M., Person, P., and Gordon, A. S. Renal lysosomes: role in biogenesis of erythropoietin. Science 185:1174-1176, 1974.
38. Rodgers, G. M., Fisher, J. W., and George, W. J. Renal cyclic GMP and cholinergic mechanisms in erythropoietin production. Life Sci. 17: 1807-1814, 1976.
39. Fehér, I., and Gidáli, J. Prostaglandin E_2 as stimulator of haemopoietic stem cell proliferation. Nature (Lond.) 247:550-551, 1974.
40. Byron, J. W. Manipulation of the cell cycle of the hemopoietic stem cell. Exp. Hematol. 3:44-53, 1975.
41. Gidáli, J., and Fehér, I. The effect of E type prostaglandins on the proliferation of haemopoietic stem cells in vivo. Cell Tissue Kinet. 10:365-373, 1977.
42. Dukes, P. P. Erythropoietic effects of prostaglandins. Adv. Biosci. 9:183-188, 1973.
43. Dukes, P. P., Datta, M. C., Ortega, J. A., Shore, N. A., and Polk, C. Heme synthesis of marrow cells in culture increased by prostaglandin E_2. Fed. Proc. 35:1627, 1976.
44. Friend, C., Scher, W., Holland, J. G., and Sato, T. Hemoglobin synthesis in murine virus-induced leukemic cells in vitro: stimulation of erythroid differentiation by dimethylsulfoxide. Proc. Natl. Acad. Sci. USA 68:378-382, 1971.
45. Tabuse, Y., Furusawa, M., Eisen, H., and Shibata, K. Prostaglandin E_1, an inducer of erythroid differentiation of Friend erythroleukemia cells. Exp. Cell Res. 108:41-45, 1977.
46. Djaldetti, M., Bessler, H., and Levi, J. Effect of prostaglandin A_2 on RNA synthesis in embryonic mouse erythroid cells. Nephron 21:345-349, 1978.
47. Chan, H. S. L., Freedman, M. H., and Saunders, E. F. Opposite effects on human erythropoiesis and granulopoiesis in vitro of prostaglandins and lithium chloride. Clin. Res. 26:343A, 1978.
48. Chan, H. S. L., Freedman, M. H., and Saunders, E. F. Prostaglandins, cyclic AMP and lithium chloride: their regulatory roles in an experimental model of human hematopoiesis. Exp. Hematol. 6(Suppl. 3): 35, 1978.
49. Hoffman, R., Zanjani, E. D., Lutton, J. D., Zalusky, R., and Wasserman, L. R. Suppression of erythroid-colony formation by lymphocytes from patients with aplastic anemia. N. Engl. J. Med. 296: 10-13, 1977.
50. Kurland, J., and Moore, M. A. S. Modulation of hemopoiesis by prostaglandins. Exp. Hematol. 5:357-373, 1977.
51. Allen, J. E., and Rasmussen, H. Human red blood cells: prostaglandin E_2, epinephrine, and isoproterenol alter deformability. Science 174: 512-514, 1971.
52. Rasmussen, H., Lake, W., and Allen, J. E. The effect of catecholamines and prostaglandins upon human and rat erythrocytes. Biochim. Biophys. Acta 411:63-73, 1975.

53. Kury, P. G., Ramwell, P. O., and McConnell, H. M. The effect of prostaglandins E_1 and E_2 on the human erythrocyte as monitored by spin labels. Biochem. Biophys. Res. Commun. 56:478-483, 1974.
54. Jay, A. W. L., Rowlands, S., and Skibo, L. Red blood cell deformability and the prostaglandins. Prostaglandins 3:871-877, 1973.

Part III
PROSTAGLANDINS AND NONVASCULAR FUNCTIONS

12 The Actions of Prostaglandins on Uterine and Gastrointestinal Smooth Muscle in Vitro

JOHN H. SANNER / G. D. Searle and Company, Chicago, Illinois

The smooth muscle-stimulating activities of prostaglandins (PGs) played an important role in their discovery and early development. The story has been told many times of how Kurzrok and Lieb (1) discovered in 1930 that human seminal fluid could cause stimulation or relaxation of human isolated myometrium. Effects on isolated smooth muscle were instrumental in the early work of Goldblatt (2,3) and Euler (4-8) in characterizing the constituents known as "prostaglandin" from seminal fluid and extracts of accessory sex organs.

As different types of prostaglandins were isolated and identified in the 1960s, much biological work was aimed at characterizing their effects on smooth muscles. It was found that the effects of the various prostaglandins varied both qualitatively and quantitatively in different tissues. Differential effects of E and F prostaglandins on various isolated smooth muscle preparations were published by Bergström et al. (9) in 1959, and Horton (10) reviewed the literature on prostaglandin activities that was available in 1965, with emphasis on comparisons of smooth muscle activities of E and F prostaglandins. At that time it was known that prostaglandins could cause contractions of isolated preparations of guinea pig ileum, chicken jejunum, cow iris, rat jejunum, hamster colon, guinea pig uterus, rabbit jejunum, and rat uterus. Both E and F prostaglandins were thought to relax bronchial smooth muscle, but it is now known that the F prostaglandins stimulate this muscle.

Differential activities of prostaglandins on smooth muscles played an important role in detecting prostaglandin release and levels of prostaglandins in biological fluids. Gilmore and coworkers (11) pioneered the use of the cascade superfusion technique to determine the release of prostaglandins. This technique made use of several different tissues with different sensitivities superfused by the same solution to detect individual prostaglandins and to differentiate these from other smooth muscle stimulants. This method was used to detect the inhibition of prostaglandin biosynthesis by nonsteroidal anti-inflammatory agents (12-14).

By the late 1960s the smooth muscle activities of the primary prostaglandins had been established quite well, and the smooth muscle pharmacology of prostaglandins progressed to more advanced studies on mechanisms by which the prostaglandins produce their effects. The emphasis of this chapter is on the more recent mechanistic studies, with special attention to areas in which discrepancies have been found or to areas that appear to warrant further investigation.

UTERINE SMOOTH MUSCLE

Species Differences

Prostaglandins are well known for their stimulant effects on human myometrium in vivo, thereby making them useful for the induction of labor and abortion. In vitro, however, they are not universally stimulatory; there is a divergence between in vivo and in vitro effects of the E prostaglandins on human myometrium. The early findings quoted by Bygdeman (15) showed prostaglandins E_1, E_2, and E_3 to decrease the tone and the frequency and amplitude of contractions on isolated nonpregnant human myometrium, whereas the F prostaglandins universally produced stimulation. Even on pregnant human uterus, where the stimulant and abortifacient effects of E prostaglandins are well established, these substances do not always have a stimulant effect in vitro (15).

Unlike the effects on human isolated uterus, prostaglandins of both the E and F series stimulate isolated uterine preparations from guinea pigs, rats, and rabbits. Exceptions have been noted, however. Some of these might be explained by the small number of animals that were used or the relatively crude materials that were used in early observations. Recently, it was found that fresh myometrial tissue from rats responded to PGE_1 by relaxation, but it caused stimulation of tissue that had been maintained in the bathing solution for several hours (16). It was thought that adrenergic nerves contribute to the early relaxation because this early effect could be changed to one of stimulation by treatment with bretylium. These observations, however, do not seem to explain the different effects of E prostaglandins on human and animal isolated myometrium because it is hard to imagine that preparations of human uterus would be fresher than those of animal uterus; if anything, the opposite might be expected.

Hormonal Influences

Early studies (17, 18) indicated that the effects of crude prostaglandins on human isolated uterus varied with the menstrual cycle and the state of pregnancy. It was also observed that uterine strips from postmenopausal women were less sensitive to the relaxant effect of crude prostaglandins. These observations suggested that the ovarian hormones influence prostaglandin responses on the uterus.

Studies conducted with pure prostaglandins have sometimes conflicted with one another and their interpretation has been complicated because the E prostaglandins ordinarily produce relaxation of nonpregnant human uteri in vitro and stimulation of pregnant human uteri and uteri from other animals. The subject of hormonal influences on uterine responses to prostaglandins was covered in a 1970 review by Speroff and Ramwell (19), but it is apparent from their discussion that the subject had not been systematically investigated. Our knowledge is not much better today.

Progesterone added to the bath at high concentrations (20 μg/ml or more) inhibits the stimulatory effects of oxytocin as well as E and F prostaglandins on isolated rat uteri (20, 21), and estradiol (20 μg/ml) was found to completely block PGE_1- and oxytocin-induced contractions (21).

Sullivan (20) pretreated rats and guinea pigs with estradiol and then tested responses to prostaglandins on isolated, electrically stimulated strips of their uteri. He found no significant differences in the stimulatory effects of PGE_1 and $PGF_{2\alpha}$ between diestrous rats and those treated with estradiol. Hawkins et al. (21), however, found that estradiol pretreatment of ovariectomized rats markedly reduced the sensitivity of their isolated uteri to PGE_1 and $PGF_{2\alpha}$, whereas responses to oxytocin were enhanced.

These in vitro results may be compared to in vivo findings: Fuchs (22) reported that estradiol pretreatment reduced prostaglandin-induced uterine stimulation when tested in ovariectomized rats. Similar to the in vitro results of Hawkins et al. (21), estradiol potentiated uterine responses produced by oxytocin; estrogens potentiated spontaneous uterine activity as well (23). These results suggest that estrogen pretreatment may specifically suppress prostaglandin-induced uterine stimulation in rats.

The effect of progesterone on prostaglandin-induced uterine stimulation is not clear. Fuchs (22) found that progesterone pretreatment increased prostaglandin responses on isolated rat uterus, but Porter and Behrman (24) found that it decreases $PGF_{2\alpha}$ responses on rabbit uterus in vivo. Hawkins et al. (21) reported that progesterone pretreatment had little effect on the responses produced by prostaglandins, serotonin, bradykinin, or oxytocin.

Tachyphylaxis

Tachyphylaxis to prostaglandins has been observed on several isolated smooth muscle preparations, but it seems to have been the most frequently observed and the most extensively studied on isolated uteri. Tachyphylaxis to prostaglandins on isolated myometrium was first reported by Eliasson in 1959 (25). Since the effect has been observed primarily in vitro, it may not be an important factor in the physiological or pharmacological activities of prostaglandins.

The different prostaglandins appear to have different potentials for the development of tachyphylaxis. Adamson et al. (26) observed tachyphylaxis in rat uterus in 11 of 11 experiments with PGE_1 and six of eight experiments with $PGF_{1\alpha}$. It was observed in only two of six experiments with PGE_2. Tachyphylaxis to PGA_1, PGA_2 (27), $PGF_{1\beta}$, and $PGF_{2\beta}$ (28) has also been reported on estrogen-dominated uterus, but no tachyphylaxis was obtained with $PGF_{2\alpha}$, nor were the F_β prostaglandins tachyphylactic on progesterone-dominated uterus. Other studies have also shown that hormonal influences are important factors in the development of tachyphylaxis.

Cross-tachyphylaxis between different prostaglandins is not common, suggesting a multiplicity of prostaglandin receptor sites. Indeed, tachyphylaxis to PGE_1 can be reduced by administration of PGE_2 or $PGF_{2\alpha}$ (29). It can also be prevented or eliminated by administering oxytocin, but other stimulating agents are not generally effective.

The ionic concentration of the bathing solution is also an important determinant in the development of tachyphylaxis. It may or may not develop with different ratios of calcium, potassium, and magnesium. This ionic influence appears to be interrelated with hormonal influences and the characteristics of different prostaglandins, so it is difficult to make generalizations about it.

Tachyphylaxis may also be temperature-dependent since it was not observed with PGE_1 on isolated rat uterus maintained at 17-20°C instead of the warmer temperatures that are commonly used (30).

Despite tachyphylaxis seen with repeated doses, prostaglandins of the E series have a long-lasting enhancing effect on contractions produced by other stimulants, such as vasopressin (31, 32), norepinephrine, 5-hydroxytryptamine (33), and oxytocin (34, 35). This enhancing activity is distinct from the potentiating activity also displayed by E prostaglandins. Clegg et al. (32) described enhancement as a long-lasting effect which increases contractile responses to nonspecific stimulation, either chemical or electrical, after the prostaglandin has been washed out of the bath. It is not associated with changes in electrical or mechanical tension, and it is not influenced by moderate changes in magnesium, calcium, or potassium concentrations.

Cyclic Nucleotides

There has been much work done recently on the relationship between levels of cyclic adenosine 3',5'-monophosphate (cyclic AMP), cyclic guanosine 3',5'-monophosphate (cyclic GMP), and smooth muscle contractility. This general subject has been covered recently in excellent reviews (36, 37). Much of this work has concentrated on relationships between the cyclic nucleotides and adrenergic and cholinergic mechanisms. Increased cyclic AMP levels are generally associated with smooth muscle relaxation and there is evidence that increased cyclic GMP levels are associated with cholinergic stimulation. Although prostaglandins influence cyclic nucleotide levels and may cause smooth muscle contraction or relaxation, these relationships have not been studied as extensively as those involved with the autonomic transmitters.

Kuehl et al. (38) cited experiments in which $PGF_{2\alpha}$ (as well as oxytocin) raised cyclic GMP levels in the rat uterus and they proposed that the actions of F prostaglandins may be related to cyclic GMP levels and that the actions of E prostaglandins may be related to cyclic AMP levels, but no clear relationships have been established to support this suggestion.

E prostaglandins stimulate the production of cyclic AMP in rat (39,40) and rabbit (41) uterus, presumably through activation of adenylate cyclase. Epinephrine and isoproterenol similarly potentiate cyclic AMP production in uterine tissue (39,40). $PGF_{2\alpha}$ and oxytocin, however, are weak or inactive in raising uterine cyclic AMP levels (37,39-41). Since the E prostaglandins, oxytocin, and the F prostaglandins all stimulate the rat uterus in vitro whereas epinephrine and isoproterenol relax uterine muscle, there is no simple correlation between cyclic AMP levels and uterine stimulation or relaxation.

$PGF_{2\alpha}$ was found to stimulate production of uterine cyclic GMP by some investigators (37,42) but not by others (43). Increased production of cyclic GMP, however, does not appear to explain the stimulant action of this prostaglandin in any case because 8-bromo cyclic GMP, like dibutyryl cyclic AMP, decreases uterine contractions (44) instead of stimulating them.

As pointed out by Anderson et al. (37), cyclic AMP and cyclic GMP levels do change during smooth muscle contraction, but these changes are complex, and they cannot be related to the contractions in a simple way. If they do indeed influence smooth muscle contractions, it may be through some mechanism such as negative feedback, inhibiting or promoting the release of neurotransmitters, increasing or decreasing the sensitivity of the muscle cells, or regulation of calcium release and binding. A consideration of prostaglandin influences on cyclic nucleotide levels adds another complicating step in the scheme.

Inorganic Ions

Concentrations of calcium, magnesium, and potassium in the bathing medium affect responses to prostaglandins perhaps to a greater extent than responses to other uterine stimulants. Stimulant actions of prostaglandins on isolated rat uterus are abolished in a calcium-free medium (30,45). Responses to prostaglandins were restored by the addition of Ca^{2+}, but not as efficiently as were responses to acetylcholine. Osa et al. (46), on the other hand, found a reciprocal activity of Ca^{2+} and Na^{+} on PGE_2-induced depolarization of isolated pregnant mouse myometrium such that a relative dominance of Ca^{2+} over Na^{+} tends to depress the electrical and mechanical activities of the tissue, and vice versa.

Prostaglandins appear to have important effects on intracellular calcium that might account for their actions on smooth muscle. Carsten has investigated the effects of prostaglandins on bovine (47) and human (48) myometrial cell fractions. She found that PGE_2 and $PGF_{2\alpha}$ inhibit ATP-dependent calcium binding in a subcellular fraction containing elements characteristic of endoplasmic reticulum. Oxytocin also inhibited this binding with the potency increasing during pregnancy, but $PGF_{2\beta}$, which has little uterine activity, had no effect on the binding. By this mechanism, oxytocic agents could cause uterine stimulation by making bound intracellular calcium available to serve in the excitation-activation coupling process. It has been stated, however, that PGE_1 itself will bind calcium (49). If this is the case, it seems that the prostaglandins might compete for intracellularly bound calcium, thereby decreasing the amount of calcium bound by cell constituents but not freeing it for activation of the contraction process because it would then be bound by the prostaglandin.

The concentration of magnesium in the bathing medium has an important influence on the actions of prostaglandins on isolated myometrium. The absence of Mg^{2+} potentiates responses to E prostaglandins on rat or guinea pig myometrium (30, 32, 50), but responses to $PGF_{2\alpha}$ do not appear to be altered by changing the Mg^{2+} concentration (50). This potentiating effect is not specific for E prostaglandins, however, because the absence of magnesium also potentiates responses induced by acetylcholine (30).

Although the direct stimulant activities of prostaglandins are influenced by variations in calcium, magnesium, and potassium, prostaglandin enhancement of vasopressin responses is not influenced by changes in these ions (32).

Prostaglandin Receptors

Pickles concluded in 1967 (51) that prostaglandins must exert their actions on myometrium through several different types of pharmacological receptors. The idea of prostaglandin receptors being limited to only two types, one for E and one for F prostaglandins, did not seem to explain the different actions of prostaglandins, so he concluded that there are probably more than two types of pharmacological receptors for prostaglandins, and that the prostaglandins may also work in other ways, such as influencing calcium movement or metabolic activities that do not involve receptor activation in the true sense.

Johnson and coworkers investigated the nature of prostaglandin receptors. They found that sulfhydryl reducing agents (52) and ultraviolet light (53) will inhibit responses produced on uterine smooth muscle by both E and F prostaglandins. The inhibition could be reversed by the sulfhydryl oxidizing agent, 5,5'-dithio-bis(2-nitrobenzoic acid). Similar effects were seen in relation to PGE_1 inhibition of ADP-induced platelet aggregation. These results indicate that sulfhydryl bonds play important roles in E prostaglandin receptors in platelets and in both E and F prostaglandin receptors in uterine smooth muscle.

Proteins with specific binding affinities for prostaglandins have been found in rabbit (54), hamster (55-57), monkey, and human (57) myometrial preparations. Prostaglandins were irreversibly bound to membrane fractions of myometrial homogenates (56, 57) but not to monkey endometrial fractions (57). Prostaglandins E_1, E_2, and $F_{2\alpha}$ specifically bound to the sites, with the E prostaglandins showing greater affinity, but the specific binding capacity of $PGF_{1\alpha}$ on hamster uterus was very low. PGE_1 and PGE_2 appeared to bind at the same sites since they had similar binding properties. The concentration of binding sites on these hamster preparations varied with the estrous cycle and with hormone treatment.

Prostaglandin binding studies on low-speed supernatant fractions from human myometrial homogenates (58) showed relative affinities for different prostaglandins in the following order: $PGE_1 > PGE_2 > PGF_{2\alpha} > PGB_2 \geq PGA_1 \geq PGA_2 > PGB_1 > PGD_2$. The order of binding-site affinities of these natural prostaglandins, some PGE_1 metabolites, and 15-methyl prostaglandin analogs appeared to correlate with uterine stimulatory potencies determined in monkeys or humans. Unfortunately, however, $PGF_{1\alpha}$, which has low binding affinity on hamster uterine slices (57), was not tested in this study. On low-speed supernatant from hamster myometrial homogenates the order of relative affinites was $PGE_2 > PGE_1 > PGA_1 > PGF_{2\alpha}$ (59).

Prostaglandin Involvement in Normal Uterine Contractility

Homogenates of guinea pig uterus (60) or rat uterine strips (61) have the ability to synthesize prostaglandins, and this synthesis by rat uterus is stimulated by oxytocin. Other studies on the mechanism of uterine contractions have led to proposals that normal uterine contractility and the contractile effect of oxytocin are mediated through the actions of prostaglandins (62, 63).

Csapo and Csapo (62) studied the action of naproxen, a prostaglandin synthetase inhibitor, on uterine strips from postpartum rabbits and found that it would greatly inhibit electrically-induced contractions and spontaneous contractions. These could be restored by administration of $PGF_{2\alpha}$, but not oxytocin. Vane and Williams (63) found that the prostaglandin synthetase inhibitors indomethacin and meclofenamate antagonize oxytocin-induced contractions of isolated uteri from nonpregnant rats, but acetylcholine-induced contractions were potentiated. Furthermore, Brummer (34, 35) has demonstrated potentiation of oxytocin-induced responses by prostaglandins on pregnant human uterus.

The interaction of oxytocin and prostaglandins may vary, however, with different hormonal influences. Baudouin-Legros et al. (64) found that the effects of indomethacin and the prostaglandin antagonist polyphloretin phosphate vary with different stages of estrus. They found that indomethacin shifted angiotensin- and oxytocin-induced dose-response curves to the right on diestrous and proestrous rat uteri, but it was inactive on metestrous uteri. Also, a higher concentration of polyphloretin phosphate was required on metestrous than on diestrous or proestrous uteri to reduce the sensitivity of the tissue to angiotensin and oxytocin. Furthermore, Vane and Williams

(63) observed that indomethacin and meclofenamate inhibited spontaneous contractions on uteri from pregnant rats, but they did not inhibit oxytocin-induced contractions on these preparations.

The interactions of prostaglandin synthetase inhibitors with oxytocin suggest that the prostaglandins are involved in oxytocin-induced contractions of the uterus. Since stretching and releasing the uterus will stimulate release of prostaglandins (65, 66), it seems that prostaglandins released in the contractile process may potentiate the response to stimulants in general. A good argument can be made against this generalization, however, because synthetase inhibitors do not inhibit responses to acetylcholine or $PGF_{2\alpha}$ (62), and therefore the release of potentiating E prostaglandins does not appear to play a role in the stimulant activities of these agents. Instead, a specific relationship between oxytocin stimulation and prostaglandin release is indicated.

GASTROINTESTINAL SMOOTH MUSCLE

General Activities

It first seemed that prostaglandins were universal stimulants of gastrointestinal smooth muscle (67, 68), and that the individual prostaglandins varied from one another only quantitatively. The E and F prostaglandins were judged to be potent stimulators, whereas the A prostaglandins were much weaker (69, 70). Metabolic products of PGE_1 had less stimulating activity than did the parent compound (71), and the unnatural isomer, $PGF_{2\beta}$, had low stimulating activity (72).

It soon became apparent, however, that the first prostaglandin assays used measurements derived from contractions of longitudinal muscle, and when the activities were tested on circular muscle it was found that the E prostaglandins are relaxants of these muscles. This has been demonstrated on circular muscle preparations from human stomach (73) and from the colon of humans, guinea pigs, and rats (74, 75).

A recent study (76) showed that the B prostaglandins (especially PGB_2) have considerable stimulating activity on both longitudinal and circular muscle from human stomach. The A prostaglandins also had significant effects. This study additionally showed that $PGF_{2\alpha}$ produced either stimulation or relaxation of human gastric circular muscle, depending on previous stimulation induced by PGA_2 or PGB_2 and on the tension applied to the muscle. The weak activities of prostaglandins A_1, A_2, B_1, and B_2 on longitudinal gastrointestinal muscle from laboratory animals were confirmed, thus indicating an important species difference for these prostaglandins. It was originally concluded that prostaglandins must act on gastrointestinal smooth muscle only as local agents because E and F prostaglandins are very rapidly metabolized and the A and B compounds had little effect on the functions of smooth muscle from laboratory animals. This recent finding suggests, however, that circulating A and B prostaglandins, which are not metabolized as rapidly as E and F prostaglandins, may have significant influences on smooth muscle activity in humans.

Another recent study (77) demonstrated that the endoperoxide intermediates PGG_2 and PGH_2 are comparable to PGE_2 and $PGF_{2\alpha}$ as stimulators of isolated gerbil colon and rat stomach preparations. Thus the total action of the prostaglandin system does not lie in the primary E and F prostaglandins.

Interactions with Cholinergic Mechanisms

The stimulatory actions of prostaglandins on smooth muscles are generally due to direct action on the smooth muscle cells, but in guinea pig ileum longitudinal muscle, cholinergic neurons appear to play a significant role in prostaglandin-induced stimulation (75,78). This is indicated by partial inhibition of the stimulation by the cholinergic antagonist atropine and by morphine (79,80), which inhibits the release of acetylcholine (81,82). Evidence for cholinergic involvement in prostaglandin stimulation has also been seen on guinea pig duodenum and jejunum (83).

There have been several hypotheses advanced concerning a modulator role of prostaglandins in the release of autonomic neurotransmitters. The one with the best basis is a negative feedback mechanism on the sympathetic system (84,85). This has been extensively studied on isolated guinea pig vas deferens, which is stimulated by sympathetic neural activation. In this case the E prostaglandins appear to play a dual role; they inhibit the release of norepinephrine but potentiate the effect of exogenous norepinephrine. It is proposed that sympathetic stimulation causes increased synthesis of E prostaglandins and that they serve a negative feedback function, limiting the further release of norepinephrine and thereby shutting off the sympathetic influence. A similar negative feedback mechanism has been proposed for parasympathetic innervation (86). This hypothesis was based on experiments on isolated rabbit hearts in which the negative chronotropic response to vagal stimulation was reduced by PGE_1 but the effect of exogenous acetylcholine was unchanged. Ehrenpries et al. (87), on the other hand, proposed that E prostaglandins perform an essential role to promote the release of acetylcholine from electrically stimulated cholinergic nerves. This hypothesis was based on experiments performed on isolated guinea pig ileum, in which electrically induced contractions were reduced by indomethacin and the inhibition was reversed by prostaglandins. The prostaglandin synthetase inhibitor 5,8,11,14-eicosatetraynoic acid (TYA) also inhibits cholinergic stimulation of bovine iris sphincter muscle, and this is reversed by PGE_1 (88). This hypothesis seems to be supported by prostaglandin reversal of the inhibitory effect that morphine has on electrically stimulated guinea pig ileum (87). Morphine inhibits acetylcholine release from the guinea pig ileum (81,82). It also inhibits prostaglandin-induced cyclic AMP production by brain tissue (89) and cultured neuroblastoma and gliomal cells (90) as well as prostaglandin-induced platelet aggregation (91). It is therefore attractive to propose that morphine inhibits the normal acetylcholine-releasing function of prostaglandins, thus accounting for the inhibitory effect that morphine has on the guinea pig ileum that is stimulated either electrically or with prostaglandins.

It is obvious that the hypothesis that prostaglandins play a negative feedback role to limit the release of acetylcholine and the hypothesis that they are mediators that promote the release of acetylcholine are incompatible if they are applied to the same tissue, and objections have been raised to both hypotheses. If E prostaglandins serve a negative feedback function, they would be expected to decrease acetylcholine release and prostaglandin synthetase inhibitors would be expected to increase acetylcholine release. Several studies on acetylcholine release from the guinea pig ileum have been reported (92-97), and, if anything, the opposite may be true; acetylcholine release is either increased or unchanged in response to PGE administration, and synthetase inhibition has resulted in either no change or a decrease. These acetylcholine release studies have been conducted on isolated guinea pig ilea, however, and the negative feedback hypothesis was based on experiments conducted on isolated rabbit hearts. The same mechanism may not apply to both organs.

The hypothesis that prostaglandins are necessary for the physiological release of acetylcholine has been controversial because of several conflicting results. There is general agreement that morphine and prostaglandin synthetase inhibitors decrease the twitch response of electrically stimulated guinea pig ileum (87, 92, 93, 95-100), although Botting and Salzmann (94) reported only a small, transient reduction caused by 10 μg/ml indomethacin in two experiments.

There is some agreement that inhibition can be overcome by addition of PGE_1 or PGE_2 if the inhibition is not maximal (87, 96, 99, 100). High doses of inhibitor or a long contact time tend to produce an irreversible blockade (87, 100), and this might account for some failures to overcome indomethacin blockade with prostaglandins (98). There is also general agreement that low concentrations of E prostaglandins augment responses to electrical stimulation (87, 96, 98, 99), but there is disagreement about whether this augmentation and the reversal of depressed contractions is a specific effect on acetylcholine release. Some investigators report that the augmentation and reversal of inhibition may be due to sensitization of the muscle cells to acetylcholine (and other spasmogens) (97, 100), whereas others find no such sensitization (96). Some workers report that prostaglandins can overcome the inhibitory effects of substances other than morphine and synthetase inhibitors (97, 98, 100), and that nicotine as well as prostaglandins can overcome morphine and synthetase inhibitor blockades (100). These reports suggest nonspecific depressant effects of synthetase inhibitors and nonspecific stimulant effects of prostaglandins rather than specific effects on prostaglandin release.

Increased release of acetylcholine induced by prostaglandins and inhibition of acetylcholine release by synthetase inhibitors would point toward prostaglandins being essential for release of the cholinergic transmitter. Several studies have been conducted on the isolated guinea pig ileum in which acetylcholine release was measured. There seems to be a general trend toward the reduction of acetylcholine release by prostaglandin synthetase inhibitors, but several investigators have failed to find statistically significant reductions. Thus Hazra (92) did not find significant reductions in acetylcholine release induced by indomethacin on either electrically stimulated or resting guinea pig ilea. An abstract by Benz and Salzmann (93) reported that 10 μg/ml indomethacin did not produce a significant change in acetylcholine output from normal resting or electrically stimulated guinea pig ilea, but they found a slight reduction from ilea of reserpine-treated guinea pigs. Another report by Botting and Salzmann (94) indicated that indomethacin (10 and 20 μg/ml) had no significant effect on acetylcholine release from electrically stimulated ilea, but it reduced the output of acetylcholine from resting tissue in some experiments. On the positive side, Kadlec et al. (95) found that the output of acetylcholine was reduced by indomethacin at the low concentration of 1.0 μM (0.36 μg/ml) on both resting and stimulated ilea, and Hall et al. (96) found that a high concentration of aspirin (75 μg/ml) decreased acetylcholine output. The E prostaglandins generally do not seem to increase acetylcholine output from normal ilea (93,95), but there are some reports that they do increase acetylcholine release after it has been depressed by morphine (97) or by synthetase inhibitors (95,96).

The involvement of prostaglandins as either positive or negative factors in cholinergic transmission is an unsettled problem. If it is true that prostaglandins do not promote the release of acetylcholine even under nonphysiological conditions, this would negate the widely accepted idea (75,78,80) that they produce stimulation of the isolated guinea pig ileum partially through activation of cholinergic neurons. Instead, it would suggest that the primary interaction of E prostaglandins with the cholinergic system in this tissue is through potentiation of the musculotropic action of acetylcholine, and there is disagreement about whether or not this occurs.

Prostaglandin Antagonists

Pharmacological antagonists are generally thought of as being substances that inhibit the actions of other substances (agonists) by competing with the agonists for their receptor sites. Studies of the actions of natural substances such as acetylcholine, histamine, and catecholamines have been greatly aided by the availability of specific, competitive pharmacological antagonists of these substances, and isolated smooth muscle preparations are powerful tools for studying such antagonists. Three main types of substances have been advanced as pharmacological antagonists of prostaglandins. The antiprostaglandin activities of each of these classes of compounds was first demonstrated on isolated preparations of gastrointestinal smooth muscle.

In 1969, Fried and coworkers (101) reported that they had synthesized a series of 7-oxaprostaglandin analogs that would inhibit the stimulating activity of prostaglandin E_1 on isolated guinea pig ileum, rabbit duodenum, and gerbil colon. Eight of these compounds with six-membered rings were tested and each of them inhibited PGE_1-induced contractions of guinea pig ileum at concentrations that produced little or no inhibition of contractions produced by histamine or acetylcholine. Only the compounds with triple bonds in the 13,14-position, however, demonstrated specific prostaglandin antagonism on the isolated gerbil colon. Compounds with 15-hydroxy constituents were later reported to be mixed agonists and antagonists (102), and the 15-nor compound with a 13,14-triple bond (7-oxa-13-prostynoic acid) has become known as the prototype prostaglandin antagonist of this series. Flack (103) found that 7-oxa-13-prostynoic acid was the only 7-oxaprostaglandin analog out of 15 that he tested that would specifically inhibit prostaglandin-induced contractions on isolated gerbil colon. It did not, however, specifically inhibit prostaglandin-induced contractions on isolated guinea pig ileum (103,104), rabbit jejunum (103), or on human stomach, ileum, or colon (104). On isolated rat stomach strips 7-oxa-13-prostynoic acid produced contractions, a prostaglandin-like activity (104).

Baudouin-Legros et al. (105) concluded that the effect of 7-oxa-13-prostynoic acid was different on proestrous rat uteri than on metestrous uteri. They found that on the proestrous uterus the compound inhibited $PGF_{2\alpha}$-induced stimulation without reducing the maximum response, but on the metestrous uterus it reduced the maximum response to $PGF_{2\alpha}$. This suggests competitive antagonism on the proestrous uterus and noncompetitive inhibition on the metestrous uterus. 7-Oxa-13-prostynoic acid also inhibited spontaneous contractions and those produced by angiotensin II on the proestrous uterus, thus indicating either a nonspecific inhibitory effect of the compound or that prostaglandins are involved in these contractions.

Prostaglandin antagonism with 7-oxa-13-prostynoic acid has been demonstrated best in experiments showing inhibition of prostaglandin-stimulated formation of cyclic AMP, and it has been found to bind weakly with prostaglandin binding sites that are proposed as prostaglandin receptors. These properties have been covered in recent reviews (106-108).

Eakins and Karim (109), using isolated jird (gerbil) colon preparations, found that the polymeric compound polyphloretin phosphate (PPP) would specifically inhibit prostaglandin-induced contractions. It was thought that this compound inhibited only F prostaglandins, but it was later found to inhibit contractions produced by E prostaglandins also (110). It did not inhibit contractions produced by acetylcholine, bradykinin, angiotensin, or 5-hydroxytryptamine, indicating a specific effect against the prostaglandins. It also shifted prostaglandin dose-response curves to the right without reducing the maximum contractions, indicating competitive antagonism.

Polyphloretin phosphate had been found earlier to inhibit several enzymes, and before demonstration of its antiprostaglandin potential it was thought that its antihyaluronidase activity accounted for its ability to prevent peritoneal adhesions in rabbits (111), to prevent capillary permeability in rats and guinea pigs (112), to stabilize the blood-aqueous barrier of rabbit eyes (113), and to inhibit fertility in female mice (114).

Besides prostaglandin antagonism on the gerbil colon, PPP specifically inhibits prostaglandin-induced contractions on isolated rabbit jejunum and uterus (110), guinea pig ileum and colon (104), rat colon (115, 116), and chick rectum (116). High concentrations were required to inhibit prostaglandin-induced contractions on human isolated gastrointestinal muscle preparations. PPP, like the other antagonists, did not inhibit the relaxant effect that prostaglandins have on circular gastrointestinal smooth muscle (104). Both PPP and SC 19220 inhibit nicotine-induced contractions of isolated guinea pig ileum (106).

Despite its prostaglandin inhibitory effects on most intestinal longitudinal muscle, PPP has stimulatory activities on some smooth muscles that are also stimulated by prostaglandins. Thus PPP was found to stimulate rather than inhibit contractions of rat isolated stomach strips (104, 117). It also produced contractions or increased pendular movements of rabbit jejunum (110). Low concentrations of PPP increased spontaneous contractions of human isolated jejunum, while high concentrations inhibited them (117). Since PPP inhibits metabolism of prostaglandins by 15-hydroxyprostaglandin dehydrogenase (118), this may account for its stimulatory effect on these tissues.

Polyphloretin phosphate is a mixture of different-weight polymers, and the prostaglandin inhibitory activity lies in the low molecular weight fractions, while the enzyme inhibitory activity is generally associated with the higher molecular weight fractions (119, 120). The dimer, di-4-phloretin phosphate, is considerably more active as a prostaglandin antagonist than is the mixture, polyphloretin phosphate (121). Unfortunately, di-4-phloretin phosphate is also a more potent inhibitor of 15-hydroxyprostaglandin dehydrogenase (122).

Inhibition of prostaglandin E_2-induced stimulation on isolated guinea pig ileum by a debenzooxazepine compound known as SC 19200 was reported by Sanner in 1969 (123). Since contractions produced by bradykinin and acetylcholine were not inhibited, the compound was considered to be a specific prostaglandin antagonist. Like polyphloretin phosphate, low concentrations produced parallel shifts of prostaglandin dose-response curves, indicating competitive antagonism, but higher concentrations flattened the curve and reduced the maximum contractions. SC 19220 is equipotent against PGE_2 and $PGF_{2\alpha}$ on guinea pig isolated ileum (104, 123); PGE_2-induced contractions are inhibited somewhat more than contractions produced by PGE_1 (80). Unpublished results obtained by Eakins and Miller show that SC 19200 has the same potency against PGE_2 on the isolated gerbil colon as it does on the guinea pig ileum, but it is essentially inactive against the F prostaglandins on the gerbil colon.

Contractions produced on isolated guinea pig ilea by nicotine are inhibited by SC 19220 (104), and 5-hydroxytryptamine (5-HT)-induced contractions are also inhibited, but to a lesser extent than are prostaglandin-induced contractions (80). These results suggest inhibition of neural stimulation of the guinea pig ileum, but the antiprostaglandin activity does not appear to be due to morphinelike inhibition of the release of acetylcholine because SC 19220 can completely inhibit prostaglandin-induced contractions of guinea pig ileum whereas morphine cannot (80). SC 19220 is also effective on cooled tissue in which the cholinergic nerves are inactivated, and it is also active in the presence of atropine. Furthermore, SC 19220 inhibits contractions produced by E prostaglandins on isolated gerbil colon and rat fundus strips upon which our unpublished experiments show that morphine has no inhibitory activity.

The inhibition of prostaglandin-induced contractions on rat fundus strips (104) is in contrast to stimulation of this tissue produced by 7-oxa-13-prostynoic acid and by polyphloretin phosphate. The difference is probably due to the lack of inhibitory effect of SC 19220 against 15-hydroxyprostaglandin dehydrogenase that was seen with both 7-oxa-13-prostynoic acid and polyphloretin phosphate (118).

SC 19220 inhibits contractions produced by arachidonic acid as well as prostaglandins on isolated rat stomach strips (124) and on isolated guinea pig ileum preparations (125). Inhibition of both agents appeared to have similar dynamics, offering support to the conclusion that arachidonic acid-induced contractions are due to formation of prostaglandins.

Prostaglandin Involvement in Normal Intestinal Muscle Functions

Strips of intestine left unstimulated in an organ bath develop increased tone after several minutes of incubation. Ferreira et al. (126) tested the bathing fluid after strips of rabbit jejunum had been incubated for various times and found significant amounts of prostaglandin-like activity which was demonstrated in superfusion assays. The rate of generation of prostaglandin-like substances increased with longer incubation times. Inhibition of prostaglandin synthetase by indomethacin progressively diminished the prostaglandin release so that none was detectable after 1-3 hr. The resting tone of the jejunum decreased over the same time and the preparations became more sensitive to stimulation produced by PGE_2 or acetylcholine. This study suggests that normal intestinal tone is maintained by the release of prostaglandins, but the authors point out that it is also possible that the prostaglandin release is due to the trauma of removing the tissue and suspending it in an organ bath. Willis and coworkers (127) found that the prostaglandin synthetase inhibitor TYA produced similar results on isolated guinea pig ileum, and their in vitro observations were confirmed in vivo.

In keeping with the relaxant effects of E prostaglandins on circular intestinal muscle, Bennett et al. (128) observed that aspirin and indomethacin increase the resting tone of these muscles and potentiate electrically induced contractions. These effects could be reversed by prostaglandin E_2, suggesting prostaglandin involvement in the activity of circular as well as longitudinal muscle.

Several studies have suggested that prostaglandins play a functional role in intestinal peristalsis, but the observations have been complicated by several extraneous factors. These involve different sites of administration, different effects on the various prostaglandins, time and concentration factors, species and tissue differences, and in vitro versus in vivo results. The findings and conclusions frequently conflict with one another.

Bennett et al. (129) found that serosal applications of prostaglandins E_1 and E_2 inhibit intraluminal pressure increases and intestinal propulsion in isolated guinea pig ilea, but intraluminally administered prostaglandins did not have a consistent effect. Radmonović (130) reported that low concentrations (10-50 ng/ml) of PGE_1 applied to the serosal surface slightly stimulated peristaltic activity in the guinea pig isolated ileum, but this was followed by a long-lasting (about 30 min) abolition of peristalsis after the prostaglandin was washed out of the chamber. Higher concentrations of PGE_1 (0.5-1.0 μg/ml) only inhibited peristalsis and the author concluded that the predominant activity of PGE_1 on peristalsis was inhibitory. The prolonged inhibition appeared to be at least partially mediated by an adrenergic mechanism because it was shortened if the guinea pigs had been pretreated with reserpine to deplete catecholamines.

Ishizawa and Miyazaki (131) found that $PGF_{2\alpha}$ increased propulsive activity in isolated guinea pig colon. This increased propulsion was accompanied by stimulation of both longitudinal and circular muscle. Atropine and tetrodotoxin inhibited the increased propulsive activity, implicating a cholinergic neural component associated with peristalsis. Curiously, however, these agents did not inhibit prostaglandin-induced smooth muscle contractions.

Reports of the effects of prostaglandin synthetase inhibitors on peristalsis are not complete. Yagasaki et al. (132) found, contrary to the previously discussed reports, that both E and F prostaglandins stimulate peristalsis, but since this was published in abstract form, the details of their methods are not available. They also reported that peristalsis was inhibited by 0.1 μg/ml indomethacin and it could be restored by prostaglandins. This was at odds with an unpublished observation by Kuhn and Willis (quoted by Willis et al.) (127), who did not find suppression of the peristaltic reflex in guinea pig intestine by microgram quantities of ETYA, indomethacin, or aspirin.

In contrast to the inhibition of intraluminal pressure and intestinal propulsion with E prostaglandins in vitro, Bennett et al. (129) found that when prostaglandins E_1 and E_2 were injected into the bloodstream of live rats, they increased intraluminal pressure in the small intestine. In vivo responses in guinea pigs were variable (129), but when the prostaglandins were added to Tyrode solution bathing guinea pig intestine in situ, marked increases in intestinal activity were observed (127). Furthermore, the prostaglandin synthetase inhibitor ETYA inhibited normal motility under the same conditions, suggesting prostaglandin involvement in normal motility, but the prostaglandin influence was judged to occur following local formation rather than delivery by means of the bloodstream.

As discussed previously, morphine inhibits prostaglandin-induced stimulation of longitudinal muscle in the isolated guinea pig ileum, but its effect on dog (and human) intestine in vivo is to increase tone and interfere with propulsive movements, apparently due primarily to stimulation of the circular muscle layers. Prostaglandin E_1 inhibits morphine-induced increases in tone or circular muscle stimulation (133, 134), an activity that is consistent with the relaxant effect on circular muscle observed in vitro (74, 75). Since prostaglandins produce diarrhea and morphine inhibits diarrhea, it seems that diarrhea may be associated with relaxation of circular muscles and constipation with contractions of circular muscles.

ENDOPEROXIDES, THROMBOXANES, AND PROSTACYCLIN

Prostaglandin endoperoxides, thromboxanes, and prostacyclin have potent effects on platelet aggregation and vascular smooth muscle, and they appear to be more important than E and F prostaglandins in these systems. In gastrointestinal and uterine smooth muscle, however, these labile arachidonic acid products are generally much less active than E and F prostaglandins, suggesting that the E and F prostaglandins are more important in gastrointestinal and uterine smooth muscle mechanisms.

The first reports of the biological activities of the prostaglandin endoperoxides came from Hamberg et al. Their first studies (135) showed that PGG_2 was 50-200 times more active than PGE_2, and that PGH_2 was 100-450 times more active than PGE_2 as stimulators of contractions in superfused rabbit aortic strips. The endoperoxides were also more active than $PGF_{2\alpha}$ (77). However, Bunting et al. (136) found the endoperoxides to be two to three times less potent than PGE_2 on rat stomach strips and chick rectum. They found the endoperoxides to be 12 to 15 times less potent than $PGF_{2\alpha}$ on rat colon. The endoperoxides break down rapidly in aqueous solutions to PGD_2 and PGE_2 (77), so in cases in which they are less active than PGE_2, it may be difficult to ascribe how much of the activity is due to the endoperoxides and how much is due to their degradation products. This difficulty may be helped by the availability of stable endoperoxide analogs (137) that have properties similar to the endoperoxides themselves.

Thromboxane A_2 is a potent stimulant of platelet aggregation and vascular smooth muscle, but it has considerably less stimulant activity on most gastrointestinal smooth muscles. Needleman et al. (138) found that when PGG_2 or PGH_2 was incubated with horse or human platelet microsomes the contractions produced on rabbit aortas were greatly augmented, but rat stomach strip contractions were reduced or eliminated, thus indicating the production of thromboxane A_2. Thromboxane A_2 has been found to be 10 times less potent than PGE_2 on rat stomach strips, four times less potent than PGE_2 on chick rectum, and inactive on rat colon (136).

Prostacyclin (PGI_2) is generated by incubating microsomes from arteries (139) or rat stomach fundus (140) with endoperoxides. Prostacyclin is a potent inhibitor of platelet aggregation, and it relaxes most arterial smooth muscles. In contrast, it causes contractions of several gastrointestinal smooth muscle preparations. Gryglewski et al. (141) found it to be less active than PGG_2 or PGH_2 in stimulating rat fundus strips, chicken rectum, or guinea pig ileum. Omini et al. (142) found PGI_2 to be less potent than PGE_2 or $PGF_{2\alpha}$ on rat and hamster stomach strips and chick rectum. PGI_2 also contracted the rat uterus with a potency of about 1/25 that of $PGF_{2\alpha}$ or 1/2 to 1/4 the potency of PGE_2. It was inactive on the cat terminal ileum. 6-Keto-$PGF_{1\alpha}$, the degradation product of PGI_2, was found to be inactive on all the tissues that were tested. Crane et al. (143) also found a low stimulating activity of PGI_2 on gerbil colon and rat uterus, with a potency about 1/10 that of PGE_1. PGD_2 had a potency similar to PGI_2.

DIRECTIONS OF FUTURE RESEARCH

The smooth muscle effects of prostaglandins are basic activities of these agents, and they have important physiological and pharmacological ramifications. Many experiments have been conducted on these activities, but there are still many gaps and inconsistencies in our knowledge. The foregoing review has pointed out many areas where there are inconsistencies, lack of complete understanding, or hypotheses that have not been adequately tested. Studies in these areas utilizing more advanced techniques should prove profitable in the future.

The endoperoxides, thromboxanes, and prostacyclin have not yet been studied extensively on gastrointestinal and uterine smooth muscle. Although these newer members of the prostaglandin family are generally less active than E and F prostaglandins on gastrointestinal and uterine smooth muscle, they may have important specialized activities that have not yet been discovered. The metabolites of thromboxane A_2 and prostacyclin (TxB_2 and 6-keto-$PGF_{1\alpha}$) are generally considered to be inert, but perhaps they have undetected activities. Other members of the prostaglandin family, such as PGD_2 and HETE, deserve further study on gastrointestinal and uterine smooth muscle. It is also likely that more new products of fatty acid metabolism will be discovered and explored in the future.

Differences between in vitro and in vivo effects of some of the prostaglandins have not been resolved. These may at first seem perplexing and seem to indicate that in vitro activities cannot be used as true indicators of in vivo effects. There must be reasons for these discrepancies however, and these reasons have usually not been examined. The observation of the relaxant effects of the E prostaglandins on circular intestinal muscle (74,

75) did much to explain why these agents are considered to be intestinal muscle stimulants in vitro, but may cause intestinal flaccidity in vivo. The previously quoted study on rat myometrium (16) suggests that the in vitro relaxant effects of E prostaglandins may be due to stimulation of adrenergic nerves which degenerate after the tissue has been removed from the animal. Perhaps some neural or humoral mechanism inhibits this adrenergic stimulation in vivo.

Prostaglandin-adrenergic interactions on vascular smooth muscle have attracted considerable attention (85), and these interactions have been carefully studied on isolated vas deferens (84) where adrenergic stimulation causes muscle contraction, but interactions between prostaglandins and adrenergic-induced relaxation of gastrointestinal muscle have not been studied extensively.

Adrenergic neurotransmitters and prostaglandins both have potent effects on cyclic nucleotide production, and it is quite likely that these activities are highly interrelated. Isolated smooth muscles are well suited to studying interrelationships between prostaglandins and cyclic nucleotides. More work is called for to confirm or reject the second messenger hypothesis as it has been applied to the contractility of smooth muscle. The effects that newer members of the prostaglandin family (endoperoxides, thromboxanes, prostacyclin, etc.) have on cyclic nucleotide production should also be studied.

Isolated smooth muscle preparations are ideally suited to studies of prostaglandin receptors. Considerable progress has been made in finding substances that specifically bind prostaglandins, but the binding studies do not differentiate between stimulant and relaxant receptors, nor do they tell if the compound is an agonist or an antagonist. There will probably be more studies correlating prostaglandin binding with smooth muscle activities. The discovery of more active, more specific prostaglandin antagonists which compete with prostaglandins at their receptors would be of great value in defining prostaglandins in normal or pathologic physiology. Studies on agonist-antagonist kinetics call for in vitro investigations on preparations such as isolated smooth muscle.

More knowledge about tachyphylaxis to prostaglandins could add considerably to general knowledge about the actions of prostaglandins. Cross-tachyphylaxis between two prostaglandins, or a prostaglandin and a thromboxane, for instance, can be used as evidence to indicate that both agents are acting through the same receptor. Is tachyphylaxis due to depletion of some substance that is needed for prostaglandins to produce their effects? It seems unlikely that a pituitary hormone such as oxytocin should be required for prostaglandins to produce uterine stimulation, but this substance can restore sensitivity to prostaglandins (29). Perhaps this is weak support for the concept that a primary activity of prostaglandins is augmentation of the action of other substances. Ionic concentrations also appear to play a part in prostaglandin tachyphylaxis. Perhaps this aspect can be valuable for studying ion fluxes such as calcium translocation in relation to smooth muscle contractions.

The possible involvement of prostaglandins in cholinergic transmission needs much clarification. The isolated guinea pig ileum may be an excellent preparation for studying such interactions, but any conclusions should be checked in other systems before generalizations are made.

More information is needed on prostaglandin involvement in normal and pathological intestinal motility. In this case in vitro activities may not be true indicators of in vivo activities, but correlations between the two are sorely needed, or at least reasons for lack of correlations may help explain the basic functions of prostaglandins.

There are hints that the many pharmacological properties of prostaglandins can be separated to achieve higher ratios of beneficial therapeutic effects to undesirable effects. Many analogs of prostaglandins have been synthesized with this dream in mind. Basic studies are called for to determine if this is an achievable goal. For instance, it may be desirable to obtain compounds with high stimulating activities on the myometrium compared to their effects on intestinal smooth muscle. Such compounds may retain their abortifacient or labor-induction properties with fewer gastrointestinal side effects. Isolated smooth muscle preparations may provide means for studying such separations of activities.

Finally, studies on the actions of prostaglandins may well lead to more basic understanding of the normal functions of smooth muscles. The prostaglandins appear to be intimately involved in several very basic mechanisms of muscle function. They also seem to be involved in one way or another with the actions of many other substances, such as the neural transmitters, cyclic nucleotides, kinins, oxytocin, and the steroid hormones. Reflections of all these interactions are visible in smooth muscle activities. Investigations of the basic activities of prostaglandins will most likely yield valuable information on basic smooth muscle mechanisms and knowledge of the mechanisms involved in the actions of other substances.

REFERENCES

1. Kurzrok, R., and Lieb, C. C. Biochemical studies of human semen: II. The action of semen on the human uterus. Proc. Soc. Exp. Biol. Med. 28:268-272, 1930.
2. Goldblatt, M. W. A depressor substance in seminal fluid. J. Soc. Chem. Ind. Lond. 52:1056-1057, 1933.
3. Goldblatt, M. W. Properties of human seminal plasma. J. Physiol. (Lond.) 84:208-218, 1935.
4. Euler, U. S. von. Zur Kenntnis der pharmakologischen Wirkung von nativsekreten und extracten männlicher accessorischer Geschlechtsdrüsen. Arch. Exp. Pathol. Pharmakol. 175:78-84, 1934.
5. Euler, U.S. von. An adrenaline-like action in extracts from the prostatic and related glands. J. Physiol. (Lond.) 81:102-112, 1934.
6. Euler, U. S. von. A depressor substance in the vesicular gland. J. Physiol. (Lond.) 84:21P-22P, 1935.

7. Euler, U. S. von. Über die spezifische blutdrucksenkende Substanz des menschlichen Prostata—und Samenblasensckretes. Klin. Wochenschr. 14:1182-1183, 1935.
8. Euler, U. S. von. On the specific vaso-dilating and plain muscle stimulating substances from accessory genital glands in man and certain animals (prostaglandin and vesiglandin). J. Physiol. (Lond.) 88:213-234, 1936.
9. Bergström, S., Eliasson, R., Euler, U. S. von, and Sjovall, J. Some biological effects of two crystalline prostaglandin factors. Acta Physiol. Scand. 45:133-144, 1959.
10. Horton, E. W. Biological activities of pure prostaglandins. Experientia 21:113-118, 1965.
11. Gilmore, N., Vane, J. R., and Wyllie, J. H. Prostaglandins released by the spleen. Nature (Lond.) 218:1135-1140, 1968.
12. Vane, J. R. Inhibition of prostaglandin synthesis as a mechanism of action for aspirin-like drugs. Nature (New Biol.) 231:232-235, 1971.
13. Smith, J. B., and Willis, A. L. Aspirin selectively inhibits prostaglandin production in human platelets. Nature (New Biol.) 231:235-237, 1971.
14. Ferreira, S. H., Moncada, S., and Vane, J. R. Indomethacin and aspirin abolish prostaglandin release from the spleen. Nature (New Biol.) 231:237-239, 1971.
15. Bygdeman, M. Studies of the effects of prostaglandins in seminal plasma on human myometrium in vitro. In Nobel Symposium 2: Prostaglandins, S. Bergstrom and B. Samuelsson (Eds.). Almqvist & Wiksell, Stockholm, pp. 71-77, 1967.
16. Osa, T., and Kuriyama, H. Electrophysiological and mechanical investigations on the dual action of prostaglandin E_1 in the pregnant rat myometrium in vitro. Jap. J. Physiol. 25:357-369, 1975.
17. Bygdeman, M., and Eliasson, R. The effect of prostaglandin from human seminal fluid on the motility of the non-pregnant human uterus in vitro. Acta Physiol. Scand. 59:43-51, 1963.
18. Bygdeman, M. The effect of different prostaglandins on human myometrium in vitro. Acta Physiol. Scand. 63(Suppl. 242):1-78, 1964.
19. Speroff, L., and Ramwell, P. W. Prostaglandins in reproductive physiology. Am. J. Obstet. Gynecol. 107:1111-1130, 1970.
20. Sullivan, T. J. Response of the mammalian uterus to prostaglandins under differing hormonal conditions. Br. J. Pharmacol. 26:678-685, 1966.
21. Hawkins, R. A., Jessup, R., and Ramwell, P. W. Effect of ovarian hormones on response of the isolated rat uterus to prostaglandins. In Prostaglandin Symposium of the Worcester Foundation for Experimental Biology, P. W. Ramwell and J. E. Shaw (Eds.). Interscience, New York, pp. 11-19, 1968.
22. Fuchs, A. R. Myometrial response to prostaglandins enhanced by progesterone. Am. J. Obstet. Gynecol. 118:1093-1098, 1974.

23. Harney, P. J., Sneddon, J. M., and Williams, K. I. The influence of ovarian hormones upon the motility and prostaglandin production of the pregnant rat uterus in vitro. J. Endocrinol. 60:343-351, 1974.
24. Porter, D. G., and Behrman, H. R. Prostaglandin-induced myometrial activity inhibited by progesterone. Nature (Lond.) 232:627-628, 1971.
25. Eliasson, R. Studies on prostaglandin. Occurrence, formation and biological actions. Acta Physiol. Scand. 46(Suppl. 158):1-73, 1959.
26. Adamson, U., Eliasson, R., and Wiklund, B. Tachyphylaxis in rat uterus to some prostaglandins. Acta Physiol. Scand. 70:451-452, 1967.
27. Eliasson, R., and Brzdekiewcz, Z. Tachyphylactic response of the isolated rat uterus to prostaglandins A. Pharmacol. Res. Commun. 1: 391-396, 1969.
28. Eliasson, R., and Brzdekiewcz, Z. Tachyphylactic response of the isolated rat uterus to prostaglandins F. Pharmacol. Res. Commun. 1: 397-402, 1969.
29. Eliasson, R., and Brzdekiewcz, Z. Effects of various agonists on the tachyphylactic response of the isolated rat uterus to prostaglandin E_1. Life Sci. 9:925-930, 1970.
30. Paton, D. M., and Daniel, E. E. On the contractile response of the isolated rat uterus to prostaglandin E_1. Can. J. Physiol. Pharmacol. 45:795-804, 1967.
31. Hall, W. J., and Pickles, V. R. The dual action of menstrual stimulant A_2 (prostaglandin E_2). J. Physiol. (Lond.) 169:90-91P, 1963.
32. Clegg, P. C., Hall, W. J., and Pickles, V. R. The action of ketonic prostaglandins on the guinea pig myometrium. J. Physiol. (Lond.) 183: 123-144, 1966.
33. Paton, W. D. M. The contractile response of the isolated rat uterus to noradrenaline and 5-hydroxytryptamine. Eur. J. Pharmacol. 3:310-315, 1968.
34. Brummer, H. C. Interaction of E prostaglandins and syntocinon on the pregnant human myometrium. J. Obstet. Gynaecol. Br. Commonw. 78:305-309, 1971.
35. Brummer, H. C. Further studies on the interaction between prostaglandins and syntocinon on the isolated pregnant human myometrium. J. Obstet. Gynaecol. Br. Commonw. 79:526-530, 1972.
36. Bär, H. P. Cyclic nucleotides and smooth muscle. Adv. Cyclic Nucleotide Res. 4:195-237, 1974.
37. Anderson, R., Nilsson, K., Wikberg, J., Johansson, S., Mohme-Lundholm, E., and Lundholm, L. Cyclic nucleotides and the contraction of smooth muscle. Adv. Cyclic Nucleotide Res. 5:492-517, 1975.
38. Kuehl, F. A., Cirillo, V. J., Ham, E. A., and Humes, J. L. The regulatory role of the prostaglandins on the cyclic 3',5'-AMP system. Adv. Biosci. 9:155-172, 1973.
39. Harbon, S., and Clauser, H. Cyclic adenosine 3',5'-monophosphate levels in rat myometrium under the influence of epinephrine, prosta-

glandins and oxytocin. Correlations with uterus and motility. Biochem. Biophys. Res. Commun. 44:1496-1503, 1971.
40. Zor, U., Koch, Y., Lamprecht, S. A., Ausher, J., and Lindner, H. R. Mechanism of oestradiol action on the rat uterus: independence of cyclic AMP, prostaglandin E_2 and β-adrenergic mediation. J. Endocrinol. 58:525-533, 1973.
41. Lerner, L. J., Carminati, P., and Rubin, B. L. Effects of prostaglandins PGE_2 and $PGF_{2\alpha}$ on the adenyl cyclase activity of various segments of the immature rabbit oviduct and uterus. Proc. Soc. Exp. Biol. Med. 143:536-539, 1973.
42. Kuehl, F. A. Prostaglandins, cyclic nucleotides and cell function. Prostaglandins 9:325-340, 1974.
43. Angles d'Auriac, G., and Worcel, M. Variations in cGMP and cAMP levels in rat uterine smooth muscle induced by carbachol, $PGF_{2\alpha}$ and changes in ionic composition. Br. J. Pharmacol. 54:236P-237P, 1975.
44. Buckle, J. W., and Nathanielz, P. W. Modification of myometrial activity in vivo by administration of cyclic nucleotides and theophylline to the pregnant rat. J. Endocrinol. 66:339-347, 1975.
45. Teraki, Y., Miyasaka, M., and Tsunoo, S. The mechanism of action of prostaglandins on contraction of the uterus. Jap. J. Pharmacol. 24 (Suppl.):30, 1974.
46. Osa, T., Suzuki, H., Katase, T., and Kuriyama, H. Excitatory action of synthetic prostaglandin E_2 on the electrical activity of pregnant mouse myometrium in relation to temperature changes and external sodium and calcium concentrations. Jap. J. Physiol. 24:233-248, 1974.
47. Carsten, M. E. Prostaglandins and oxytocin: their effects on uterine smooth muscle. Prostaglandins 5:33-40, 1974.
48. Carsten, M. E. Prostaglandins and cellular calcium transport in the pregnant human uterus. Am. J. Obstet. Gynecol. 117:824-832, 1973.
49. Eagling, E. M., Lovell, H. G., and Pickles, V. R. Interaction of prostaglandin E_1 and calcium in the guinea-pig myometrium. Br. J. Pharmacol. 44:510-516, 1972.
50. Chan, W. Y., Hruby, V. J., and Vigneaud, V. Effects of magnesium ion and oxytocin inhibitors on the uterotonic activity of oxytocin and prostaglandins E_2 and $F_{2\alpha}$. J. Pharmacol. Exp. Ther. 190:77-87, 1974.
51. Pickles, V. R. The myometrial actions of six prostaglandins: consideration of a receptor hypothesis. In Nobel Symposium 2: Prostaglandins, S. Bergstrom and B. Samuelsson (Eds.). Almqvist & Wiksell, Stockholm, pp. 79-83, 1967.
52. Johnson, M., Jessup, R., and Ramwell, P. The significance of protein disulfide and sulfhydryl groups in prostaglandin action. Prostaglandins 5:125-136, 1974.
53. Johnson, M., Jessup, R., and Ramwell, P. Ultraviolet light modification of the prostaglandin receptor. Prostaglandins 4:593-605, 1973.

54. Bito, L. Z. Accumulation and apparent active transport of prostaglandins by some rabbit tissue in vitro. J. Physiol. (Lond.) 221:371-387, 1972.
55. Wakeling, A. E., Kirton, K. T., and Wyngarden, L. J. Prostaglandin receptors in the hamster uterus during the estrous cycle. Prostaglandins 4:1-8, 1973.
56. Wakeling, A. E., and Wyngarden, L. J. In vitro studies on the nature of prostaglandin E_1 binding in the hamster uterus. Prostaglandins 5: 291-300, 1974.
57. Wakeling, A. E., and Wyngarden, L. J. Prostaglandin receptors in the human, monkey and hamster uterus. Endocrinology 5:55-64, 1974.
58. Kimball, F. A., Kirton, K. T., Spilman, C. H., and Wyngarden, L. J. Prostaglandin E_1 specific binding in human myometrium. Biol. Reprod. 13:482-489, 1975.
59. Kimball, F. A., and Wyngarden, L. J. Prostaglandin specific binding in hamster myometrial low speed supernatant. Prostaglandins 9:413-429, 1975.
60. Poyser, N. L. Production of prostaglandins by the guinea-pig uterus. J. Endocrinol. 54:147-159, 1972.
61. Chan, W. Y. Oxytocin-induced release of prostaglandin-like substance in isolated rat uterus. Life Sci. 14:2385-2392, 1974.
62. Csapo, A. I., and Csapo, E. E. The "prostaglandin step," a bottleneck in the activation of the uterus. Life Sci. 14:719-724, 1974.
63. Vane, J. R., and Williams, K. I. The contribution of prostaglandin production to contractions of the isolated uterus of the rat. Br. J. Pharmacol. 48:629-639, 1973.
64. Baudouin-Legros, M., Meyer, P., and Worcel, M. Influence of prostaglandins and oestrus cycle on the spasmogenic action of angiotensin II and oxytocin on rat uterus. Eur. J. Clin. Invest. 4:327, 1974.
65. Csapo, A. I. On the mechanism of the abortifacient action of prostaglandin $F_{2\alpha}$. J. Reprod. Med. 9:400-412, 1972.
66. Csapo, A. I. The prospects of PGs in postconceptional therapy. Prostaglandins 3:245-289, 1973.
67. Bergström, S., and Euler, U. S. von. The biological activity of prostaglandin E_1, E_2 and E_3. Acta Physiol. Scand. 59:493-494, 1963.
68. Horton, E. W., and Main, I. H. M. A comparison of the biological activities of four prostaglandins. Br. J. Pharmacol. 21:182-189, 1963.
69. Horton, E. W., and Jones, R. L. Prostaglandins A_1, A_2 and 19-hydroxy A_1; their actions on smooth muscle and their inactivation on passage through the pulmonary and hepatic portal vascular beds. Br. J. Pharmacol. 37:705-722, 1969.
70. Weeks, J. R., Sekhar, G., and Ducharme, D. W. Relative activity of prostaglandins E_1, A_1, E_2 and A_2 on lipolysis, platelet aggregation, smooth muscle and the cardiovascular system. J. Pharm. Pharmacol. 21:103-108, 1969.

71. Änggård, E. The biological activities of three metabolites of prostaglandin E_1. Acta Physiol. Scand. 66:509-510, 1966.
72. Sanner, J. H., Rozek, L. F., and Cammarata, P. S. Comparative smooth muscle and cardiovascular actions of prostaglandin E_2, $F_{2\alpha}$, and $F_{2\beta}$. In Prostaglandin Symposium of the Worcester Foundation for Experimental Biology, P. W. Ramwell and J. E. Shaw (Eds.). Interscience, New York, pp. 215-224, 1968.
73. Bennett, A., Murray, J. G., and Wyllie, J. H. Occurrence of prostaglandin E_2 in the human stomach, and a study of its effects on human isolated gastric muscle. Br. J. Pharmacol. 32:339-349, 1968.
74. Fleshler, B., and Bennett, A. Responses of human, guinea pig and rat colonic circular muscle to prostaglandins. J. Lab. Clin. Med. 74:872-873, 1969.
75. Bennett, A., Eley, K. G., and Scholes, G. B. Effects of prostaglandins E_1 and E_2 on human, guinea-pig and rat isolated small intestine. Br. J. Pharmacol. 34:630-638, 1968.
76. Adaikan, P. G., and Karim, S. M. M. Effects of PGA and PGB compounds on gastrointestinal tract smooth muscle from man and laboratory animals. Prostaglandins 11:15-22, 1976.
77. Hamberg, M., Hedqvist, P., Strandberg, K., Svensson, J., and Samuelsson, B. Prostaglandin endoperoxides: IV. Effects on smooth muscle. Life Sci. 16:451-462, 1975.
78. Harry, J. D. The action of prostaglandin E_1 on the guinea-pig isolated intestine. Br. J. Pharmacol. 33:213P-214P, 1968.
79. Jaques, R. Morphine as inhibitor of prostaglandin E_1 on the isolated guinea-pig intestine. Experientia 25:1059-1060, 1969.
80. Sanner, J. Prostaglandin inhibition with a dibenzoxazepine hydrazide derivative and morphine. Ann. N.Y. Acad. Sci. 180:396-409, 1971.
81. Paton, W. D. M. The action of morphine and related substances on contraction and on acetylcholine output of coaxially stimulated guinea-pig ileum. Br. J. Pharmacol. 12:119-127, 1957.
82. Schaumann, W. Inhibition by morphine of the release of acetylcholine from the intestine of the guinea-pig. Br. J. Pharmacol. 12:115-118, 1957.
83. Akanuma, M. Modes of the stimulating action of prostaglandin E_1 on the gastrointestinal tract of the guinea-pig. Sapporo Med. J. 38:41-52, 1970.
84. Hedqvist, P. Autonomic neurotransmission. In The Prostaglandins, P. W. Ramwell (Ed.). Plenum Press, New York, pp. 101-131, 1973.
85. Brody, M. J., and Kadowitz, P. J. Prostaglandins as modulators of the autonomic nervous system. Fed. Proc. 33:48-60, 1974.
86. Wennmalm, A., and Hedqvist, P. Inhibition by prostaglandin E_1 of parasympathetic neurotransmission in the rabbit heart. Life Sci. 10:465-470, 1971.
87. Ehrenpreis, S., Greenberg, J., and Belman, S. Prostaglandins reverse inhibition of electrically induced contractions of guinea pig ileum by

morphine, indomethacin and acetylsalicylic acid. Nature (New Biol.) 245:280-282, 1973.
88. Gustafsson, L., Hedqvist, P., and Langercrantz, H. Prostaglandin mediated enhancement of effector response to cholinergic nerve stimulation. Acta Physiol. Scand. (Suppl. 396):106, 1973.
89. Collier, H. O. J., and Roy, A. C. Morphine-like drugs inhibit the stimulation by E prostaglandins of cyclic AMP formation by rat brain homogenate. Nature (Lond.) 248:24-27, 1974.
90. Traber, J., Fischer, K., Latzin, S., and Hamprecht, B. Morphine antagonizes action of prostaglandin neuroblastoma and neuroblastoma X glioma hybrid cells. Nature (Lond.) 253:120-122, 1975.
91. Gryglewski, R. J., Szczeklik, A., and Bieron, K. Morphine antagonizes prostaglandin E_1-mediated inhibition of human platelet aggregation. Nature (Lond.) 256:56-57, 1975.
92. Hazra, J. Evidence against prostaglandin E having a physiological role in acetylcholine liberation from Auerbach's plexus of guinea-pig ileum. Experientia 15:565-566, 1975.
93. Benz, M., and Salzmann, R. The effect of PGE_1, PGE_2 and $PGF_{2\alpha}$ on parasympathetic transmission. Arch. Pharmacol. 282(Suppl.):R7, 1974.
94. Botting, J. H., and Salzmann, R. The effect of indomethacin on the release of prostaglandin E_2 and acetylcholine from guinea-pig isolated ileum at rest and during field stimulation. Br. J. Pharmacol. 50: 119-124, 1974.
95. Kadlec, O., Mašek, K., and Šeferna, I. The role of prostaglandins in the output of neurotransmitters from the isolated guinea-pig ileum. Abstr. 6th Int. Congr. Pharmacol., p. 156, 1975.
96. Hall, W. J., O'Neill, P., and Sheehan, J. D. The role of prostaglandins in cholinergic neural transmission in the guinea pig. Eur. J. Pharmacol. 34:39-47, 1975.
97. Schulz, R., and Cartwright, C. Sensitization of the smooth muscle by prostaglandin E_1 contributes to reversal of drug-induced inhibition of the guinea-pig ileum. Naunyn Schmiedeberg's Arch. Pharmacol. 294: 257-260, 1976.
98. Gintzler, A., and Musacchio, J. M. Failure of prostaglandins to participate in the inhibitory response of the guinea-pig ileum to morphine. Fed. Proc. 33:502, 1974.
99. Kadlec, O., Mašek, K., and Šeferna, I. A modulating role of prostaglandins in contractions of the guinea-pig ileum. Br. J. Pharmacol. 51:565-570, 1974.
100. Fameay, J. P., Fontaine, J., and Reuse, J. Inhibiting effects of morphine, chloroquine, nonsteroidal and steroidal anti-inflammatory drugs on electrically induced contractions of guinea-pig ileum and the reversing effect of prostaglandins. Agents Actions 5:354-358, 1975.

101. Fried, J., Santhanakrishnan, T. S., Himizu, J., Lin, C. H., Ford, S. H., Rubin, B., and Gringas, E. O. Prostaglandin antagonists: synthesis and smooth muscle activity. Nature (Lond.) 223:208-210, 1969.
102. Fried, J., Lin, C. H., Mehra, M. M., Kao, W. L., and Dalven, P. Synthesis and biological activity of prostaglandins and prostaglandin antagonists. Ann. N.Y. Acad. Sci. 180:38-63, 1971.
103. Flack, J. D. In Ramwell, P. W., and Shaw, J. E. Biological significance of the prostaglandins. Recent Prog. Horm. Res. 26:174-179 1970.
104. Bennett, A., and Posner, J. Studies on prostaglandin antagonists. Br. J. Pharmacol. 42:584-594, 1971.
105. Baudouin-Legros, M., Meyer, P., and Worcel, M. Action of 7-oxa-13-prostynoic acid on rat uterine contractility and sensitivity to $PGF_{2\alpha}$ and angiotensin II. Prostaglandins 9:203-209, 1975.
106. Bennett, A. Prostaglandin antagonists. Adv. Drug Res. 8:83-118, 1974.
107. Sanner, J. H. Substances that inhibit the actions of prostaglandins. Arch. Intern. Med. 133:133-146, 1974.
108. Sanner, J. H., and Eakins, K. E. Prostaglandin antagonists. In Prostaglandins: Chemical and Biochemical Aspects, S. M. M. Karim (Ed.). MTP Press, Lancaster, England, pp. 139-189.
109. Eakins, K. E., and Karim, S. M. M. Polyphloretin phosphate—a selective antagonist for prostaglandin $F_{1\alpha}$ and $F_{2\alpha}$. Life Sci. 9:1-5, 1970.
110. Eakins, K. E., Karim, S. M. M., and Miller, J. D. Antagonism of some smooth muscle actions of prostaglandins by polyphloretin phosphate. Br. J. Pharmacol. 39:556-563, 1970.
111. Fries, B. Polyphloretin phosphate—a hyaluronidase inhibitor—and hyaluronidase in prevention of intra-peritoneal adhesions. An experimental study in the rabbit. Acta Chir. Scand. (Suppl. 217), 1956.
112. Fries, B. The edema-inhibiting action of polyphloretin phosphate (PPP) in some types of capillary damage. Acta Chir. Scand. 119:1-7, 1960.
113. Beitch, B. R., and Eakins, K. E. The effects of prostaglandins on the intraocular pressure of the rabbit. Br. J. Pharmacol. 37:158-167, 1969.
114. Wohlzogen, F. X. Reduction of fertility in rats by an enzyme inhibitor. Acta Endocrinol. (Kbh.) 37:298-300, 1961.
115. Gagnon, D. J., and Sirois, P. The rat isolated colon as a specific assay organ for angiotensin. Br. J. Pharmacol. 45:89-93, 1972.
116. Somova, L. Inhibition of prostaglandin synthesis in the kidneys by aspirin-like drugs. Adv. Biosci. 9:155-172, 1973.
117. Adaiken, P. G., and Karim, S. M. M. Polyphloretin phosphate temporarily potentiates prostaglandin E_2 on the rat fundus, probably by inhibiting PG 15-hydroxydehydrogenase. J. Pharm. Pharmacol. 25: 229-233, 1973.

118. Marrazzi, M. A., and Matschinsky, F. M. Properties of 15-hydroxy prostaglandin dehydrogenase: structural requirements for substrate binding. Prostaglandins 1:373-387, 1972.
119. Eakins, K. E. Prostaglandin antagonism by polymeric phosphates of phloretin and related compounds. Ann. N.Y. Acad. Sci. 180:386-395, 1971.
120. Bethel, R. A., and Eakins, K. E. The mechanism of the antagonism of experimentally induced ocular hypertension by polyphloretin phosphate. Exp. Eye Res. 13:83-91, 1971.
121. Eakins, K. E., Fex, H., Fredholm, B., Högberg, B., and Veige, S. On the prostaglandin inhibitory action of polyphloretin phosphate. Adv. Biosci. 9:135-138, 1973.
122. Crutchley, D. J., and Piper, P. J. Inhibition of the inactivation of prostaglandins in guinea pig lungs. Naunyn Schmiedeberg's Arch. Pharmacol. 279(Suppl. R):20, 1973.
123. Sanner, J. H. Antagonism of prostaglandin E_2 by 1-acetyl-2-(8-chloro-10,11-dihydrodibenz[b,f][1,4]oxazepine-10-carbonyl) hydrazine (SC-19220). Arch. Int. Pharmacodyn. Ther. 180:46-56, 1969.
124. Splawinski, J. A., Nies, A. S., Sweetman, B., and Oates, J. A. The effects of arachidonic acid, prostaglandin E_2 and prostaglandin $F_{2\alpha}$ on the longitudinal stomach strip of the rat. J. Pharmacol. Exp. Ther. 187:501-510, 1973.
125. Tsai, T. H., Parmeter, L., White, H. L., and Maxwell, R. A. Effect of indomethacin and aspirin on the response of isolated guinea-pig ileum to arachidonic acid, a precursor of prostaglandin E_2. Abstr. 5th Int. Congr. Pharmacol., p. 237, 1972.
126. Ferreira, S. H., Herman, A., and Vane, J. R. Prostaglandin generation maintains the smooth muscle tone of the rabbit isolated jejunum. Br. J. Pharmacol. 44:328P-330P, 1972.
127. Willis, A. L., Davison, P., and Ramwell, P. W. Inhibition of intestinal tone, motility and prostaglandin biosynthesis by 5,8,11,14-eicosatetraynoic acid (TYA). Prostaglandins 5:355-368, 1974.
128. Bennett, A., Eley, K. G., and Stockley, H. L. The effects of prostaglandins on guinea-pig isolated intestine and their possible contribution to muscle activity and tone. Br. J. Pharmacol. 54:197-204, 1975.
129. Bennett, A., Eley, K. G., and Scholes, G. B. Effect of prostaglandins E_1 and E_2 on intestinal motility in the guinea pig and rat. Br. J. Pharmacol. 34:639-647, 1968.
130. Radmonović, B. Z. Effect of prostaglandin E_1 on the peristaltic activity of the guinea-pig isolated ileum. Arch. Int. Pharmacodyn. Ther. 200:396-404, 1972.
131. Ishizawa, M., and Miyazaki, E. Effect of prostaglandin $F_{2\alpha}$ on propulsive activity of the isolated segmental colon of the guinea-pig. Prostaglandins 10:759-768, 1975.

132. Yagasaki, O., Matsuyama, S., and Takai, M. The release of prostaglandins from the passively distended wall of guinea pig intestine. Jap. J. Pharmacol. 24(Suppl.):31, 1974.
133. Grubb, M. N., and Burks, T. F. Selective antagonism of the intestinal stimulatory effects of morphine by isoproterenol, prostaglandin E_1 and theophylline. J. Pharmacol. Exp. Ther. 193:884-891, 1975.
134. Dajani, E. Z., Roge, E. A. W., and Bertermann, R. E. Effects of E prostaglandins, diphenoxylate and morphine on intestinal motility in vivo. Eur. J. Pharmacol. 34:105-113, 1975.
135. Hamberg, M., Svensson, J., Wakabayashi, T., and Samuelsson, B. Isolation and structure of two prostaglandin endoperoxides that cause platelet aggregation. Proc. Natl. Acad. Sci. USA 71:345-349, 1974.
136. Bunting, S., Moncada, S., and Vane, J. R. The effects of prostaglandin endoperoxides and thromboxane A_2 on strips of rabbit coeliac artery and certain other smooth muscle preparations. Br. J. Pharmacol. 57:462P-463P, 1976.
137. Bundy, G. L. The synthesis of prostaglandin endoperoxide analogs. Tetrahedron Lett. No. 24:1957-1960, 1975.
138. Needleman, P., Moncada, S., Bunting, S., Vane, J. R., Hamberg, M., and Samuelsson, B. Identification of an enzyme in platelet microsomes which generates thromboxane A_2 from prostaglandin endoperoxides. Nature (Lond.) 261:558-560, 1976.
139. Moncada, S., Gryglewski, R., Bunting, S., and Vane, J. R. An enzyme isolated from arteries transforms prostaglandin endoperoxides to an unstable substance that inhibits platelet aggregation. Nature (Lond.) 263:663-665, 1976.
140. Moncada, S., Gryglewski, R. J., Bunting, S., and Vane, J. R. A lipid peroxide inhibits the enzyme in blood vessel microsomes that generates from prostaglandin endoperoxides the substance (prostaglandin X) which prevents platelet aggregation. Prostaglandins 12:715-737, 1976.
141. Gryglewski, R. J., Bunting, S., Moncada, S., Flower, R. J., and Vane, J. R. Arterial walls are protected against deposition of platelet thrombi by a substance (prostaglandin X) which they make from prostaglandin endoperoxides. Prostaglandins 12:685-713, 1976.
142. Omini, C., Moncada, S., and Vane, J. R. The effects of prostacyclin (PGI_2) on tissues which detect prostaglandins (PG's). Prostaglandins 14:625-632, 1977.
143. Crane, B. H., Maish, T. L., Maddox, Y. T., Corey, E. J., Székely, I., and Ramwell, P. W. Effect of prostaglandin I_2 and analogs on platelet aggregation and smooth muscle contraction. J. Pharmacol. Exp. Ther. 206:132-138, 1978.

13 Prostaglandin Actions on the Gastrointestinal Tract

THOMAS F. BURKS / University of Arizona College of Medicine, Tucson, Arizona

MARGARET G. NORTHWAY* / Uniformed Services University of the Health Sciences, Bethesda, Maryland

Prostaglandins and related prostanoid substances exert a variety of profound effects on the functions of the digestive system. Endogenously produced and exogenously administered prostaglandins affect both contractile activity and fluid and electrolyte transport. The ability of certain nonsteroidal anti-inflammatory agents to damage gastrointestinal mucosa may be related, in part, to inhibition of prostaglandin synthesis. Prostaglandins are thought to exert nonspecific cytoprotective effects on certain portions of gastrointestinal mucosa.

GASTROINTESTINAL MOTILITY

In general, stomach and intestinal longitudinal smooth muscle is contracted by most PGs, whereas circular smooth muscle is contracted by $PGF_{2\alpha}$ but relaxed by PGEs (1). Longitudinal strips of rat forestomach were thus contracted by PGE_2, $PGF_{2\alpha}$, and by arachidonic acid (2). Similar relative maximum effects and sensitivity to blockade by a putative PG receptor antagonist (SC 19,220) suggested stimulation of a common receptor site by both PGE and PGF to induce longitudinal muscle contractions. PGE_2 inhibited contractions of circular muscle in dog isolated stomach (3). In accord with results obtain in animal preparations, prostaglandins E and F were found to contract longitudinal muscle of human stomach in vitro (4). In circular muscle strips of human stomach, $PGF_{2\alpha}$ caused contractions and PGE_2 induced relaxation (4).

PGE and PGF contract longitudinal muscle of guinea pig isolated ileum and colon; PGF contracts circular muscle and PGE relaxes or inhibits

---

*Present Affiliation: King's Hospital Medical School, London, England

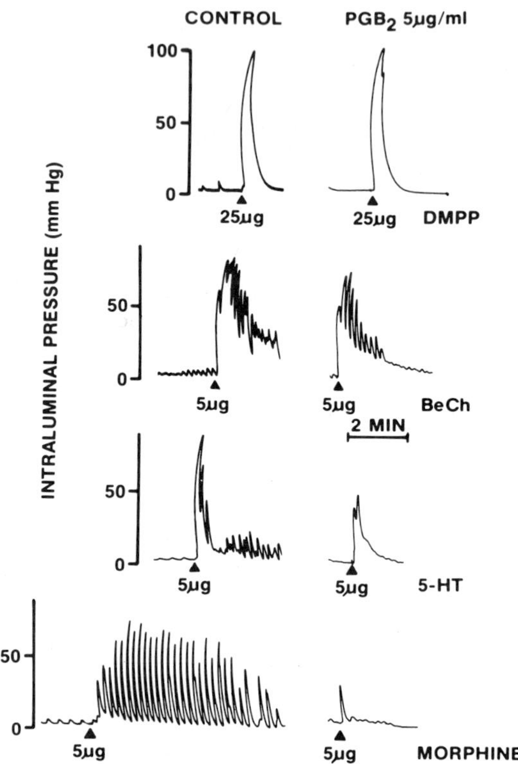

FIG. 1. Contractions of vascularly perfused dog isolated intestine induced by dimethylphenylpiperazinium (DMPP), bethanechol (BeCh), 5-hydroxytryptamine (5-HT), and morphine given as bolus intraarterial injections in the doses indicated. Responses on the left side were obtained during perfusion of an intestinal segment with plain Krebs solution (control); responses on the right were obtained during perfusion with Krebs solution containing 5 μg/ml of prostaglandin B_2. Note that PGB_2 diminished responses to 5-HT and morphine without significantly affecting responses to DMPP and BeCh.

contractions of intestinal circular muscle (5). The ability of PGs to contract intestinal smooth muscle appears to be partly direct and partly as a result of neural interactions. Contractions of guinea pig ileum longitudinal muscle induced by $PGF_{1\alpha}$, $PGF_{2\alpha}$, and PGE_2 were reduced 16-32% by application of tetrodotoxin. Anticholinergic drugs reduced responses to these PGs by 52-67%. As the effects of tetrodotoxin and anticholinergic drugs were not additive, it seems that the neurons affected by the PGs are cholinergic (6). These experiments demonstrate that the excitatory effects of the prostaglandins on intestinal smooth muscle are partially mediated by actions on cholinergic neurons. In the same series of experiments, it was found that PGE_2 inhibited contractions of ileal circular muscle induced by electrical stimulation (6). Treatment of the isolated tissue with aspirin or indomethacin produced small increases in tone of the smooth muscle and enhanced electrically induced contractions (6). These results suggest that blockade of prostaglandin production in vitro can enhance responses to contractile stimuli. The observations raise the possibility that responses to drugs could be altered by endogenous production of PGs. The following experiments illustrate the interactions between endogenous PGs and drugs.

The effects of several PG compounds were evaluated on responses of dog isolated intestine to four types of stimulatory drugs: bethanechol, dimethylphenylpiperazinium (DMPP), 5-hydroxytryptamine (5-HT), and morphine. Bethanechol acts directly on intestinal smooth muscle, DMPP is a ganglion stimulant, 5-HT has both cholinergic and noncholinergic intestinal stimulatory effects, and morphine causes stimulation of the dog intestine mainly through release of 5-HT (7). The arterial vasculature of isolated

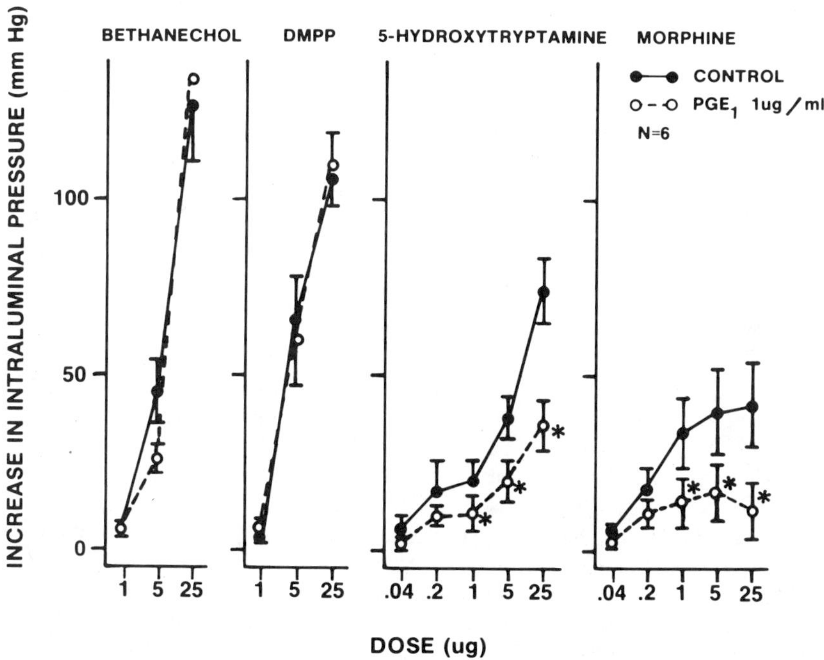

FIG. 2. Dose-response curves for bethanechol, dimethylphenylpiperazinium (DMPP), 5-hydroxytryptamine, and morphine in dog isolated intestine during perfusion with plain Krebs solution (control) or Krebs solution containing 1 μg/ml of prostaglandin E_1. Asterisks indicate responses in presence of PGE_1 significantly different ($p < 0.05$) from control responses. Values shown are means (± SE) of responses in preparations from six animals.

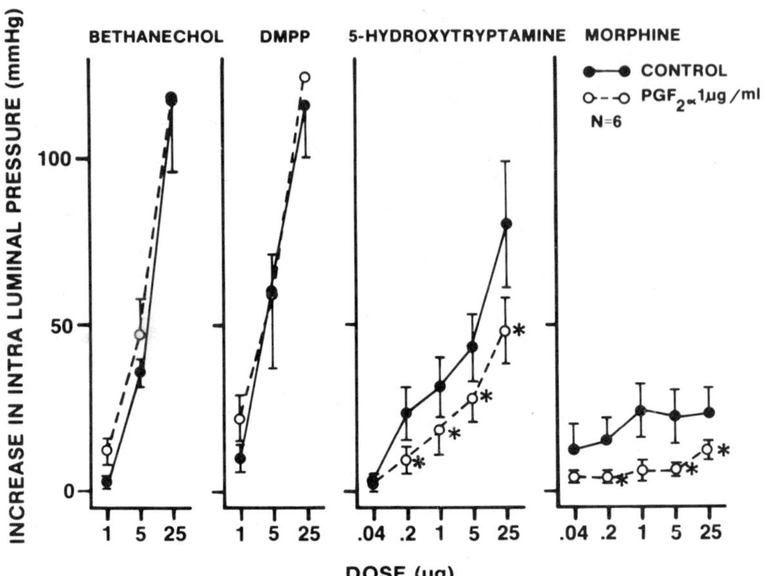

FIG. 3. Dose-response curves for bethanechol, dimethylphenylpiperazinium (DMPP), 5-hydroxytryptamine, and morphine in dog isolated intestine during perfusion with plain Krebs solution (control) or Krebs solution containing 1 μg/ml of prostaglandin $F_{2\alpha}$. Asterisks indicate responses in the presence of $PGF_{2\alpha}$ significantly different ($p < 0.05$) from control responses. Values shown are means ($\pm$ SE) of responses in preparations from six animals.

intestinal segments was perfused with a physiological salt solution (Krebs solution). Contractions were measured as increases in intraluminal pressure. The four stimulatory drugs were administered as intraarterial bolus injections. Responses were obtained to each of the four stimulatory agents during perfusion with control Krebs solution or during perfusion with various concentrations of PG. Examples of the types of response obtained are illustrated in Fig. 1. As the contractions measured by this technique reflect mainly those of circular muscle, bolus intraarterial doses of PGE_1, PGE_2, PGA_2, and PGB_2 either caused relaxation or inhibited ongoing spontaneous contractions. Bolus intraarterial injections of $PGF_{2\alpha}$ caused contractions.

Perfusion of isolated intestinal segments with PGE_1 selectively inhibited contractile responses to 5-HT and morphine, without significant inhibition of responses to the cholinergic agents bethanechol and DMPP. This result was consistent with previous studies (8,9). The PGE_1 produced a modest, but consistent, inhibition of responses to exogenously administered 5-HT or the 5-HT mobilized by morphine (Fig. 2). $PGF_{2\alpha}$ also inhibited responses to 5-HT and morphine without significant effects on responses to bethanechol or DMPP (Fig. 3).

Content of PG-like substances in the venous effluent from the perfused intestinal segments was estimated by bioassay. Strips of stomach fundus from rats treated with indomethacin (40 mg/kg) were prepared for superfusion by the venous effluent from intestinal segments. Tripelennamine, cinanserin, and atropine were added to the superfusion stream to prevent contractions of the stomach strip assay organ by histamine, 5-HT, or acetylcholine. Intraarterial administration of arachidonic acid to dog intestinal segments caused inhibition of ongoing contractile activity and resulted in contractions of the assay organ (Fig. 4), indicating conversion of arachidonic acid to PG. Prostaglandin synthesis in the isolated intestinal segments was prevented by pretreatment of the donor animals with indomethacin (2 mg/kg). Indomethacin was administered to the donor animals instead of being added to the perfusing Krebs solution because it sometimes caused nonspecific inhibition of contractions in the isolated segments. The efficacy of indomethacin pretreatment of donor animals was shown by failure of arachidonic acid to affect ongoing contractions and by lack of appearance in the venous effluent of PG-like substances after arachidonic acid administration in segments removed from indomethacin-treated animals (Fig. 4).

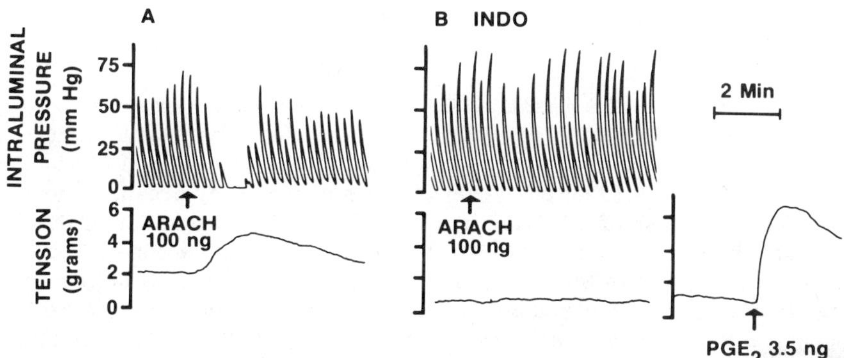

FIG. 4. Contractions of dog isolated intestinal segments (top tracing) and rat stomach strip (bottom tracing) superfused with venous effluent from the vascularly perfused intestinal segment. In panel A, arachidonic acid (100 ng) was injected as an intraarterial bolus to the perfused intestinal segment. The injection caused brief inhibition of ongoing intestinal contractions and the appearance in the intestinal venous perfusate of a PG-like material, which contracted the bioassay organ. In panel B, the donor dog was treated with indomethacin (2 mg/kg) 30 min before removal of the intestinal segment. Administration of arachidonic acid to the intestinal segment after indomethacin treatment failed to inhibit ongoing contractions and did not produce contractions of the assay organ. The assay organ itself was still responsive to PGE_2 (3.5 ng) added directly.

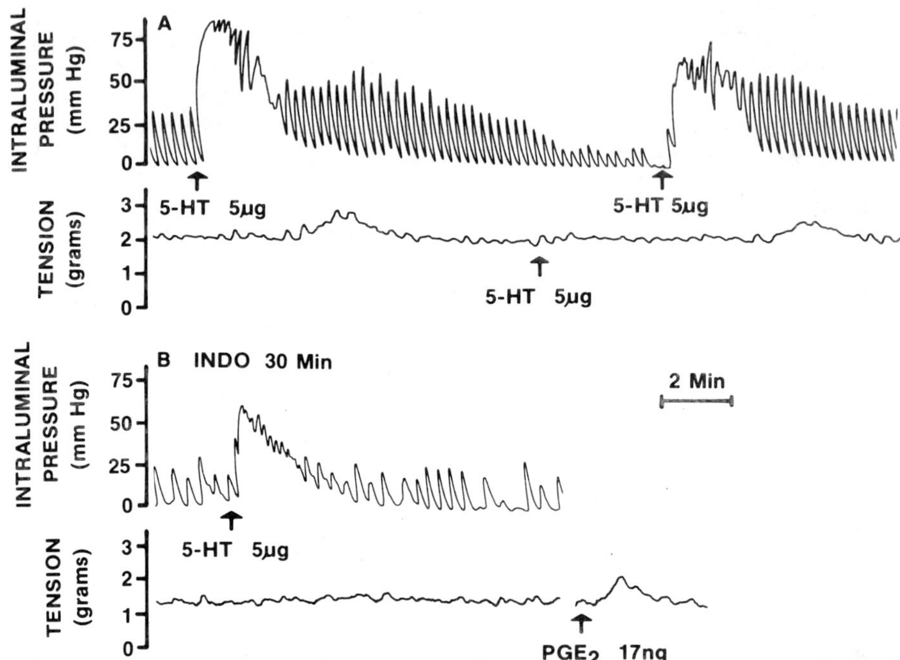

FIG. 5. Contractions of dog isolated intestinal segment (top tracing) and rat stomach strip bioassay organ (bottom tracing) superfused with venous effluent from the vascularly perfused intestinal segment. The contractions induced by 5-HT were followed by contractions of the assay organ, indicating formation and release of a PG-like material by 5-HT. Contraction of the assay organ could not be due to 5-HT, because direct application of 5 μg of 5-HT to the assay organ (middle of tracing) did not cause a contraction. In an intestinal segment removed 30 min after administration of indomethacin (2 mg/kg) to the donor animal, administration of 5-HT did not induce release of PG-like material (panel B). The assay organ was still sensitive to directly applied PGE_2 (17 ng).

Intraarterially injected 5-HT and morphine caused contractions of the dog intestinal segments and the appearance in the venous perfusate of PG-like activity (Fig. 5). Intestinal segments removed from indomethacin-treated animals responded with contractions to intraarterially administered 5-HT but did not form PG-like substances (Fig. 5). As the PGs tested caused inhibition of intestinal motor responses to 5-HT and morphine, it was reasoned that endogenous PG production might modulate intestinal responses to these substances. Contractile responses to bethanechol, DMPP, 5-HT, and morphine were compared in preparations taken before and after indomethacin treatment of donor animals. Treatment with indomethacin caused small but consistent enhancement of responses to 5-HT and morphine without producing significant shifts in dose-response curves for bethanechol or DMPP (Fig. 6). These experiments suggest that prostaglandins may exert a regulatory influence on dog intestinal motility. Prevention of prostaglandin synthesis with indomethacin augments motor responses to 5-HT and to drugs that release 5-HT. The magnitude of the increase in responsiveness to 5-HT and morphine produced by indomethacin was similar to the degree of inhibition produced by the PGs.

This type of study has been extended into examinations of the effect of indomethacin on tone and contractions of human small intestine. Burleigh has found that indomethacin decreased tone and spontaneous activity in longi-

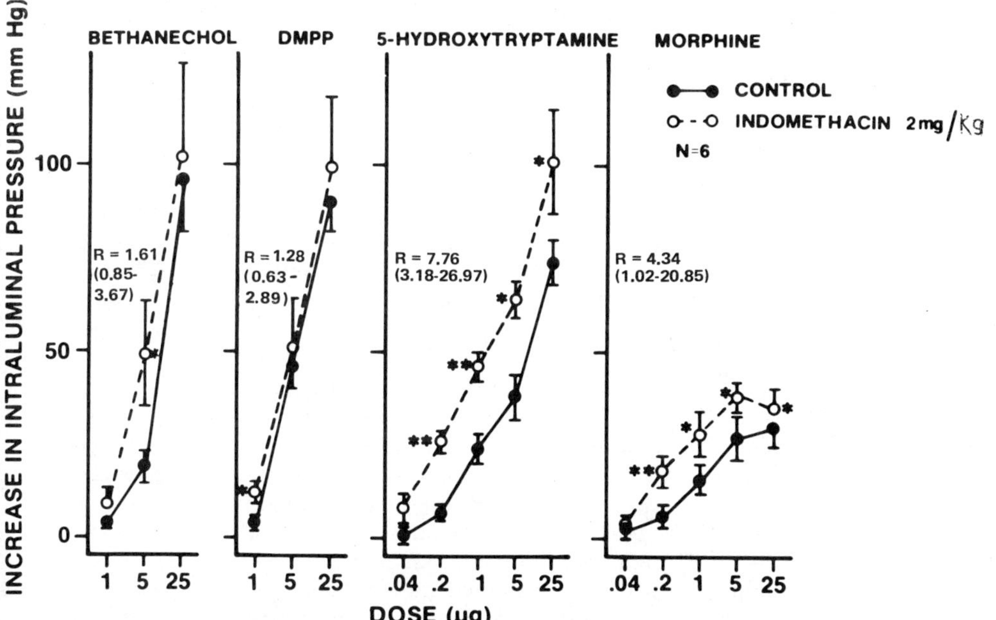

FIG. 6. Dose-response curves to bethanechol, dimethylphenylpiperazinium (DMPP), 5-hydroxytryptamine, and morphine in dog isolated intestinal segments removed from the donor animals before (control) or after administration of 2 mg/kg of indomethacin. Points are means (± SE) of values in preparations from six dogs. Asterisks indicate that indomethacin treatment differs significantly from control ($p < 0.05$). R values refer to potency ratio (±95% confidence limits) for control versus indomethacin groups. R values for bethanechol and DMPP do not differ from control.

tudinal muscle strips of human terminal ileum (10). This observation suggests ongoing synthesis and release of a PG-like material which continuously stimulates the longitudinal muscle; inhibition of synthesis by indomethacin would eliminate the stimulus. On strips of circular muscle, indomethacin either initiated or markedly increased spontaneous activity. As PGE_2 was found to inhibit circular muscle and $PGF_{2\alpha}$ was found to stimulate the circular muscle, the effect of indomethacin suggests that a PGE_2-like substance may be responsible in vitro for inhibition of circular muscle contractions. In contrast to other results, one report suggests that indomethacin enhances longitudinal muscle contractile responses to a variety of agonists as a result of its direct effects upon intestinal smooth muscle (11). Other workers, however, have observed specificity of indomethacin effects (8-10). Consistent with other in vitro effects, prostaglandins have been found to increase peristaltic activity in isolated segments of guinea pig intestine (12, 13). Brisk formation of PG-like substance in vitro may be an artifact caused by isolation of gastrointestinal tissues. A study of the effects of aspirin on gastric emptying, duodenal-gastric reflux, and small bowel propulsion in vivo in rats revealed no effect of aspirin on these parameters (14). Prostaglandins themselves certainly affect intestinal contractions in vivo, in laboratory animals and in humans (15). The often dramatic inhibition of contractions of the longitudinal muscle of guinea pig ileum by prostaglandin synthetase inhibitors may imply a direct role of prostaglandins in the release of acetylcholine or other excitatory neurotransmitters (16-19).

GASTRIC ANTISECRETORY ACTIVITY

Following the initial observation by Robert and colleagues in 1967 (20) that PGs inhibited food or histamine-stimulated gastric secretion in dogs, the gastric antisecretory effects of the PGs have been subjects of many reports (1, 21, 22). Natural prostaglandins administered orally exhibit only weak antisecretory actions, presumably because of rapid inactivation by prostaglandin 15-OH-dehydrogenase. Prostaglandin metabolism occurs very rapidly and the resulting compounds possess greatly reduced biological activity. A number of prostaglandin analogs have been prepared with modifications at carbons 15 or 16 to protect against enzymatic degradation by prostaglandin 15-OH-dehydrogenase. The two most widely tested analogs have been 15(S)-methylprostaglandin E_2-methyl ester and 16, 16-dimethylprostaglandin E_2-methyl ester. As summarized in Table 1, these two prostaglandin analogs have been found to inhibit basal or stimulated gastric acid secretion in a variety of species. Interestingly, the PG analogs appear to be more effective as inhibitors of gastric acid secretion after intragastric than after intraintestinal administration (26, 29). Unfortunately, oral or intragastric administration in humans is frequently complicated by serious side effects (24, 26).

TABLE 1 Gastric Antisecretory Studies with Two Synthetic Prostaglandin Analogs

Species	Secretory stimulus	Route of administration	Effective doses	Side effects	Reference
		15(S)-methylprostaglandin E_2-methyl ester			
Rat	None	s.c.	500 μg/kg	None	23
Rat	None	p.o.	250 μg/kg	None	23
Dog	Histamine	i.v.	0.25 μg/kg	None	23
Dog	Histamine	p.o.	5 μg/kg	Emesis	23
Monkey	Histamine	i.v.	3-10 μg/kg	Emesis, diarrhea	24
Human	None	p.o.	25-50 μg	Nausea, borborygmi	25
		16,16-dimethylprostaglandin E_2-methyl ester			
Rat	None	s.c.	75 μg/kg	None	23
Rat	None	p.o.	250 μg/kg	None	23
Dog	Histamine	i.v.	0.1 μg/kg	None	23
Dog	Histamine	p.o.	7.5 μg/kg	Emesis	23
Dog	Histamine	i.v.	0.4 μg/kg/hr	None	26
Human	Pentagastrin	i.v.	12-50 μg	None	27
Human	Pentagastrin	p.o.	25-200 μg	None	27
Human	Meal	p.o.	1.0-1.77 μg/kg	Cramps, diarrhea	28

CYTOPROTECTIVE EFFECTS

In addition to their ability to inhibit gastric acid secretion, many natural and synthetic PGs have been shown to prevent the formation of gastric and duodenal ulcers in animals (30). The antiulcer effects of PGs have usually been attributed to their antisecretory actions. More recently, however, the gastric and intestinal lesions produced in animals by nonsteroidal anti-inflammatory compounds were found to be inhibited by a variety of PGs, some of which have not been shown to inhibit either gastric secretion or development of ulcers (30). As a result of these findings, gastric and intestinal ulceration produced by the nonsteroidal anti-inflammatory compounds has been attributed to a local PG deficiency in mucosal tissues (31). Treatment with PGs, according to this hypothesis, prevents the local deficiency and thus protects the animal against ulceration. Although the precise mechanism of the cytoprotective action of PGs is not clear, they have been shown to protect against ulcers induced by ligation of the pylorus, stress, glucocorticoids, reserpine, 5-hydroxytryptamine, ethanol, hydrochloric acid, sodium hydroxide, sodium chloride, and even boiling water (32)!

The cytoprotective effects of PGs occur at low dosages, which may allow effective therapeutic use without inducing the side effects (nausea, emesis, diarrhea) that often accompany administration of PGs at antisecretory dosages.

ACKNOWLEDGMENT

This work has been supported in part by U.S. Public Health Service Grant DA-02163.

REFERENCES

1. Weeks, J. R. Prostaglandins. Annu. Rev. Pharmacol. Toxicol. 12: 317-336, 1972.
2. Splawinski, J. A., Nies, A. S., Sweetman, B., and Oates, J. A. The effects of arachidonic acid, prostaglandin E_2 and prostaglandin $F_{2\alpha}$ on the longitudinal stomach strip of the rat. J. Pharmacol. Exp. Ther. 187:501-510, 1973.
3. Kowalewski, K., and Kolodej, A. Effect of prostaglandin E_2 on myoelectrical and mechanical activity of totally isolated, ex vivo-perfused, canine stomach. Pharmacology 13:325-339, 1975.
4. Adaikan, P. G., and Karim, S. M. M. Effects of PGA and PGB compounds on gastrointestinal tract smooth muscle from man and laboratory animals. Prostaglandins 11:15-22, 1976.
5. Bennett, A., Eley, K. G., and Scholes, G. B. Effects of prostaglandins E_1 and E_2 on human, guinea-pig and rat isolated small intestine. Br. J. Pharmacol. 34:630-638, 1968.
6. Bennett, A., Eley, K. G., and Stockley, H. L. The effects of prostaglandins on guinea-pig isolated intestine and their possible contribution to muscle activity and tone. Br. J. Pharmacol. 54:197-204, 1975.
7. Burks, T. F. Mediation by 5-hydroxytryptamine of morphine stimulant actions in dog intestine. J. Pharmacol. Exp. Ther. 185:530-539, 1973.
8. Grubb, M. N., and Burks, T. F. Modification of intestinal stimulatory effects of 5-hydroxytryptamine by adrenergic amines, prostaglandin E_1 and theophylline. J. Pharmacol. Exp. Ther. 189:476-483, 1974.
9. Grubb, M. N., and Burks, T. F. Selective antagonism of the intestinal stimulatory effects of morphine by isoproterenol, prostaglandin E_1 and theophylline. J. Pharmacol. Exp. Ther. 193:884-891, 1975.
10. Burleigh, D. E. The effects of indomethacin on the tone and spontaneous activity of the human small intestine in vitro. Arch. Int. Pharmacodyn. Ther. 225:240-245, 1977.
11. Aboulafia, J., Mendes, G. B., Miyamoto, M. E., Paiva, A. C. M., and Paiva, T. B. Effect of indomethacin and prostaglandin on the smooth

muscle contracting activity of angiotensin and other agonists. Br. J. Pharmacol. 58:223-228, 1976.
12. Eley, K. G., Bennett, A., and Stockley, H. L. The effects of prostaglandins E_1, E_2, $F_{1\alpha}$ and $F_{2\alpha}$ on guinea-pig ileal and colonic peristalsis. J. Pharm. Pharmacol. 29:276-280, 1977.
13. Sanger, G. J., and Watt, A. J. The effect of PGE_1 on peristalsis and on perivascular nerve inhibition of peristaltic activity in guinea-pig isolated ileum. J. Pharm. Pharmacol. 30:762-765, 1978.
14. Fenning, B., Johansson, H., Nilsson, F., Ohrn, P. G., and Olazabal, A. Acetylsalicylic acid and gastrointestinal propulsion. Scand. J. Gastroenterol. 12:249-252, 1977.
15. Cummings, J. H., Newman, A., Misiewitz, J. J., Milton-Thompson, G. J., and Billings, J. A. Effect of intravenous prostaglandin $F_{2\alpha}$ on small intestinal function in man. Nature (Lond.) 243:169-171, 1973.
16. Ehrenpreis, S., Greenberg, J., and Comaty, J. E. Block of electrically induced contractions of guinea pig longitudinal muscle by prostaglandin synthetase and receptor inhibitors. Eur. J. Pharmacol. 39: 331-340, 1976.
17. Schulz, R., and Cartwright, C. Sensitization of the smooth muscle by prostaglandin E_1 contributes to reversal of drug-induced inhibition of the guinea-pig ileum. Naunyn-Schmiedeberg's Arch. Pharmacol. 294: 257-260, 1976.
18. Bennett, A., Eley, K. G., and Stockley, H. L. Inhibition of peristalsis in guinea-pig isolated ileum and colon by drugs that block prostaglandin synthesis. Br. J. Pharmacol. 57:335-340, 1976.
19. Willis, A. L., Davison, P., and Ramwell, P. W. Inhibition of intestinal tone, motility and prostaglandin biosynthesis by 5,8,11,14-eicosatetraynoic acid (TYA). Prostaglandins 5:355-368, 1974.
20. Robert, A., Nezamis, J. E., and Phillips, J. P. Inhibition of gastric secretion by prostaglandins. Am. J. Dig. Dis. 12:1073-1076, 1967.
21. Wilson, D. E. Prostaglandins and the gastrointestinal tract. Prostaglandins 1:281-293, 1972.
22. Bass, P. Gastric antisecretory and antiulcer agents. Adv. Drug Res. 8: 205-328, 1974.
23. Robert, A., Schultz, J. R., Nezamis, J. E., and Lancaster, C. Gastric antisecretory and antiulcer properties of PGE_2, 15-methyl PGE_2, and 16,16-dimethyl PGE_2. Gastroenterology 70:359-370, 1976.
24. Dajani, E. Z., and Callison, D. A. Gastric antisecretory actions of (15S)-15-methyl prostaglandin E_2 methyl ester and natural prostaglandin E_2 in rhesus monkeys. Prostaglandins 11: 799-808, 1976.
25. Karim, S. M. M., Carter, D. C., Bhana, D., and Ganesan, P. A. Effect of orally administered prostaglandin E_2 and its 15-methyl analogues on gastric secretion. Br. Med. J. 1:143-146, 1973.
26. Mihas, A. A., Gibson, R. G., and Hirschowitz, B. I. Inhibition of gastric secretion in the dog by 16,16-dimethyl prostaglandin E_2. Am. J. Physiol. 230:351-356, 1976.

27. Karim, S. M. M., Carter, D. C., Bhana, D., and Ganesan, P. A. The effect of orally and intravenously administered prostaglandin 16:16 dimethyl E_2 methyl ester on human gastric acid secretion. Prostaglandins 4:71-83, 1973.
28. Ippoliti, A. F., Isenberg, J. I., Maxwell, V., and Walsh, J. H. The effect of 16,16-dimethyl prostaglandin E_2 on meal-stimulated gastric acid secretion and serum gastrin in duodenal ulcer patients. Gastroenterology 70:488-491, 1976.
29. Nylander, B., Robert, A., and Andersson, S. Gastric secretory inhibition by certain methyl analogs of prostaglandin E_2 following intestinal administration in man. Scand. J. Gastroenterol. 9:759-762, 1974.
30. Robert, A. Antisecretory, antiulcer, cytoprotective and diarrheogenic properties of prostaglandins. Adv. Prostaglandin Thromboxane Res. 2: 507-520, 1976.
31. Robert, A. An intestinal disease produced experimentally by a prostaglandin deficiency. Gastroenterology 69:1045-1047, 1975.
32. Robert, A., Nezamis, J. E., and Lancaster, C. Gastric cytoprotective property of prostaglandins. Gastroenterology 72:1121, 1977.

Part IV
PROSTAGLANDINS AND PATHOPHYSIOLOGIC PROCESSES

14 Prostaglandins and Cerebral Vasospasm

RICHARD P. WHITE / University of Tennessee Center for the Health Sciences, Memphis, Tennessee

CLINICAL CONSIDERATIONS

Cerebral vasospasm commonly occurs in individuals following a subarachnoid hemorrhage (SAH), usually caused by a ruptured aneurysm, and affects as many as two-thirds of such patients (1). The vasospasm may develop immediately after rupture or, more commonly, several days later (1, 2). The spasm is usually limited to the artery hemorrhaged but may spread over the arterial tree and involve other arteries, even contralateral ones. Cerebral vasospasm may also follow head trauma (1-3) and hemorrhage from malformed vessels (1), but this is not common.

Many believe that cerebral vasospasm is a major cause of mortality and morbidity among patients who initially survive rupture of an aneurysm (4). However, some patients may show impaired consciousness and infarct (edema) of cerebral tissue (1, 5, 6) without arteriographic evidence of vasospasm. Conversely, patients may be normal neurologically with vasospasm (1, 5). Moreover, cerebral blood flow may be normal to an area supplied by a spastic artery or reduced in patients without vasospasm (1). Some question, therefore, whether cerebral vasospasm is a clinically significant phenomenon. Nevertheless, cerebral vasospasm is a clinical entity which increases mortality (7) and most investigators have reported that cerebral blood flow falls after subarachnoid hemorrhage, in patients and in laboratory animals. It is certainly abnormal and may be considered one index of a SAH complex that is interrelated. That is, substances responsible for vasospasm may also be responsible for other clinical findings, the symptoms observed depending on concentrations in cerebrospinal fluid (CSF) and the sensitivity of the tissue affected. Responsiveness may vary, in turn, because of hypoxia, inherent tissue differences, synergism of several agents whose rate of

TABLE 1 Possible Relationship Between Clinical Findings in SAH and Known Experimental Actions of Prostaglandins

Clinical findings with references	Experimental findings[a]		References
	Action	Prostaglandin	
Cerebrovasospasm (1,2,8)	Cerebro-vasospasm	E_2, $F_{1\alpha}$, $F_{2\alpha}$	9-11
Fever (8)	Hyperthermia	E_1, E_2	12-14
CNS depression (1,4,8)	Sedation, sleep, stupor	E_1, E_2, E_3	15
Hypertension (8)	Pressor	$F_{2\alpha}$	10
Cerebral edema, hydrocephalus (1,6,8)	Inflammation	E_1, E_2	16,17

[a]All responses listed were elicited by means of central application of the prostaglandins except inflammation, which remains to be determined. However, E and F types are known to be released with trauma of the spinal cord (18). The pressor response was induced by application of $F_{2\alpha}$ into the chiasmatic cistern (10).

synthesis differ, and natural barriers to the offending substance. The sequelae to SAH are complex, but the information available suggests that prostaglandins could contribute to the symptomology: impaired consciousness, hypertension, fever, cerebral edema, and cerebral vasospasm. This relationship is summarized in Table 1. It is possible, therefore, that prostaglandins are associated with all of the clinical manifestations of SAH, but evidence for their involvement in cerebrovasospasm is presently available.

Hypotheses of Vasospasm

The prostaglandin hypothesis of cerebral vasospasm is only one among several (19). None explains why some patients escape and others manifest typical symptoms of SAH, or the high variability in the onset and course of this disease. Most of these hypotheses emphasize the role that blood, particularly platelets, may play in delivering stored spasmogens to the cerebral vessels (catecholamines, serotonin, and platelet spasmogenic factor). In contrast, the prostaglandin hypothesis emphasizes that these vasoactive agents are synthesized by the many tissues (brain, vessels, and blood) in response to various stimuli (11). This synthesis would explain why the most serious symptoms may appear hours or days after hemorrhage, corresponding to a slow increase in CSF levels. This increase would be facilitated by an impediment in CSF flow caused by the clot, particularly at the base of the brain, where most of the forward flow of CSF occurs. Rebleeding would intensify the symptoms and is most commonly associated with mortality among these patients (7).

Finally, prostaglandins may enhance the effects of other vasoactive agents trapped in the blood coagulum and CSF. Following hemorrhage there must be an explosive release of spasmogens from blood. In this regard, experimentally the following pure substances cause vasoconstriction of cerebral vessels: dopamine (20), serotonin (11, 21-24), prostaglandin $F_{2\alpha}$ (11, 22), prostaglandin $F_{1\alpha}$ (11), angiotensin (22), acetylcholine (25), epinephrine (23), norepinephrine (23), bradykinin (23), prostaglandin E_1 (23), prostaglandin A_1 (23), histamine (11, 20, 22, 23), and prostaglandin E_2 (11). Some of these have been tested in vivo (11, 20) but fail as vasoconstrictors (norepinephrine, prostaglandin E_1), whereas others cause constriction (histamine, prostaglandin E_2, serotonin, prostaglandin $F_{2\alpha}$, prostaglandin $F_{1\alpha}$). Also, unknown factors in platelets (26) and in hypothalamic extracts (27) and polypeptide B released during the formation of fibrin (28) may contribute to the genesis of vasospasm. The fact that substances such as histamine dilate cerebral vessels when delivered via the endothelium (21, 29, 30) but cause constriction when applied to isolated cerebral arteries (23) or topically (11, 26) in several species, compounds the problem of identifying the factors responsible. Regardless of the mechanism, the incongruent responses produced by some vasodilator substances (e.g., histamine, bradykinin, and PGE_2) must be considered in any explanation of the genesis of vasospasm.

OVERVIEW OF FINDINGS THAT IMPLICATE PROSTAGLANDINS IN CEREBRAL VASOSPASM

The early reports that $F_{2\alpha}$ constricts and E_1 dilates cerebral vessels suggested that these substances might normally modulate cerebrovascular tone, being responsible for autoregulation (21, 30-32). Moreover, it was conjectured that an excess of $F_{2\alpha}$ may cause vasospasm (21, 32). This appeared reasonable because prostaglandins are synthesized on demand (17, 18), increasing in amounts in response to a variety of stimuli (Table 2). Even careful exposure of the dura can double amounts present in the spinal cord (18).

Pharmacological studies indicate many prostaglandins ($F_{1\alpha}$, $F_{2\alpha}$, E_2) could cause spasm if present in the CSF in pathological concentrations (9-11, 20, 33). They are at least as potent as other putative spasmogens in producing prolonged vasospasm lasting hours by this route (11, 20). They are clearly synthesized ubiquitously in brain tissue, blood, and blood vessels (Table 2). Furthermore, this synthesis is enhanced by a variety of specific blood-borne substances as well as by trauma (Table 2). CSF is a suitable medium for the synthesis of prostaglandins (34), so that following hemorrhage conditions

TABLE 2 Evidence Showing Brain, Spinal Cord, Blood Vessels, and Platelets as Sources of Prostaglandins with Some Known Stimulators of Synthesis

Source with references	PGs identified	Stimulator studied
Brain		
Rat cortical slices, homogenates (38)	E_2, $F_{2\alpha}$	Dopamine, norepinephrine, adrenochrome
Cat and ox homogenates	E, $F_{2\alpha}$	None (39)
Dog ventricles (13)	E_1, E_2, $F_{1\alpha}$, $F_{2\alpha}$	Serotonin
Cat cortex (40,41)	E, F	Electrostimulation (40); strychnine, metrazol, pictrotoxin (41)
Spinal cord (18)	E, F	Trauma
Blood vessels		
Bovine mesenteric (35)	E_2, $F_{2\alpha}$	Bradykinin
Porcine cerebral (42)	E, F	None
Bovine middle cerebral (43)	PG-like	None
Platelets		
In blood (37)	E_2, $F_{2\alpha}$	None
In plasma (37)	E_2, $F_{2\alpha}$	Thrombin
In CSF (34)	$F_{2\alpha}$	None
In plasma (44)	D_2	Thrombin

are favorable for their generation. Finally, levels in CSF generally rise following hemorrhage in patients (Table 4) despite the fact that normally prostaglandins rapidly disappear from the CSF.

Known stimuli for prostaglandin synthesis are obviously numerous. These vary widely in character, from polypeptides to trauma (Table 2). Thus a barrage of stimuli would follow hemorrhage. Moreover, one stimulus can generate many prostaglandins from a single source, as illustrated with thrombin and platelets (Table 2). Each stimulus also increases synthesis at least twofold. Bradykinin increases synthesis in arteries and veins two- to threefold (35), serotonin in brain fourfold (13), and thrombin in platelets several fold (36,37). Similarly, trauma alone increases synthesis more than threefold in the spinal cord (18). Basal synthesis in brain varies fivefold (13), so that the clinical manifestations of SAH may depend on innate individual differences in synthesis. It is possible that the yield of prostaglandins may be enhanced if the stimuli were present in combination and from present evidence hemorrhage should provide such stimuli for prostaglandin synthesis in SAH.

CEREBROVASCULAR EFFECTS OF PROSTAGLANDINS

Prostaglandin $F_{2\alpha}$ and $F_{1\alpha}$

All reports agree that prostaglandin $F_{2\alpha}$ causes vasoconstriction of cerebral arteries in laboratory animals regardless of the species studied or route of administration (Table 3). Because of the paucity of substances that will induce constriction by the intravascular route (29), this prostaglandin was proposed as a spasmogen in the genesis of cerebrovasospasm (21, 31, 32). The vasoconstrictor mechanism is independent of those caused by serotonin or norepinephrine in monkeys (21). Prostaglandin $F_{1\alpha}$ is also a vasoconstrictor agent (Table 3) but is not as potent as $F_{2\alpha}$ (9, 11, 45).

TABLE 3 Prostaglandins and Cerebral Responses[a]

PG	Species	Route	Main target arteries	Constriction	Dilation	None or equivocal
$F_{2\alpha}$	Dog	IC	Brain	(30, 32)		
		ICV	Brain	(49)		
		ChC	Basilar	(10)		
		CM	Basilar	(9, 11, 20)		
		CC	Brain, pial	(50)		
		Bath	Basilar	(23)		
	Cat	IV	Basilar	(48)		
		Top	Basilar	(48, 51)		
		Top	Pial	(45)		
		EC	Pial			(45)
	Mouse	Top	Pial	(52)		
	Monkey	IC	Brain	(21, 53)		
$F_{1\alpha}$	Dog	CM	Basilar	(9, 11, 20)		
	Cat	Top	Pial	(45)		
		EC	Pial			(45)
	Monkey	IC	Brain			(53)

(continued)

TABLE 3 (continued)

PG	Species	Route	Main target arteries	Constriction	Dilation	None or equivocal
E_1	Dog	IC	Brain		(30)	
		CC	Brain, pial	(50)		
		Top	Pial		(54)	
		CM	Basilar			(9, 11)
		Bath	Basilar	(23)		
	Cat	EC	Pial		(45)	
		Top	Pial		(45)	
		IV	Basilar		(48)	
		Top	Basilar	(48)		
	Monkey	IC	Brain			(21, 30, 53)
		CC	Brain, pial	(50, 55)		
	Baboon	IC	Brain		(47)	
	Humans	IC	Brain			(46)
E_2	Dog	CM	Basilar	(9, 11, 33)		
	Cat	Top	Basilar	(48)		
		IV	Basilar		(48)	
A_1	Dog	IC	Brain			(30, 32)
		Bath	Basilar	(23)		
	Cat	Top	Basilar	(48)		
		IV	Basilar		(48)	

[a]Abbreviations: IC, internal carotid; ICV, intracerebroventricular; ChC, chiasmatic cistern; CM, cisterna magna; CC, common carotid; IV, intravenous; Top, topical; EC, external carotid. "Bath" refers to studies of isolated artery in chamber. "Brain" refers to total cerebrovascular tone or flow studies. Numbers in parentheses are references.

Prostaglandin E_1

In contrast to prostaglandin $F_{2\alpha}$, variable effects have been reported for prostaglandin E_1. The ability of E_1 to vasodilate, together with platelet inhibitition, prompted some to suggest that E_1 might be useful as a treatment for cerebrovasospasm (30, 31). Consequently, it was tried in patients without obvious clinical benefit and with equivocal effects on blood flow (46). However, the flow studies were performed approximately 5 min after the termination of an infusion of E_1, at which time some animal studies indicate that vasodilation would have ceased (21,47). In addition, the drug was not deleterious, one patient given the highest dose improved remarkably, and in some vasodilation was documented arteriographically following treatment (46). Final judgment of its precise effect in humans, therefore, awaits further investigation. In general, it appears that vasodilator responses are more likely if this drug is administered intravascularly to animals with intact skulls, whereas craniotomy seems to favor a vasoconstrictor effect (Table 3). Nevertheless, variable effects appear to be characteristic of this compound and in critical concentrations may contribute to the pathophysiology of cerebral vasospasm.

Prostaglandins E_2 and A_1

The cerebrovascular effects of the remaining prostaglandins shown in Table 3 also present an enigma. Prostaglandin E_2 and A_1 given intravenously causes vasodilation of the basilar artery which far outlasts their systemic depressor effect, indicating that this dilation is not simply due to autoregulatory mechanisms (48). However, applied topically to this same artery these induce vasoconstriction (48) and E_2 given intrathecally will generate a vasospasm that lasts for hours (9,11,20). Indeed, it appears that when prostaglandins are applied to the outside surface of the arteries at the base of the brain (whether to isolated vessels, added to CSF or topically), they will induce vasoconstriction (Table 3). These findings suggest that in sufficient CSF concentrations, all prostaglandins might produce cerebrovasospasm at the base of the brain, where the majority of ruptured aneurysms occur in humans. The pial arteries, however, appear to be more selective, constricting with $F_{2\alpha}$ and dilating with E_1 when applied topically (Table 3).

THE INCONGRUENT PRINCIPLE AND CEREBROVASOSPASM

The incongruent effects of prostaglandins must be emphasized when analyzing the role these agents play in cerebrovasospasm. That is, many that cause vasodilation via access to the endothelial surface will cause constriction via the adventitial surface. Conventional studies fail to reveal this phenomenon. Given intravenously or intracarotidly, for example, prostaglandins E_1, E_2, A_1, and A_2 clearly increase blood flow in the common carotid artery and increase CSF pressure indicative of cerebral vasodilation (56). Yet under different conditions or applied topically, these vasodilator prostaglandins will cause constriction (Table 3).

This principle also applies to other vasoactive agents. By all accounts acetylcholine dilates the cerebral vessels of cats when given intravascularly (29). Yet when applied topically to isolated middle cerebral arteries (25) of cats, acetylcholine causes constriction. Opposite effects are also obtained with histamine, dilating cerebral vessels by intravascular injection (21, 29, 30) and constricting when applied topically via the CSF (11), to arteries in isolated baths (23), or to exposed basilar arteries (22). Similarly, vasodilators as isoproterenol and bradykinin by conventional studies cause contraction of isolated cerebral vessels (23, 25). The principle also applies to other vascular beds, such as the spleen (57). It is possible that different receptors are involved when drugs penetrate from the adventitial than from the endothelial surface of blood vessels. Interestingly, the rate of penetration is greater from the adventitia (58). Also, it has been suggested the salt moiety of commercially available drugs might alter an effect (11). However, this would not be the case with prostaglandins (e.g., E_2) (11). Finally, the principle seems to apply only to vasodilators that became constrictors upon topical application. That is, substances such as serotonin and prostaglandin $F_{2\alpha}$ produce constriction of cerebral arteries by any route of application (11, 21). Regardless of the mechanisms involved, evidence for the incongruent principle is sufficient to warrant its consideration as a factor contributing to the pathogenesis of cerebrovascular accidents.

PROLONGED EFFECTS OF PROSTAGLANDINS

Since the symptoms associated with subarachnoid hemorrhage persist for days and even weeks, any substance(s) that might account for these must either be synthesized or produce prolonged effects. The evidence clearly indicates that prostaglandins fulfill both of these criteria. Studies demonstrating synthesis are numerous, but examples of prolonged action are sparse. Apparently, prolonged vascular effects are best observed following topical administration, as would be the case following a subarachnoid hemorrhage. Added to the CSF of dogs, $F_{2\alpha}$, $F_{1\alpha}$, and E_2 generate vasospasm persisting for hours (9-11, 20, 33), yet $F_{2\alpha}$ infused intracarotidly produces cerebral vasoconstriction that persists only for minutes in dogs (30) and monkeys (21). Applications of $F_{2\alpha}$ to the basilar artery of the cat for 5 min causes vasospasm lasting at least 1 hr (59). Similarly, the action of E_1 applied topically on vascular responses evoked by norepinephrine persist for at least 1 hr even with repeated washing of the tissue studied (60). Behaviorally, prostaglandins of the E type produce sedation to stupor in a wide variety of animals (15). Stupor was produced in cats, for example, for 4-24 hr by the administration of 3-20 μg into the lateral ventricle, and sedation was often evident thereafter for 24 hr. E_2 and E_3 had similar effects, although $F_{2\alpha}$ was inactive. The amount of prostaglandin responsible for these prolonged effects could be minute because of the circulation of CSF, diffusion into the parenchyma, and the prolonged time during which catabolism of the substances could occur. Prolonged effects are also noted in the production of fever and symptoms of inflammation caused by E-type prostaglandins (16, 17). The data available, therefore, indicate that specific prostaglandins may account for the different symptoms of subarachnoid hemorrhage (Table 1) and that these symptoms might persist long after prostaglandin synthesis has been terminated.

ELIMINATION OF PROSTAGLANDINS BY THE CSF AND CEREBRAL VASOSPASM

Reports indicate that normally, prostaglandins are removed from the brain by the circulating CSF. Prostaglandin E_1 infused into the hypothalamus is recovered in the CSF (14) and when added to fluid perfusing the ventricular system is recovered from the cisterna magna (13). Hence the brain does not normally absorb prostaglandins significantly, so that the CSF must provide an egress for these substances. Evidently, the choroid plexus is one tissue that removes prostaglandins from CSF (61-63), and presumably the arachnoid villi and large cerebral veins could do likewise (64). Regardless of the mechanism, normally the disappearance of prostaglandin from CSF is rapid. When mixed in 2 ml of CSF and injected into the cisterna magna, 200 μg of tritiated $F_{2\alpha}$ (containing 1 μCi) has a half-life of 8 min (A. A. Hagen, J. T. Robertson, and R. P. White, unpublished findings). When mixed with blood prior to injection, concentrations detected in CSF are less, presumably because of binding with blood elements. The fact that radioactive material is present in external jugular blood after these cisternal injections clearly indicates that prostaglandins in CSF may eventually rely on the systemic circulation for final removal. This rapid elimination would appear essential, for the best data available indicate that the cortical surface of the brain normally produces 1.2 ng/cm^2 per min of prostaglandins (40), that 1 g of cat brain produces about 496 (400-677) ng (65), that 1 g of porcine cerebral arteries produces about 198 (160-250) ng (42), and that 1 g of bovine middle cerebral artery produces about 220 ng (43) in 1 hr of incubation. Without this removal by circulation the CSF might become a cesspool for prostaglandins (Table 4). From the data available it is possible to estimate that far less than 33 ng/ml of one prostaglandin is sufficient to cause spasm for hours. Hence a total of 730 ng in 2 ml of CSF (1×10^{-6} M) injected intracisternally (11, 20) may diffuse throughout the CSF of approximately 20 ml (64) in dogs. Since prostaglandins rapidly egress from the CSF, this exogenous concentration should be further reduced within minutes after the injection. Blood, on the other hand, generates prostaglandins when given intracisternally, reaching levels of 63 ng/ml (66). Originally, these substances were given intracisternally to establish which would be spasmogenic by this route (9, 11, 20) and how they compare dose-wise with other putative cerebrovascular spasmogens (11, 20). The results show they are very potent compounds which can cause prolonged vascular effects in CSF. In this respect, the original concentration injection (e.g., 1×10^{-6} M) is of little moment. This is not the concentration in CSF responsible for the effect as some suggest, nor is the concentration found in lumbar or ventricular fluid proof of concentration at the site of production, as some imply. In this regard,

TABLE 4 Some Average Concentrations of Prostaglandins in CSF of Patients[a]

References	Method	Normal amount/ml	Condition	Number of patients	Amount/ml $F_{2\alpha}$	Amount/ml E_2
67	RID	NA	Disc hernia	20 (LP)	8 ng	2 ng
			Hypopituitism	1 (LP)	1 ng	20 ng
			Lumbar sprain	1 (LP)	12 ng	Trace
			Cerebral infarct	5 (LP)	14 ng	11 ng
			Cerebral hemorrhage	4 (LP)	14 ng	12 ng
68	RIA	38 pg	Brain damage	6 (LP)	196 pg	NA
			SAH	4 (LP)	406 pg	NA
			Aneurysmal SAH	8 (LP)	666 pg (> 50-1300)	NA
			Aneurysmal SAH	1 (C)	1120 pg	NA
69	GC/MS	72 pg (30-139)	Epilepsy	11 (LP)	559 pg (124-1230)	NA
			Postoperative	5 (LP)	1195 pg	NA
			Meningo-encephalitis	5 (LP)	954 pg	NA
			Aneurysmal SAH	1 (V)	720 pg	NA
			SAH	2 (LP)	1118 pg	NA
70,71	GC/MS	$\geq$79 pg	Aneurysmal SAH	11 (LP)	1979 pg (> 100-7500)	NA

[a]Abbreviations: NA, not available; RID, radioisotope dilution; RIA, radioimmunoassay; GC/MS, gas column-mass spectrometry; (LP), lumbar spinal fluid; (V), ventricle fluid, (C), cisternal fluid. Numbers in parentheses show range associated with preceding average.

procaine injected intrathecally in the lumbar region was not detectable at the cervical level, although the metabolite is present in blood and dyes injected intraventricularly may not reach the lumbar area (64). Therefore, the interaction of blood with intracranial tissue (Tables 2 and 4) could provide the milieu for high local concentrations not evident by sampling CSF from distant sites.

ROLE OF BLOOD IN CEREBROVASOSPASM

Some investigators have considered blood to be an agent for delivering a single spasmogen to the central vessels. The fact that vasospasm is most commonly seen clinically several days after hemorrhage (1, 2, 8) indicates it does more. It is a source for many spasmogens which can generate vasospasm experimentally (11, 72). These may account for the observation that experimentally introducing blood intrathecally will induce an immediate spasm. However, this spasm commonly lyses within 90 min but returns later (11, 73–76). This delayed spasm may be more related to the clinical situation. In chronic experiments (77) this delayed spasm did differ from the early findings in that solutions of saline or phenoxybenzamine given intracisternally relieves temporarily vasospasm of the basilar artery initially but fails to do so the day after (S. P. Huang and R. P. White, unpublished findings). Possible relationships of blood and prostaglandins may involve at least the following: blood is a source of many spasmogens, including prostaglandins which may interact; it synthesizes prostaglandins, which could accumulate with time; it provides stimulators of synthesis (Table 2); it impedes CSF flow and removal of prostaglandins; and it envelops vessels for the entrapment of spasmogens (78). This entrapment accounts for the fact that vasospasm is most commonly associated with the hemorrhaged vessel; is most commonly seen at the base of the brain (75), where CSF flow would most likely be affected (64); and explains why an intrathecal wash fails to relieve spasm in areas where the coagulum is marked (79). In addition, blood would release thrombin adhering to fibrin during fibrinolysis. This thrombin apparently stimulates synthesis in a variety of tissues—platelets (Table 2), fibroblasts (80), and brain tissue (81)—and may account for the delayed spasm phenomenon. Blood destroys intracranial sympathetic nerve fibers (82), which may in turn change the sensitivity of the vessels to spasmogens. In this regard, blood still induces spasm in such animals (82) and sympathectomy increases the vasoactivity of cerebral vessels to $F_{2\alpha}$ (19). Blood releases polypeptides, which can enhance smooth muscle effects of autacoids (28). Certainly, the contributions of blood elements in the genesis of vasospasm require more careful study (78), but the evidence available to date supports the hypothesis that one contribution is that of enhancing the production and levels of prostaglandins at sites of injury.

SPECIAL BIOCHEMICAL ASPECTS OF VASOSPASM

New information concerning the actions and biochemistry of prostaglandins appears consonant with the prostaglandin hypothesis of vasospasm. These substances apparently effect contraction of smooth muscle by facilitating the influx or inhibiting efflux of calcium (65, 83, 84). Calcium also stimulates cyclase activity, which in turn can modify metabolism of prostaglandins. One can serve as a precursor for another (e.g., E_2 to $F_{2\alpha}$ via 9-ketoreductase) whose conversion is accelerated by cyclic GMP (85), reactions that are reversible. Prostaglandins may even serve as substrates for endoperoxides, the common precursor of both thromboxanes and prostaglandins (86), so that a vicious cycle could be established in pathophysiological conditions. Such findings may explain some of the aforementioned long-term effects of prostaglandins. Moreover, as the number of known stimulators of synthetase increases, many of which are present in blood and brain (Table 2), it becomes more likely that prostaglandin synthesis must occur at the site of hemorrhage and even distant ones. Recently, stimulators have been described which, in contrast to most, increase the rate of formation of prostaglandins as a linear function of time. These stimulators vary in nature from norepinephrine on brain homogenates (38) to serum on fibroblasts (80) and illustrate the importance of considering the types of stimulators that might contribute to the pathogenesis of cerebrovasospasm. Each stimulator may differ in its contribution to this synthesis, with norepinephrine serving as a hydrogen donor (38) as an example. Finally, there are families of enzymes that synthesize prostaglandins and some of these respond to only certain agents; for instance, bradykinin stimulates blood vessels (35) but not brain (38). Conversely, some synthetase enzymes are inhibited preferentially by certain agents (87). Indeed, some inhibitors even inhibit the synthesis of one prostaglandin by brain more than another (38), and the same tissues from different species show different sensitivity to inhibitors (88). Such new knowledge helps explain the complex of symptoms observed in patients following subarachnoid hemorrhage and why the management of these patients has been generally unsuccessful. Concerning the latter, several synthetase inhibitors may be required for prevention or control of the symptoms in view of the large number of stimulators and variety of prostaglandin synthetases. In this regard, the number of known inhibitors increase yearly and include some psychotropic agents (88), so that an effective combination of drugs of low toxicity may ultimately be found. On the other hand, until a rapid procedure is developed for determining total prostaglandin in biological fluid, it is difficult to screen for potential agents to prevent and treat symptoms of subarachnoid hemorrhage in patients. Any one of 18 prostaglandins may be responsible for the subarachnoid complex, and studying one or two, as is now done, only samples what must transpire.

CRITIQUE OF HYPOTHESIS

Many arguments advanced for the prostaglandin hypothesis of cerebral vasospasm could also apply to other spasmogens: incongruent effects; local synthesis of spasmogens alone or in combination could cause fever, edema, and other features of subarachnoid hemorrhage. The hypothesis does not explain why reserpinization of dogs will prevent the development of an experimentally induced vasospasm (19,89), or why patients with subarachnoid hemorrhage reportedly benefit from prolonged intravenous infusions of lidocaine and isoproterenol (90). Moreover, indomethacin in doses (20 mg/kg) sufficient to cause bleeding from surgical sites in anesthetized dogs, and which should inhibit prostaglandin synthesis by platelets (16), blood vessels (35), and very likely brain, fails to prevent the production of vasospasm (11). Finally, the hypothesis is not compatible with the findings that CSF levels of prostaglandins are not well correlated with the symptoms patients manifest (Table 4).

NEEDED RESEARCH

More Sensitive Methods and Drug Effects

The greatest need for the advancement of exploratory studies on the role prostaglandins may play in the genesis of the subarachnoid hemorrhage complex is a rapid sensitive method for determining total prostaglandin content in biological fluids. Hopefully, this method would also register the total content of related substances: thromboxanes and endoperoxides. At present one or two prostaglandins are measured at great expense, long after treatment or trauma, and the sample for analysis is taken at an arbitrary time. Also, relatively large amounts of CSF are collected and concentrated to fit the sensitivity of the method. A rapid, sensitive method for total prostaglandins would enable investigators to ascertain moment-to-moment changes in prostoglandin content and to correlate readily drug effects and pathology to these changes. This is particularly important in exploratory studies of pathophysiological conditions because total content is almost certain to rise if prostaglandins participate, and this knowledge would avoid the mistake of dismissing such participation if determinations of one correlated poorly with the pathology. In brief, it would enable the investigator to look for other prostaglandins if total content rose but a particular one did not. In this regard, Aizawa and Yamada (67) clearly showed that CSF $F_{2\alpha}$ and E_2 levels vary independently in patients of similar diagnostic categories (Table 4). Also, one can be converted to others. Low values for one, therefore, would not prove that prostaglandins, as a group, are not involved in the condition studied. Perhaps all prostaglandins are involved, whose values might fluctuate independently with time. With present methods knowledge grows slowly: for years it has been known that platelets synthesize E_2 and $F_{2\alpha}$; recently, D_2 has been added to this list (44). Also, it was recently shown that reserpine and chlorpromazine inhibit the synthesis of prostaglandins in seminal vesicles and conjectured to do so in brain (88). If so, perhaps this effect of reserpine, together with its ability to inhibit prostaglandin penetration into cells (91) and to inhibit the potentiated responses among $F_{2\alpha}$, serotonin, and angiotensin (92), may account for its prophylaxis in cerebral vasospasm. Indeed, reserpine has multifarious pharmacologic actions that may affect vasospasm (11). Perhaps the benefit derived from the antifibrinogenic ϵ-aminocaproic acid in such patients (7) may prove to be related to effects on prostaglandin levels. Numerous drugs may modify prostaglandin synthesis and activity, but with present methods it could take years to reveal these relationships. A rapid, sensitive method for determining total content would permit the rapid screening for effective drugs and facilitate the monitoring of clinical progress of patients suffering from subarachnoid hemorrhage.

Relationship Between Synthetase Stimulators and Inhibitors

The effectiveness of prostaglandin synthetase inhibitors varies greatly and depends upon the tissue as well as the drug studied (87, 88). Another variable, which at present is unknown, is how well these inhibitors work in the presence of multiple stimulators of prostaglandin synthesis. In SAH a plethora of potential stimulators are released and may explain why a single inhibitor failed to prevent the appearance of vasospasm (11). A similar situation may prevail in asthma, where indomethacin failed to modify the symptoms (93) and other clinical entities. Some stimulators may be more effective than others in antagonizing inhibitors; in combination they may enhance this antagonism. Information as to such relationships would help define the magnitude of the problem associated with the management of the subarachnoid hemorrhage complex and perhaps yield clues in the design of better inhibitors and the mechanism by which stimulators activate the synthetase system. Concerning the latter, it appears that each system is selectively sensitive to a particular stimulator; e.g., norepinephrine stimulates isolated brain tissue (38) but fails to increase CSF levels of prostaglandins, whereas serotonin does when given intracisternally (13). Thus in combating the symptoms of subarachnoid hemorrhage, controlling the mechanism by which stimulators increase prostaglandin synthesis could be more important than attempts to inhibit multiple synthetase system.

Search for Prostaglandin Antagonists

There are scattered reports of substances blocking the effects of prostaglandins. Meclofenamic acid is one such substance (94) which is also a synthetase inhibitor. Polyphloretin phosphate (PPP) is another reported to inhibit some prostaglandins directly and was proposed as being potentially useful in the treatment of vasospasm because it changed the pressor effect of $F_{2\alpha}$ into a depressor effect and prolonged the vasodilator actions of other prostaglandins (95). However, exploratory studies indicate neither of these substances given intravenously 30 min prior to hemorrhage will prevent cerebral vasospasm (R. P. White, A. A. Hagen, H. Morgan, and J. T. Robertson, unpublished findings). Compounds of diverse structure, such as phenoxybenzamine (96) and dibutyryl cyclic AMP (59), appear to inhibit physiologically the vasoconstriction of cerebral arteries induced by prostaglandin $F_{2\alpha}$. Whether such findings bear on the pathphysiological processes described here awaits discovery. Regardless, if the mechanism by which prostaglandins in CSF initiate vasospasm were elucidated, antagonists to this response might be efficacious in lysing vasospasm.

Relationship Between Cerebrovascular Effects of Prostaglandins and Other Putative Spasmogens

The prostaglandins produce effects by acting on specific receptors and also by modifying responses induced by a wide variety of vasoactive agents (78). Although much is known about these interrelationships on extracranial smooth muscle, little is known concerning the interactions between prostaglandins and other spasmogens on cerebral vessels. In one study, $F_{2\alpha}$ when applied topically to the pial vessels of mice in combination with serotonin or norepinephrine produced a simple additive effect (52). On extracerebral vessels the vasoconstriction caused by these biogenic amines and angiotensin were potentiated by $F_{2\alpha}$ (92). It is likely, therefore, that prostaglandins act in concert with other spasmogens in the genesis of cerebrovasospasm. Studies to establish this point are needed and might help avoid a prolonged search for a single spasmogen (including a single prostaglandin) to account for this phenomenon.

Systematic Clinical Studies

The problems inherent in attempts to correlate the symptoms of subarachnoid hemorrhage with prostaglandins are enormous. Some of these have been mentioned: the large volume of CSF required, restrictions imposed by the detection of only one or two prostaglandins, and the lack of moment-to-moment analysis. The patient's clinical history is also presented, by necessity, simplistically in the literature. For one thing, patients are administered numerous drugs. Some of these, given in various combinations for arteriography and successful therapy during hospitalization of four patients, are pentobarbital, atropine, codeine, meperidine, hydroxyzine, hypaque, phenytoin, acetaminophen, aspirin, ϵ-aminocaproic acid, acetophenetidin, diazepam, chlordiazepoxide, propoxyphene, thiethylperazine, methyl predmisolone, dexamethosone, pentazocine, ampicillin, cephalothin, bacitracin, gentamicine, vitamin B_{12}, iron, multiple vitamins, electrolytes, laxatives, premarin, and oxygen. However, reports fail to disclose such details, although several experimental drugs may be mentioned, or that a common treatment for such patients is spinal drainage. It is not possible, therefore, to assess precisely what factors may attend the success or failure of treatment. Many procedures may affect CSF production, pH, and other factors, which in turn might alter prostaglandin synthesis and CSF levels throughout the neuraxis. As previously stated, prostaglandins have prolonged actions locally which cannot be judged by CSF levels generally. However, from the clinical data available (Table 4), such levels may be expected to fluctuate, and these fluctuations may have predictive value if a rigorous history were taken throughout the course of illness. This involves the cooperation of many professionals and was tried in one very limited study with suggestive results (70). Such studies would be obviously enhanced by more sensitive, less expensive methods for determining prostaglandins.

Chronic Animal Experiments

These experiments would facilitate the determination of drug effects and better define the role prostaglandins play in the genesis of cerebral vasospasm. For this purpose, multiple cannulae could be implanted so that samples of CSF may be obtained throughout the observation period, an invasive technique not possible in humans. As important, neurological assessment of the animal, arteriography, and other evaluations should be conducted before and after the injection of blood into the subarachnoid space to produce experimentally the signs and symptoms of subarachnoid hemorrhage. Many have demonstrated experimentally that the introduction of blood intrathecally will produce chronic spasm (2, 3, 73-75) but to date all completed drug studies have been conducted in acute experiments. Only one used an indwelling (subarachnoid) cannula (75) through which blood and/or saline was given. In this experiment it was reported that the widespread spasm induced by blood was relieved by saline irrigation, a result interpreted by others to mean that the spasm was caused by spasmogens (11). Such experiments illustrate the advantage of using multiple indwelling cannulae: samples of CSF may be obtained from various parts of the subarachnoid space for analysis, substances may be injected to ascertain whether they produce effects similar to the clinical features of subarachnoid hemorrhage, and injected to answer questions that may be theoretically and clinically important. Concerning the latter, it appears that saline would be an excellent irrigant during neurosurgery and that solutions of thrombin should be avoided because saline dilates (75) and thrombin constricts (11) cerebral vessels. Such experiments may also reveal the nature of the "biphasic" phenomenon of vasospasm, i.e., the common report that the spasm observed initially lessens or disappears within several hours only to return again the following day (73-76). Hence experiments designed to study the initial spasm may fail to bear on the delayed spasm, the latter being more likely related to the clinical situation. The initial spasm could be due largely to blood-borne substances, the delayed mainly to prostaglandin synthesis. If so, synthetase inhibitors may have little effect initially, which is certainly the case with indomethacin (11). Also, the report that irrigation of the cisterna magna with solutions of phenoxybenzamine relieves spasm in acute experiments in dogs (79) has been extended to include more chronic experiments. The findings indicate that solutions of either phenoxybenzamine or saline (infused at 0.4 ml/min) reverses the initial spasm but fails in the same dog manifesting spasm the next day (S. P. Huang and R. P. White, unpublished findings). It is apparent, therefore, that chronic experimentation is necessary if the nature of the phenomenon of cerebral vasospasm is to be understood (77).

CONCLUSION

The prostaglandin hypothesis of cerebral vasospasm is based on a plethora of data acquired within the past six years. Subarachnoid blood, which initiates this spasm experimentally and clinically, is known to contain serotonin, thrombin, and other stimulators of prostaglandin synthesis. The three main tissues associated with the site of hemorrhage are known to synthesize prostaglandins: blood, cerebral blood vessels, and ubiquitously, brain. The coagulum formed should impede the flow of CSF which is normally necessary for the local egress of prostaglandins. Because local elimination is reduced and synthesis is increased, prostaglandins should rise to pathophysiological levels within the subarachnoid space and generate the symptoms of subarachnoid hemorrhage. That CSF levels do rise is supported by clinical and experimental observations. That they could produce the symptoms has been shown experimentally.

By any standard, prostaglandins must be considered as spasmogens in the genesis of cerebral vasospasm. In minute amounts they produce spasm of long duration. The outstanding pharmacodynamic effect of prostaglandins on cerebral arteries when given topically, in CSF, and via isolated baths is vasoconstriction. These include prostaglandins of the E type, which by an intravascular route cause vasodilation but paradoxically produce cerebrovasospasm otherwise. Prostaglandins also act in concert with other vasoconstrictors, so that subarachnoid hemorrhage should convert the areas of hemorrhage into spasmogen factories.

The ultimate worth of this or other hypotheses of vasospasm requires further observation. At present, correlations between reported levels of prostaglandins and the symptoms manifested by patients are tenuous. This relationship should be strengthened if methods were available for readily detecting all prostaglandins in biological fluids and by in-depth studies of patients. Rational therapy may ultimately depend on new knowledge concerning the mechanism by which different stimulators act on many different synthetase systems, interact with inhibitors of these systems, and are influenced by numerous drugs. Nevertheless, the available data clearly indicate that prostaglandins must contribute to the pathogenesis of subarachnoid hemorrhage.

ADDENDUM

A recent study (97) demonstrated chemically that bovine cerebral arteries synthesize $PGF_{2\alpha}$, PGE_2, PGD_2, TxB_2, and 6-keto-$PGF_{1\alpha}$ (the metabolite of PGI_2). All of these substances in sufficient concentrations will cause constriction of cerebral arteries in vivo (98) and in vitro (99). However, PGI_2 (prostacyclin) is the only known prostaglandin which relaxes isolated cerebral arteries in low concentrations and may therefore exert this effect physiologically (99, 100). Since PGI_2 is synthesized mainly by the endothelium (101), this source of PGI_2 would be damaged in cerebral hemorrhage and its deficiency might contribute to cerebral vasospasm (100). The fact that certain long-acting inhibitors of prostaglandin synthesis significantly reduced the incidence and magnitude of an experimentally induced cerebral vasospasm (102) suggests that such drugs may have value in treating this vasospasm clinically. Moreover, several inhibitors of PG synthesis, but not aspirin, will also prevent the usual contractions induced in isolated cerebral arteries by serotonin, $PGF_{2\alpha}$, and arachidonic acid (103, 104), further indicating that some nonsteroidal anti-inflammatory agents directly modify contractile mechanisms.

REFERENCES

1. Martins, A. N., and Wiley, J. K. Cerebral vasospasm: a review. Mil. Med. 141:482-485, 1974.
2. Arutiunov, A. I., Baron, M. A., and Majorova, N. A. Experimental and clinical study of the development of spasm of the cerebral arteries related to subarachnoid hemorrhage. J. Neurosurg. 32:617-625, 1970.
3. Wilkins, R. H., and Odom, G. L. Intracranial arterial spasm associated with craniocerebral trauma. J. Neurosurg. 32:626-633, 1970.
4. Echlin, F. A. Current concepts in the etiology and treatment of vasospasm. Clin. Neurosurg. 15:133-159, 1968.
5. Millikan, C. H. Cerebral vasospasm and ruptured intracranial aneurysm. Arch. Neurol. 32:433-449, 1975.
6. Nornes, H. Monitoring of patients with intracranial aneurysms. Clin. Neurosurg. 22:321-331, 1975.
7. Nibbelink, D. W., Torner, J. C., and Henderson, W. G. Intracranial aneurysm and subarachnoid hemorrhage: a cooperative study. Antifibrinolytic therapy in recent onset subarachnoid hemorrhage. Stroke 6:622-629, 1975.
8. Van Der Werf, A. J. M. Clinical aspects of subarachnoid hemorrhage and significance of vasospasm. Psychiatr. Neurol. Neurochir. 75: 411-415, 1972.
9. Morgan, H., White, R. P., Pennink, M., and Robertson, J. T. Prostaglandins and experimental cerebral vasospasm. Surg. Forum 23:447-448, 1972.
10. Pennink, M., White, R. P., Crockarell, J. R., and Robertson, J. T. Role of prostaglandin $F_{2\alpha}$ in the genesis of experimental cerebral vasospasm. Angiographic study in dogs. J. Neurosurg. 37:398-406, 1972.
11. White, R. P., Hagen, A. A., Morgan, H., Dawson, W. N., and Robertson, J. T. Experimental study on the genesis of cerebral vasospasm. Stroke 6:52-57, 1975.
12. Feldberg, W. Fever, prostaglandins, and antipyretics. In Prostaglandin Synthetase Inhibitors, H. J. Robinson and J. R. Vane (Eds.). Raven Press, New York, pp. 197-203, 1974.
13. Holmes, S. W. The spontaneous release of prostaglandins into the cerebral ventricles of the dog and the effect of external factors on this release. Br. J. Pharmacol. 38:653-658, 1970.
14. Veale, W. L., and Cooper, K. E. Prostaglandin in cerebrospinal fluid

following perfusion of hypothalamic tissue. J. Appl. Physiol. 37:942-945, 1974.

15. Horton, E. W. Prostaglandins: Monographs on Endocrinology, F. Gross, A. Labhart, T. Mann, L. T. Samuels, and J. Zander (Eds.). Springer-Verlag, New York, pp. 117-149, 1972.
16. Vane, J. R. Mode of action of aspirin and similar compounds. In Prostaglandin Synthetase Inhibitors, H. J. Robinson and J. R. Vane (Eds.). Raven Press, New York, pp. 155-163, 1974.
17. Vane, J. R. Prostaglandins as mediators of inflammation. Adv. Prostaglandin Thromboxane Res. 2:791-801, 1974.
18. Jonsson, H. T., and Daniell, H. B. Altered levels of PGF in cat spinal cord tissue following traumatic injury. Prostaglandins 11:51-61, 1976.
19. Robertson, J. T. Cerebral arterial spasm: current concepts. Clin. Neurosurg. 21:100-106, 1975.
20. White, R. P., Hagen, A. A., and Robertson, J. T. Experimental evaluation of the spasmogenicity of dopamine on the basilar artery. J. Neurosurg. 44:45-49, 1976.
21. White, R. P., Heaton, J. A., and Denton, I. C. Pharmacological comparison of prostaglandin $F_{2\alpha}$, serotonin and norepinephrine on cerebrovascular tone of monkey. Eur. J. Pharmacol. 15:300-309, 1971.
22. Kapp, J., Mahaley, M. S., and Odom, G. L. Cerebral arterial spasm: Part 2. Experimental evaluation of mechanical and humoral factors in pathogenesis. J. Neurosurg. 29:339-349, 1968.
23. Allen, G. S., Henderson, L. M., Chou, S. N., and French, L. A. Cerebral arterial spasm: Part 1. In vitro contractile activity of vasoactive agents on canine basilar and middle cerebral arteries. J. Neurosurg. 40:433-441, 1974.
24. Raynor, R. B., and McMurty, J. G. Prevention of serotonin-produced cerebral vasospasm. J. Neurosurg. 20:94-96, 1963.
25. Nielsen, K. C., and Owman, C. Contractile response and amine receptor mechanisms in isolated middle cerebral artery of the cat. Brain Res. 27:33-42, 1971.
26. Kapp, J., Mahaley, M. S., and Odom, G. L. Cerebral arterial spasm: Part 3. Partial purification and characterization of a spasmogenic substance in feline platelets. J. Neurosurg. 29:350-356, 1968.
27. Wilson, J. L., and Feild, J. R. The production of intracranial vascular spasm by hypothalamic extract. J. Neurosurg. 40:473-479, 1974.
28. Osbahr, A. J., Gladner, J. A., and Laki, K. Studies on the physiological activity of the peptide released during the fibrinogen-fibrin conversion. Biochim. Biophys. Acta 86:535-542, 1964.
29. Sokoloff, L. The action of drugs on the cerebral circulation. Pharmacol. Rev. 11:1-85, 1959.
30. Denton, I. C., White, R. P., and Robertson, J. T. The effects of prostaglandins E_1, A_1 and $F_{2\alpha}$ on the cerebral circulation of dogs and monkeys. J. Neurosurg. 36:34-42, 1972.

31. Denton, I. C., White, R. P., and Robertson, J. T. Effects of some prostaglandins on cerebral circulation in dogs. Program abstr., 38th Ann. Meet. Am. Assoc. Neurol. Surg., Washington, D.C., April, 1970.

32. White, R. P., Denton, I. C., and Robertson, J. T. Differential effects of prostaglandins A_1, E_1, and $F_{2\alpha}$ on the cerebrovascular tone in dogs and rhesus monkeys. Fed. Proc. 30:625, 1971 (abstr.).

33. Morgan, H., White, R. P., Pennink, M., and Robertson, J. T. Prostaglandin activity in canine experimental cerebral vasospasm: an angiographic study. In Subarachnoid Hemorrhage and Cerebrovascular Spasm, R. R. Smith and J. T. Robertson (Eds.). Charles C. Thomas, Springfield, Ill., pp. 55-62, 1975.

34. Hagen, A. A., Sweeley, C. C., White, R. P., and Robertson, J. T. Prostaglandin $F_{2\alpha}$ levels in dog cerebral spinal fluid in the presence of blood or platelets. Pharmacologist 16:197, 1974 (abstr.).

35. Terragno, D. A., Crowshaw, K., Terragno, N. A., and McGiff, J. C. Prostaglandin synthesis by bovine mesenteric arteries and veins. Circ. Res. 36/37(Suppl. I):76-80, 1975.

36. Smith, J. B., and Willis, A. L. Formation and release of prostaglandins in response to thrombin. Br. J. Pharmacol. 40:545, 1970 (abstr.).

37. Silver, M. J., Smith, J. B., Ingerman, C., and Kocsis, J. J. Human blood prostaglandins: formation during clotting. Prostaglandins 1:429-436, 1972.

38. Wolfe, L. S., Pappius, H. M., and Marion, J. The biosynthesis of prostaglandins by brain in vitro. Adv. Prostaglandin Thromboxane Res. 1:345-355, 1976.

39. Coceani, F., Dreifuss, J. J., Puglisi, L., and Wolfe, L. S. Prostaglandins and membrane function. In Prostaglandins, Peptides and Amines, P. Mantegazza and E. W. Horton (Eds.). Academic Press, New York, pp. 73-84, 1969.

40. Bradley, P. B., Samuels, G. M. R., and Shaw, J. E. Correlation of prostaglandin release from the cerebral cortex and cats with the electrocorticogram, following stimulation of the reticular formation. Br. J. Pharmacol. 37:151-157, 1969.

41. Ramwell, P. W., and Shaw, J. E. Spontaneous and evoked release of prostaglandins from cerebral cortex of anesthetized cats. Am. J. Physiol. 211:125-134, 1966.

42. White, R. P., Terragno, D. A., Terragno, N. A., Hagen, A. A., and Robertson, J. T. Prostaglandins in porcine cerebral arteries. Stroke 8:135, 1977 (abstr.).

43. Pickard, J. D., Vinall, P. E., and Simeone, F. A. Prostaglandins and cerebral vasospasm: a problem of interpretation. Surg. Forum 26:496-498, 1975.

44. Oelez, O., Oelez, R., Knapp, H. R., Jr., Sweetman, B. J., Wilcox, H. G., Oates, J. A. Prostaglandin D_2 is formed by human platelets. Fed. Proc. 35:297, 1976 (abstr.).

45. Welch, K. M. A., Knowles, L., and Spira, P. Local effect of prostaglandins on cat pial arteries. Eur. J. Pharmacol. 25:155-158, 1974.
46. Steiner, L., Forster, D. M. C., Bergval, V., and Carlson, L. A. Effects of prostaglandin E_1 on cerebral circulatory disturbances following subarachnoid haemorrhage in man. Neuroradiology 4:20-24, 1972.
47. Pelofsky, S., Jacobson, E. D., and Fisher, R. G. Effects of prostaglandin E_1 on experimental cerebral vasospasm. J. Neurosurg. 36:634-639, 1972.
48. Handa, J., Yoneda, S., Matsuda, M., and Handa, H. Effects of prostaglandins A_1, E_1, E_2, and $F_{2\alpha}$ on the basilar artery of cats. Surg. Neurol. 2:251-255, 1974.
49. Emerson, T. E., Jr., Radawski, D., Veenendaal, M., and Daugherty, R. M., Jr. Effects of cerebral ventricular, systemic, and local administration of prostaglandin $F_{2\alpha}$ on canine cerebral hemodynamics. Prostaglandins 8:523-530, 1974.
50. Yamamoto, Y. L., Feindel, W., Wolfe, L. S., Katoh, H., and Hodge, C. P. Experimental vasoconstriction of cerebral arteries by prostaglandins. J. Neurosurg. 37:385-397, 1972.
51. Kapp, J. P., Robertson, J. T., and White, R. P. Spasmogenic qualities of prostaglandin $F_{2\alpha}$ in the cat. J. Neurosurg. 44:173-175, 1976.
52. Rosenblum, W. I. Constriction of pial arterioles produced by prostaglandin $F_{2\alpha}$. Stroke 6:293-297, 1975.
53. Welch, K. M. A., Spira, P. J., Knowles, L., and Lance, J. W. Effects of prostaglandins on the internal and external carotid flow in the monkey. Neurology 24:705-710, 1974.
54. Spira, P. J., Misbach, J., and Welch, K. M. A. Pial artery response to prostaglandin E_1 in the dog. Proc. Aust. Soc. Clin. Exp. Pharmacol., November 1973.
55. Yamamoto, Y. L., Feindel, W., Wolfe, L. S., and Hodge, C. P. Prostaglandin induced vasoconstriction of cerebral arteries and its reversal by ethanol. Adv. Biosci. 9:359-366, 1973.
56. Nakano, J., Chang, A. C., and Fisher, R. G. Effects of prostaglandins E_1, E_2, A_1, A_2, and $F_{2\alpha}$ on canine carotid arterial blood flow, cerebrospinal fluid pressure, and intraocular pressure. J. Neurosurg. 38:32-39, 1973.
57. Davies, B. N., and Withrington, P. G. The actions of drugs on the smooth muscle of the capsule and blood vessels of the spleen. Pharmacol. Rev. 25:373-413, 1973.
58. Török, J., and Bevan, J. A. Entry of ^{3}H-norepinephrine into the arterial wall. J. Pharmacol. Exp. Ther. 177:613-620, 1971.
59. Peterson, E. W., Leblanc, R., and Lebel, F. Cyclic Adenosine Monophosphate antagonism of prostaglandin induced vasospasm. Surg. Neurol. 4:490-496, 1975.
60. Siggins, G. R. Prostaglandins and the microvascular system: physiological and histochemical correlations. In Prostaglandins in Cellular

Biology, P. W. Ramwell and B. B. Pharriss (Eds.). Plenum Press, New York, pp. 451–476, 1972.
61. Bito, L. Z. Accumulation and apparent active transport of prostaglandins by some rabbit tissue in vitro. J. Physiol. 221:371-387, 1972.
62. Bito, L. Z., and Davson, H. Carrier-mediated removal of prostaglandins from cerebrospinal fluid. J. Physiol. 236:39-40, 1973.
63. Bito, L. Z., Wallenstein, M., and Baroody, R. The role of transport processes in the distribution and disposition of prostaglandins. Adv. Prostaglandin Thromboxane Res. 1:297-303, 1976.
64. Davson, H. Physiology of the Cerebrospinal Fluid, Little, Brown, Boston, 1967.
65. Wolfe, L. S., Coceani, F., and Pace-Asciak, C. Brain prostaglandins and studies on the action of prostaglandins on the isolated rat stomach. In Nobel Symposium 2: Prostaglandins, S. Bergstrom and B. Samuelsson (Eds.). Almqvist & Wiksell, Stockholm, pp. 265-276, 1967.
66. Hagen, A. A., Gerber, J. N., Sweeley, C. C., Sisco, A. B., White, R. P., and Robertson, J. T. The possible role of prostaglandin $F_{2\alpha}$ ($PGF_{2\alpha}$) in the etiology of cerebral vasospasm. Stroke 6:230-231, 1975 (abstr.).
67. Aizawa, Y., and Yamada, K. Determination of prostaglandin $F_{2\alpha}$ and E_2 in human cerebrospinal fluid by radioisotope dilution method. Prostaglandins 11:43-50, 1976.
68. La Torre, E., Patrono, C., Fortuna, A., and Grossi-Belloni, D. Role of prostaglandin F_2 in human cerebral vasospasm. J. Neurosurg. 41:293-299, 1974.
69. Wolfe, L. S., and Mamer, O. A. Measurement of prostaglandin $F_{2\alpha}$ levels in human cerebrospinal fluid in normal and pathological conditions. Prostaglandins 9:183-192, 1975.
70. Hagen, A. A., Sweeley, C. C., Gerber, J. N., White, R. P., and Robertson, J. T. The possible role of prostaglandin $F_{2\alpha}$ ($PGF_{2\alpha}$) in the etiology of cerebral vasospasm. 6th Int. Congr. Pharmacol., p. 291, 1975 (abstr.).
71. Hagen, A. A., Gerber, J. N., Sweeley, C. C., White, R. P., and Robertson, J. T. Levels and disappearance of prostaglandin $F_{2\alpha}$ in cerebral spinal fluid: A clinical and experimental study. Stroke 8:672-675, 1977.
72. White, R. P. Role of prostaglandins in cerebrovascular tone. Prostaglandins 9:405–407, 1975.
73. Brawley, B. W., Strandness, D. E., and Kelly, W. A. The biphasic response of cerebral vasospasm in experimental subarachnoid hemorrhage. J. Neurosurg. 28:1-8, 1968.
74. Kuwayama, A., Zervas, N. T., Belson, R., Shintani, A., and Pickren, K. A model for experimental cerebral arterial spasm. Stroke 3:49-56, 1972.
75. Echlin, F. Experimental vasospasm, acute and chronic, due to blood in the subarachnoid space. J. Neurosurg. 35:646-656, 1971.

76. Nagai, H., Suzuki, Y., Sugiura, M., Noda, S., and Mabe, H. Experimental cerebral vasospasm: Part 1. Factors contributing to early spasm. J. Neurosurg. 41:285-292, 1974.
77. Huang, S. P., and White, R. P. Evaluation of vasodilators on cerebral vasospasm in dogs. Fed. Proc. 35:297, 1976 (abstr.).
78. White, R. P., Morgan, H., and Robertson, J. T. Cerebrovascular effects of prostaglandins and possible role in vasospasm. In Subarachnoid Hemorrhage and Cerebrovascular Spasm, R. R. Smith and J. T. Robertson (Eds.). Charles C. Thomas, Springfield, Ill., pp. 72-85, 1975.
79. Allen, G. S., Gold, L. H. A., Chou, S. N., and French, L. A. Cerebral arterial spasm: Part 3. In vivo intracisternal production of spasm by serotonin and blood and its reversal by phenoxybenzamine. J. Neurosurg. 40:451-458, 1974.
80. Hong, S. L., Polsky-Cynkin, R., and Levin, L. Stimulation of prostaglandin biosynthesis by vasoactive substances in methylcholanthrene-transformed mouse BALB/3T3. J. Biol. Chem. 251(3):776-780, 1976.
81. Hagen, A. A., Gerber, J. N., Sweeley, C. C., White, R. P., and Robertson, J. T. Pleocytosis and elevation of prostaglandin $F_{2\alpha}$ and E_2 in cerebrospinal fluid following intracisternal injection of thrombin. Stroke 8:236-238, 1977.
82. Fraser, R. A. R., Stein, B. M., Barrett, R. E., and Pool, J. L. Noradrenergic mediation of experimental cerebrovascular spasm. Stroke 1:356-362, 1970.
83. Rubanyi, G. Interaction between exogenous prostaglandin $F_{2\alpha}$ and Ca^{2+} in the pregnant and post partum rabbit myometrium. Fed. Proc. 35: 843, 1976 (abstr.).
84. Kohn, K. I., and Anderson, G. F. The effect of prostaglandin E_2 and indomethacin on calcium activated detrusor smooth muscle. Fed. Proc. 35:843, 1976 (abstr.).
85. Wong, P. Y.-K., Terragno, N. A., and Terragno, A. Evidence of PGE-9 ketoreductase activities in human umbilical arteries. Fed. Proc. 35:854, 1976 (abstr.).
86. Kolata, G. B. Thromboxanes, the power behind the prostaglandins? Science 190:770-771, 1975.
87. Dembinska-Kiec, A., Zmuda, A., and Krupinska, J. Inhibition of prostaglandin synthesis by aspirin-like drugs in different microsomal preparations. Adv. Prostaglandin Thromboxane Res. 1:99-103, 1976.
88. Kunze, H., Bohn, E., and Bahrke, G. Effects of psychotropic drugs on prostaglandin biosynthesis in vitro. J. Pharm. Pharmacol. 27:880-881, 1975.
89. Zervas, N. T., Kuwayama, A., Rosoff, C. B., and Salzman, E. W. Cerebral vasospasm. Modifications by inhibition of platelet function. Arch. Neurol. 28:400-404, 1973.
90. Sundt, T. M. Management of ischemic complications after subarachnoid hemorrhage. J. Neurosurg. 43:418-425, 1975.

91. Gandini, A., Lualdi, P., and Bella, D. D. Influence of reserpine on release and effects of prostaglandins. Arch. Int. Pharmacodyn. Ther. 196(Suppl.):179-181, 1972.
92. Greenberg, S., Kadowitz, P. J., Dieke, F. P. J., and Long, J. P. Effect of prostaglandin $F_{2\alpha}$ on responses of vascular smooth muscle to serotonin, angiotensin and epinephrine. Arch. Int. Pharmacodyn. Ther. 206:5-18, 1973.
93. Smith, A. P., and Cuthbert, M. F. The response of normal and asthmatic subjects to prostaglandins E_2 and $F_{2\alpha}$ by different routes, and their significance in asthma. Adv. Prostaglandin Thromboxane Res. 1:449-459, 1976.
94. Koss, M. C., Nakano, J., and Rieger, J. A. Inhibition of prostaglandin $F_{2\alpha}$ induced reflex bradycardia and hypotension by meclofenamic acid. Prostaglandins 11:691-698, 1976.
95. White, R. P., and Pennink, M. Reversal of the pressor response of prostaglandin $F_{2\alpha}$ by polyphloretin phosphate in dogs. Arch. Int. Pharmacodyn. Ther. 197:274-281, 1972.
96. Allen, G. S., Henderson, L. M., Chou, S. N., and French, L. A. Cerebral arterial spasm: Part 2. In vitro contractile activity of serotonin in human serum and CSF on the canine basilar artery, and its blockage by methylsergide and phenoxybenzamine. J. Neurosurg. 40: 442-450, 1974.
97. Hagen, A. A., White, R. P., and Robertson, J. T. Synthesis of prostaglandins and thromboxane B_2 by cerebral arteries. Stroke 10(3): 306-309, 1979.
98. White, R. P. Multiplex origins of cerebral vasospasm. In Cerebrovascular Diseases, 11th Princeton Conference), T. R. Price and E. Nelson (Eds.). Raven Press, New York, pp. 307-319, 1979.
99. Chapleau, C. E., and White, R. P. Effects of prostacyclin on the canine isolated basilar artery. Prostaglandins 17:573-580, 1979.
100. Jarman, D. A., DuBoulay, G. H., Kendall, B., and Boullin, D. J. Responses of baboon cerebral and extracerebral arteries to prostacyclin and prostaglandin endoperoxide in vitro and in vivo. J. Neurol. Neurosurg. Psychiatr. 42:677-686, 1979.
101. Herman, A. G., Moncada, S., and Vane, J. R. Formation of prostacyclin (PGI_2) by different layers of the arterial wall. Arch. Int. Pharmacodyn. 227:162-163, 1977.
102. White, R. P., Hagen, A. A., and Robertson, J. T. Effect of nonsteroid anti-inflammatory drugs on subarachnoid hemorrhage in dogs. J. Neurosurg. 51:164-171, 1979.
103. Chapleau, C. E., White, R. P., and Robertson, J. T. Cerebral vasospasm: effects of prostacyclin synthetase inhibitors in vitro. Neurosurgery 6:155-159, 1980.

104. Chapleau, C. E., White, R. P., and Robertson, J. T. Effects of prostaglandin synthetase inhibitors (PSI) on contractions induced by arachidonate, prostaglandin $F_{2\alpha}$ and serotonin in basilar arteries. Fed. Proc. 38:359, 1979 (abstr.).

15 Effect of Prostaglandins on Central Nervous System Function

FREDERICK A. CURRO / Fairleigh Dickinson University, College of Dentistry, Hackensack, New Jersey, and New York University, College of Dentistry, New York, New York

STAN GREENBERG / University of South Alabama College of Medicine, Mobile, Alabama

ROBERT W. GARDIER / Wright State University College of Medicine, Dayton, Ohio

It is now generally accepted that the central nervous system contains a number of different prostaglandins. These substances are also found as normal constituents of the cerebrospinal fluid. The mammalian central nervous system contains primarily the PGF series and in some cases small amounts of PGE.

RELEASE OF PROSTAGLANDINS ON STIMULATION FROM CEREBRAL CORTEX

In a review by Coceani (1), the author suggests that a correlation exists between the release of prostaglandins from nervous tissue under physiological conditions and the general level of neuronal activity. The evoked release of neural stimulation is frequency dependent. Putative neurotransmitters may also stimulate prostaglandin release, and this action has physiological implications at some sites. The question of specificity of prostaglandin release remains a moot point. Iontophoretically applied prostaglandins suggest that neurons throughout the brain may not be evenly responsive to the prostaglandins. Furthermore, release experiments present problems since data are obtained from nonhomogeneous portions of the brain. An alternative approach is needed. The development of a histochemical localization of prostaglandin synthetase will provide the ultimate answer to the question of the special relationship of prostaglandins to certain neuronal pathways. It is true that prostaglandins may be released from neurons themselves; on the other hand, one must not overlook the possibility that prostaglandins may be capable of being released from glial cells.

Wolfe (2) has reviewed the roles of prostaglandins in the nervous system. He suggests that the spontaneous release of prostaglandins into superfusates of various brain regions is now well documented (cerebral cortex, cerebellum, spinal cord, and cerebral ventricles). In addition, Wolfe (2) states that the activation of cortical neurons by analeptic drugs also increases the prostaglandin content of cerebral cortex superfusates. Drugs such as barbiturates and chlorpromazine decrease the basal release of prostaglandins. Prostaglandin release from brain can be affected by many different stimuli, neuronal, hormonal, pharmacological, or traumatic.

Prostaglandins are not accumulated in stores and subsequently released upon stimulation. The evidence suggests a stimulated biosynthesis related to the functional state. Differences in the types of prostaglandins released from nervous tissue in the stimulated and unstimulated state have been found (3). Wolfe (2) suggests that this may be due to three possible mechanisms.

The most likely mechanism is that activities of the 15-hydroxyprostaglandin endoperoxide isomerase and reductase enzymes might be altered during stimulation.

The release of prostaglandins from the cerebral cortex was first reported by Ramwell and Shaw (4). They suggested that prostaglandin release might be connected with neuronal activity, after finding that release could be increased by stimulation of the contralateral forepaw and by the administration of analeptics. Other workers (5) have found that electrocortical desynchronization could be correlated with an increase in the level of prostaglandin release from the cerebral cortex. Conversely, drug-induced synchronization was accompanied by a decrease in prostaglandin release.

Bradley et al. (6) have indicated that high-frequency electrical stimulation of the brain stem reticular activating system is accompanied by a significant increase in prostaglandin efflux. These studies suggest that the level of prostaglandin released from the cerebral cortex appears to be more closely correlated with the pattern of electrocortical activity than with the level of behavioral arousal. Raffel et al. (7) have reported that rat brain homogenate, containing synaptosomes, synthesized and released prostaglandins F and E upon aerobic incubation. The prostaglandin of the F type was PGF_2. The amount of prostaglandins released was dependent on incubation time and temperature as well as pH and osmolarity of the incubation medium. Synaptosomes are probably not a main source of prostaglandins compared to other subcellular brain fraction. Anti-inflammatory drugs such as indomethacin, high concentrations of some local anesthetics, and Δ^1-tetrahydrocannabinol inhibited prostaglandin release. Holmes (8) has shown that serotonin will markedly stimulate the release of prostaglandins into cerebral spinal fluid in the dog and it might, therefore, be proposed that the mode of action of serotonin is via the release of prostaglandins. This suggestion would conform with the proposed role of serotonin in cholinergic pathways for cold receptors.

The significance of the findings to date that total brain homogenate releases more prostaglandins than do purified synaptosomes per milligram of protein indicates that some subcellular brain fraction other than synaptosomes are the primary sources of prostaglandins. It is interesting that anti-inflammatory drugs, local anesthetics, and Δ^1-tetrahydrocannabinol inhibit prostaglandin release. It would be interesting to explore the various mechanisms by which this effect occurs. It is also interesting that electrical cortical desynchronization rather than the level of behavioral arousal determines the level of prostaglandin release from the cerebral cortex.

The direction of future research appears to be in isolating and identifying the subcellular brain fractions, which are the main source of prostaglandin localization and release. What is needed in the studies of prostaglandin release are better and more sensitive methods for localizing prostaglandin synthetase in tissues and using gas chromatography-mass fragmentography methods for specific quantification of the indogenous biosynthetic capacity of the brain subcellular fractions from the various brain regions. This would yield better information on the localization of the synthetic enzymes. Also, a more clear-cut approach is needed to define the contributions made by neurons or glial cells to prostaglandins biosynthesis.

In summary, it appears that increased release of prostaglandins on neuronal pathway stimulation suggests that prostaglandin release is localized in the neurons rather than in the glial cells.

ADENYL CYCLASE AND GUANYL CYCLASE (CYCLIC NUCLEOTIDE SYSTEM)

A substantial amount of evidence (1) now suggests that the prostaglandin and adenyl cyclase-cyclic nucleotide system are functionally related. Depending on the tissue, prostaglandins can inhibit or stimulate the formation of cyclic AMP. Hence it has been proposed that PGEs, for example, may act as regulators of the adenyl cyclase reaction by a negative feedback mechanism or conversely as internal "messengers" or hormonal and neural humoral stimuli to the adenyl cyclase system. In the past few years, evidence of these PGE-cyclic AMP interactions in brain have accumulated. It has been suggested that the PGEs (PGE_1 and PGE_2) but not PGFs ($PGF_{1\alpha}$ and $PGF_{2\alpha}$) stimulate cyclic AMP formation in nervous tissue (1). The effect of the PGEs in stimulating cyclic AMP function is seen in rat nervous tissue.

The sensitivity of the adenyl cyclase system to PGE_1, coupled with the rapidity of the response, suggests that this system may play a central role in the events leading to neuronal activity. The same results are also compatible with the concept that PGEs may function as intermediate messengers in the activation of the adenyl cyclase by neural humoral stimuli. In addition, PGE_2 and norepinephrine potentiate cyclic AMP formation in cerebral cortex slices. PGEs may also modulate the adenyl cyclase reaction by a negative feedback mechanism.

Wolfe (2) also states that the PGEs stimulate cyclic AMP formation and increase intracellular cyclic AMP. Several laboratories have shown stimulation by PGE_1 of cyclic AMP formation in cultured neural tissues and in slices of cerebral cortex in vitro. Berti et al. (9, 10) have studied the effects of PGE_1 and PGE_2 on rat brain cortex slices and have found a stimulation of the formation of cyclic AMP from adenosine triphosphate (ATP); this activity is potentiated by theophylline. Micro iontophoretic application to neurons in the Purkinje cells evokes responses which show the central action, independent of vascular changes, of prostaglandins, suggesting that prostaglandins interfere with the processes involved in cyclic AMP formation. These authors have shown that prostaglandins may act on adenyl cyclase, preventing cyclic AMP formation induced by norepinephrine. When prostaglandins enhance the levels of cyclic AMP, the adenyl cyclase system appears to be activated, but the mechanisms involved in this process are still unknown. The brain adenyl cyclase sensitivity to various biogenic amines is reduced in broken-cell preparations; however, in sliced brain cortex preparations, the sensitivity is retained. PGE_1 and PGE_2 increase cyclic AMP formation only in the rat cerebral cortex, not in rabbit or humans. Theophylline potentiates the effect of PGE_2, suggesting that it may stimulate adenyl cyclase activity. Interestingly, morphine inhibits the stimulation by PGE_1 of cyclic AMP formation in rat brain homogenates (11). It has been suggested that morphine inhibits the action of PGE_1 on intracellular cyclic AMP.

Abdulla and McFarlane (12) reported that PGE_2 and PGE_3 control the adenyl cyclase reaction in brain. PGE_2 stimulated the enzyme, whereas PGE_3 caused the enzyme to be inhibited by adenosine diphosphate (ADP). They suggest that a sensitive system for controlling adenyl cyclase is provided by PGE_3; it switches off enzyme activity as more ADP is formed. Under the influence of PGE_3 the reaction is sensitive to the size of the ADP pool that is accessible to the enzyme. When the pool is small, the reaction proceeds uninhibited. As the pool enlarges, ADP formation gets slower until at high ADP concentrations the reaction completely stops. It is thus possible that control of adenyl cyclase by PGE_3 functions more when the enzyme is stimulated by PGE_2 (12). Furthermore, Abdulla and McFarlane (13) investigated the control of prostaglandins biosynthesis by adenine nucleotides in rat brain homogenates. They found that ADP stimulated PGE_1 formation. Cyclic AMP enhanced PGE_2 formation. The formation of PGE_3 was inhibited by ATP. The conclusions were incorporated after looking at the action of some drugs on this control system, to form a hypothesis on the mechanism of depressive illness. Wellman and Schwabe (14), after administering intravenous doses of PGE_1 and PGE_2 to rats, caused an initial increase in cyclic AMP levels in the first minute in seven discrete brain regions followed by a rapid decrease. PGE_2 was the most effective and PGE_2 produced only a slight increase in the first 30 sec after injection. The sedation and stupor produced correlated fairly well with the increase in cyclic AMP. Dismukes and Daly (15) concurred with the findings of others in that PGE_1 and PGE_2 stimulate the accumulation of cyclic AMP in brain slices of rats. The accumulation of cyclic AMP elicited by PGE_1 was not blocked by naloxone, propranolol, phentolamine, tetracaine, or theophylline. Morphine potentiated the effects of PGE_1.

Tell et al. (16) studied the effects of the E prostaglandins, morphine, and guanosine triphosphate (GTP) on brain adenyl cyclase. The nucleotide GTP, which has been shown to play an important role in regulating the stimulation of adenyl cyclase by several hormones in various tissues, inhibits the basal adenyl cyclase activity of arcuate nucleus homogenates. The inhibitory effect of GTP is reversed by dopamine. This effect of dopamine is more profound than is the stimulation of adenyl cyclase by dopamine. Neither PGE_1 nor PGE_2 nor morphine alter the activity of adenyl cyclase in brain homogenates. It has been suggested that morphine can reverse the stimulation of cyclic AMP formation induced by prostaglandins in rat brain homogenates. Tell et al. (16) attempted to compare the effects in this preparation with those obtained in the dopamine-sensitive rat caudate homogenate. Dopamine has been shown to stimulate the adenyl cyclase activity of homogenates from several neuronal preparations. The dopamine effect on the caudate of reversing the GTP inhibition of adenyl cyclase activity more than it stimulates the adenyl cyclase activity remains to be elucidated. It is not known whether these two effects are related or which one is physiologically more relevant; it is possible, however, that adenyl cyclase activity in the caudate may normally be modulated by the relative concentrations of GTP and dopamine.

Wolfe (2) states that guanyl cyclase has been found in particulate fractions of many tissues, and cyclic GMP levels are high in brain. A surprising finding is that acetylcholine elevates cyclic AMP levels in many tissues, including the perfused rat cerebral cortex. It is of great interest that $PGF_{2\alpha}$ and serotonin also promote cyclic GMP accumulation in the rat uterus. These findings have led to the speculation that cyclic GMP is involved in promoting cellular processes that are antagonistic to those mediated by cyclic AMP. Goldberg et al. (17) have formulated a "dualism theory" of biological control by opposing actions of the two nucleotides. One can propose a role for $PGF_{2\alpha}$ in facilitating excitation of acetylcholine and serotonin pathways through activation of guanyl cyclase. More research is needed to further explain the role of guanyl cyclase.

MICROCIRCULATION

Prostaglandins may play a unique role in the modulation of humoral stimuli to neurons (1). Therefore, they could be involved in the control of the microcirculation in the central nervous system. Much work has been done on the actions of prostaglandins on the central nervous system since Horton (18) first studied their effects. Hedqvist (19) has developed the concept that PGE compounds have an inhibitory feedback effect on neurotransmission. These findings may suggest a role for the prostaglandins on the control of brain microcirculation.

Indeed, some work has been reported on the effect of PGE_1 on cerebral circulatory disturbances by Steiner et al. (20). They observed that intracerebral infusions of PGE_1 induced a decrease in systemic blood pressure, and concluded that PGE_1 was an effective cerebral spasmolytic agent in dogs. In addition, they suggested that PGE_1 might be beneficial as a spasmolytic agent for cerebral vasospasm in humans. In patients who were undergoing cerebral arterial spasm, they showed that the effects of PGE_1 in the clinical state showed an improved condition on the cerebral blood flow in a few patients but indicated that the effects observed were small considering the methods used. That is, the PGE_1 produced modest changes in cerebral blood flow in the subjects and it was apparent that PGE_1 had little effect on vessels of the circle of Willis and its branches. The fact that PGE_1 did not markedly improve intracerebral spasm emphasized the complexity of the pathogenesis of spasm as well as the mechanism of adrenergic innervation of the cerebral vascular tree. It seems that adrenergic impulses are inhibited by PGE_1 but has not been proved that the action of PGE_1 is due to direct inhibition of the catecholamine effect on vascular smooth muscle or due to unrelated vasodilatory effect of PGE_1. Certain facts suggest that the release of serotonin may occur in response to the injection of PGE_1; serotonin has been shown to cause spasm when applied topically to cerebral arteries. The compound action of PGE_1 suggests an explanation of its relative ineffectiveness in improving cerebral arterial spasm.

Yamamoto et al. (21) has shown that infusion of PGE_1 causes vasodilation of the cerebral arteries of dogs, whereas PGE_2 causes vasoconstriction in these vessels. These results were based on measurement of pressures in the carotid artery and the subarachnoid space, which provides only indirect indications of cerebral blood flow and the vasomotor state of the cerebral vessels. However, changes in cerebral hemodynamics were observed directly on the exposed brain of dogs during the intracarotid infusion of PGE_1 and PGF_2. Regional blood flow measurements with the Zenon 133 clearance technique provides a means of measuring cerebral circulation transit time. Yamamoto et al. (21) concluded that intracarotid infusion of PGE_1 does not cause vasoconstriction of cerebral vessels. On the contrary, we have observed that PGE_1 has a powerful vasoconstricting effect on small cerebral arteries. Ethanol inhibits the powerful vasoconstricting effect of PGE_1. It is possible that other workers have used ethanol in preparing their prostaglandin solutions. This, together with the inhibitory action on the synthesis of prostaglandins by aspirin, indicates directions in which a search can be made for agents that block or relieve cerebral vasospasm.

Pickard (22) has studied the mechanism of action of $PGF_{2\alpha}$ on cerebral flow in a baboon. His changes following $PGF_{2\alpha}$ were a reduction in cerebral blood flow by 23%, a reduction in oxygen consumption by 31%, and an increase in cerebral vascular resistance by 38%. There was no dissociation between the effects on cerebral oxygen consumption and cerebral blood flow by varying either the dose of PGF_2 or the arterial PCO_2. These results suggested that the primary effect of PGF_2 is on the cerebral oxygen consumption and not on the cerebral vascular smooth muscle. The observation of Yamamoto et al. (21) that only the smallest visible arteries constrict after $PGF_{2\alpha}$ would also be consistent with a primary reduction in metabolism.

Pickard and Mackenzie (23) studied the inhibition of prostaglandin synthesis in the response of cerebral circulation to CO_2 and they designed their experiment to test the hypothesis that an undefined endogenous prostaglandin may provide a link between hypercapnia and cerebral vasodilation independent of any change on extracellular pH. The response of cerebral circulation to hypercapnia was compared before and during infusions of indomethacin. Because of the uncoupling of oxidative phosphorylation they found that the cerebral vascular vasoconstriction, with the maintenance of autoregulation, is contrary to what would be expected if indomethacin has a "nonspecific" depressant effect on the cerebral vascular smooth muscle. Rather, it supports the hypothesis that endogenous generation of an unspecified prostaglandin, acting as a local vasodilator, is necessary for the normal level of cerebral blood flow. That microgram doses of PGE_1 infused into the carotid artery of dogs and baboons reduce the cerebral blood flow may not reflect the physiological role of endogenous PGE compounds. The effect in brain may be analogous to that in rabbit adipose tissue, where indomethacin will block the functional vasodilation associated with ACTH-induced lipolysis. If this effect of indomethacin results from an inhibition of prostaglandin synthesis, the speed of onset of the effect on cerebral blood flow would indicate an extremely rapid turnover of the relevant prostaglandin. This complements the rapidity of onset of the change in the cerebral blood flow with hypo- and hypercapnia.

Emerson et al. (24) studied the effects of $PGF_{2\alpha}$ on cerebral blood flow, cerebral vascular resistance, and cerebral spinal and systemic arterial pressures. The infusion of 1-100 μg/ml $PGF_{2\alpha}$ into the cerebral ventricular system did not affect cerebral venous outflow but increased cerebral vascular resistance and cerebral spinal fluid pressure at the higher concentrations. Therefore, the PGF_2 increase in cerebral vascular resistance is dependent on the route of administration since systemic intraaortic arch infusion of PGF_2 decreased cerebral venous outflow and increased cerebral vascular resistance slightly. Intracarotid arterial infusion of PGF_2 had similar effects as the systemic infusion. The magnitude of this constriction is not great considering the dose used. Also, PGF_2 can increase systemic arterial blood pressure via a central effect.

Staszewska-Barczak and Vane (25) suggest that the prostaglandins play a role in the local control of circulation. They suggest further that prostaglandins, being local hormones, may influence vascular tone when synthesized and released within the vascular wall or from the nearby tissues. The vasodilation produced by prostaglandins of the E type involves all segments of the vascular tree. The vasodilator effect is long lasting and includes a direct action, a reduction of the effects of vasoconstrictor substances, and interference with the release of the adrenergic mediator. The continuous basal release of a vasodilator prostaglandin by some tissues indicates a role for prostaglandins in the maintenance of vessel tone and normal blood flow. Prostaglandins contribute to autoregulation and to reactive and functional hyperemia in various organs and tissues. Thus local prostaglandin release is an important mechanism for regional control of blood flow under physiological and pathological conditions. Wolfe (2) indicates that cerebral blood flow is generally shown to be decreased by PGE and decreased by PGF, and there is no effect or slight increase by PGA types of compounds. This is interesting when correlated with defects on adrenergic neurotransmission, in that PGE causes a decreased adrenergic neurotransmission; PGF types may increase while PGA types have no effect. There is no doubt that one of the possible physiological and pathophysiological roles of prostaglandins is the regulation of the microcirculation and tissue perfusion in the central nervous system in addition to regulating the central and autonomic neurotransmission.

In summary, the results seem to be open to speculation. However, it is significant that in these studies on the effect of prostaglandins on the cerebral microcirculation, PGE and PGF_2 generally increase cerebral vascular resistance and decrease flow. It would be interesting to examine further the effect of prostaglandin antagonists on the general effects of the prostaglandins on the microcirculation of the cerebral cortex with the possibility of finding therapeutic tools for relieving vasospasm of the cerebral arteries and cerebral anoxia due to cerebral vascular arterial spasms and circulatory disturbances.

PAIN

Collier and Roy (11) have examined the effect of morphine in rat brain homogenate on the stimulation of PGE_1 or PGE_2 of cyclic AMP formation and found that morphine inhibited this stimulation without inhibiting the basal production of cyclic AMP. Heroin was more effective and methadone was less effective than morphine and naloxone antagonized the effect of morphine. This inhibition may represent a mechanism whereby morphinelike drugs exert their analgesic effects. Collier and Roy (26) further indicate that in interacting with prostaglandin mechanisms, morphine inhibits the stimulation by PGE_1 and E_2 in cyclic AMP formation in rat brain homogenate. They suggest that this action is sereo specific and is reversed by naloxone. Prostaglandins and cyclic AMP may be the mechanism by which morphine exerts its analgesic effect, i.e., by inhibiting the stimulation by endogenous PGE of a PGE-sensitive adenyl cyclase of the appropriate neurons.

Collier et al. (27) further suggest that morphine blocks the stimulation by PGE of cyclic AMP formation by rat brain homogenate. This may be the basis of the inhibitory effects of morphine, such as analgesia and hypothermia. They indicate further that morphine has stimulant effects such as hyperthemia, emesis, and hyperglycemia that PGEs also possess. Both morphine and apomorphine stimulate the biosynthesis of prostaglandins from arachidonic acid. Morphine and apomorphine stimulated total prostaglandin production by rabbit brain homogenate (27). Morphine stimulated the production of both PGE_2 and PGF_2, and morphine does not inhibit prostaglandin dehydrogenase. The stimulation of prostaglandin synthetase in brain homogenate might explain the effects of morphine and apomorphine in causing vomiting, fever, and hyperglycemia. Injection of morphine into the rabbit lateral cerebral ventricle elicits hyperthermia and the doses used (500 μg) might be sufficient to stimulate PGE production in the anterior hypothalamus. Thus a possible explanation may exist to explain the stimulant effects of morphine and apomorphine in vivo. Ferri et al. (28) found that the administration of PGE_1 intracerebrally antagonizes morphine analgesia in rats.

Singh and Bhandari (29) studied the effect of $PGF_{2\alpha}$ for its analgesic properties and found that a high dose of 50 μg/kg exerted only weak analgesic effects. However, this dose potentiated the effect of subanalgesic doses of morphine. It would seem to be of some interest to investigate the role of prostaglandins in narcotic analgesics. After morphine injection, Singh and Bhandari (29) found that the threshold for the pain stimulus is strongly enhanced; intraventricular administration of PGE_1 after morphine administration induces a significant reduction of this threshold level. The PGE_1 effect reaches its maximum 10 min after administration intraventricularly and the analgesic threshold approaches the level of the animals treated with morphine alone. The results indicate that PGE_1 antagonizes morphine when administered directly to the brain. Although the physiological role of prostaglandins is still obscure, they may have some pharmacological effects either due to a direct action or to an indirect one.

Ferreria et al. (30) give evidence for a supporting role for the catecholamines in the pain mechanism and in the analgesic action of morphine. The antagonist effect of PGE_1 on morphine analgesia compares well with the analgesic action of aspirinlike drugs in that it might inhibit the generation of prostaglandins. It also agrees with the fact that prostaglandins are released in the spinal cord and in the sensory cortex by a noxious stimulus in frogs and cats. Kakunaga et al. (31) suggest that calcium ions decrease morphine analgesia. Prostaglandins are claimed to interfere with calcium by displacing the bound ion from both sides of the cell membrane in facilitating its penetration. This brings out yet another hypothesis for a direct action of PGE_1.

Sleep-Wakefulness

Prostaglandins of the E series cause profound sedation and stupor when administered intraventricularly to cats. A study by Haubrich et al. (32) suggests that intraperitoneal administration of PGE_1 to rats induces sedation accompanied by diminished muscular tone and an increased turnover rate of brain 5-hydroxytryptamine (5-HT). The results were interesting in that PGE_1 administered to rats induced sedation which was accompanied by a low-voltage high-frequency EEG pattern characteristic of the waking animal. Administration of PGE_1 also increased the turnover of 5-HT and raised the concentration of acetylcholine in brain. The effects of prostaglandin were blocked by prior administration of pargyline, which lowers brain concentration of 5-hydroxyindoleacetic acid (5-HIAA) and were potentiated by pretreatment with probenecid, which elevated the 5-HIAA concentrations. The results were compatible with the possibility that PGE_1 induces a state resembling paradoxical sleep through an action on 5-HT metabolism in brain. Singh and Bhandari (29) studied the effect of $PGF_{2\alpha}$ on barbiturate hypnosis and found that it potentiated the hypnosis of pentobarbital sodium by increasing the sleep time. The results showed that $PGF_{2\alpha}$ has central nervous system depressant properties, as indicated by the potentiation of pentobarbital-induced hypnosis. This potentiation of barbiturate hypnosis by PGF $PGF_{2\alpha}$ could be due to its inhibitory effect on the metabolism of pentobarbital or as a result of its hypothermic effect. The latter seems to be more convincing since $PGF_{2\alpha}$ exerted hypothermic activity as well as potentiated the hypothermia induced by reserpine.

HYPOTHALAMUS

Thermoregulation

Endogenous monoamines in the anterior hypothalamus are widely regarded as the effectors of temperature regulation in mammals (1). According to one model, thermoregulation results from a balance between opposite effects of 5-HT and norepinephrine at hypothalamic sites. For each amine the site of action is species dependent. Much work has been done to ascertain whether biogenic amines have a role in the production of pyrogen fever. The discovery that PGE_1 is a powerful pyretic agent has triggered a new phase of research in this field, and an impressive body of evidence is now available relating PGEs to fever responses. The evidence is summarized in a review by Coceani (1). According to a current model, PGEs are formed in the anterior hypothalmus following exposure of the tissue to pyrogens, and then act locally to produce fever. An open question remains as to whether PGEs have a role in the normal regulation of body temperature. The finding that intraventricular infusion of 5-HT stimulates the release of PGEs suggests that these compounds may be a general mediator of thermogenic stimuli under both physiological and pathological conditions. Support to this idea comes from the evidence that salicylate can lower body temperature in nonfebrile animals. However, an opposite view is expressed by Milton (33) since aspirin has no effect on normal body temperature, and the hypothermic action of some antipyretics such as indomethacin in nonfebrile animals can be explained without implicating a reduced rate of prostaglandin (PG) biosynthesis.

Milton and Wendlandt have shown (34) that single intraventricular injections of pyrogen-free solutions of PGE_1 or PGE_2 into cats produced a prompt elevation of body temperature associated with skin vasoconstriction, shivering, and pyloerection. These experiments triggered a new approach in the complex field of thermoregulation, and the evidence is now very convincing that the E-type PGs are natural mediators for pyrogen-induced hyperthermia. A brief summary is presented by Wolfe (2). The current hypothesis is that pyrogens (bacterial or leukocytic) and endotoxins accelerate the biosynthesis of PGEs in brain, and specifically in the anterior hypothalamus through stimulation of the rate-controlling step releasing the precursor fatty acids. The PGs formed or the endoperoxide intermediates act locally on neurons, a process that leads to fever responses, and are liberated into the cerebrospinal fluid (CSF), where they may affect behavior through actions on other brain centers. The action of the PGEs differs in a number of respects from the effects of monoamines (norepinephrine, DA, 5-HT) which are widely thought to be the effectors of temperature regulation in mammals. The PGs are about 1000 times more potent and always produce a temperature increase, which is little affected by the ambient temperature in all species studied. A current theory explains temperature regulation in terms of an antagonistic relationship between the catecholamines and 5-HT, which is that of Veale and Cooper (35). Although there is much evidence to implicate PGs in the genesis of pyrogen fever, there is little evidence that normal body temperature is maintained by a continuous release of PGs. It is possible that stimulation of the release of 5-HT from neurons in the anterior hypothalamus accelerates PGE synthesis, which would initiate the thermogenic response. However, more research is needed before PGs can be implicated in the normal physiological control of temperature or in pharmacologic or pathological thermogenic responses.

Feldberg and Saxena (36) state that microinjection of a few nanograms of PGE_1 into the anterior hypothalamus produced a rise in rectal temperature, whereas temperature was not affected by microinjections of larger doses into the posterior hypothalamus. The hyperthermia produced by injections of PGE_1 into the cerebral ventricles is therefore attributed to an action of PGE_1 on the anterior hypothalamus. During a pentobarbital anesthesia the sensitivity of cats to the hypothermic effect of PGE_1 injected into the cerebral ventricles was found to be greatly reduced, particularly during the early stage of anesthesia when body temperature was falling steeply.

Hales et al. (37) demonstrated that four PGs—E_1, E_2, $F_{1\alpha}$, and $F_{2\alpha}$—injected into the lateral cerebral ventricle of conscious sheep caused deep body temperature rise. In a cool environment, faint shivering became intensified and peripheral vasoconstriction became maximal. In a warm environment, panting was markedly reduced and there was sometimes a slight vasoconstriction. PGE_1 and PGE_2 were the most effective, $PGF_{2\alpha}$ was slightly less effective. It was concluded that PGs may be involved in transmission along brain normal pathways involved in the stimulation of heat production and increased peripheral vasomotor tone, and the inhibition of heat-loss mechanisms. It has recently been shown that PGs of the E series are generally mediators for raising body temperature in different animal species. Bligh et al. (38) viewed temperature regulation in terms of the thermoregulatory responses to 5-HT, norepinephrine (NE), and adrenocortical hormone (ACH) in sheep, goats, and rabbits. They postulated that PGEs cause a marked rise in body temperature and that the PGEs are mediators for raising body temperature. They observed that the influence of PGs on thermoregulatory mechanisms varied with peripheral thermal receptor activity. In view of this, these PGs occur naturally in the brain, upon microinjection of PGE_1 into the anterior hypothalamus, causing hyperthermia (36). It appears that PGs may play a role in the normal regulation of body temperature. Thus the PGs exert excitatory influences in the pathway between various receptors and heat production mechanisms, with an excitatory effect on peripheral vasomotor tone and in inhibitory effect on heat loss mechanisms.

Avery (39) suggests that with 5-HT causing hyperthermia in some species and hypothermia in others, any relationship between 5-HT and PGs in controlling thermal regulatory mechanisms therefore remains to be determined. Thus the precise mechanisms of action of PGs is unknown. Thermoregulatory responses quite different from those obtained would have been expected if the PGs were acting by inhibiting NE release in the central nervous system (CNS); this is so because NE appears to act as an inhibitor in both heat loss and heat production control pathways in the CNS. Lipton et al. (40) demonstrated that PGE_1 causes thermal stimulation in the rat when injected in the preoptic/anterior hypothalamic temperature control region (PO/AH) and the medulla oblongata. They compared changes in rectal temperature produced by injecting PGE_1 into the PO/AH region in the dog. The results show that PGE_1 injected into the PO/AH region caused a rise in rectal temperature. On the other hand, injection of equal amounts of PGE into the medulla lowered the rectal temperature in all rats.

The results show no clear parallel between the effects of rectal temperature produced by injecting hyperthermogenic agents into the PO/AH and medulla temperature control regions in the brain. The result is interesting since the two regions are known to respond in parallel fashion to certain chemical substances known to influence thermoregulation. This contrast suggests that the thermal regulatory mechanisms of the PO/AH region of the medulla are organized in one way with respect to responsiveness to thermal stimuli and in quite different ways with respect to responsiveness to chemical compounds. The present findings indicate that PGE_1 injected into two brain regions can influence temperature. If PGE_1 does play a role as a mediator of thermal regulation, its function in the medulla must be antagonistic to its function in the PO/AH region. The medulla normally contains small amounts of PGE_1, and this makes it plausible that PGE_1 in the medulla has a role in thermoregulation. To reiterate, PGE_1 causes hyperthermia when injected into the third ventricle of the cat and into the lateral ventricle of the rat and rabbit, and may be involved in fever, as bacterial pyrogen releases a PG-like substance into the ventrical system of the cat (41).

To study further the action of PGE_1 on thermoregulatory processes, PGE_1 has been infused into the lateral ventricle of the sheep. At 10°C ambient temperature, shivering changed from mild bursts to strong continuous shivering as the rectal temperature rose. When the infusion is stopped, respiratory frequency rose to above its preinfusion level, shivering ceased, and the temperature of the ear rose and temperature of the rectum fell. At the three ambient temperatures studied, the rise in rectal temperature produced by the infusion of PGE_1 was of the order of 2°C. These effects of PGE_1 on sheep resemble those of single intraventricular injections of acetylcholine and can likewise be interpreted as indicating an action somewhere in the pathway between cold sensors and heat production effectors before the origin of a crossed inhibitory influence on the pathways between warm sensors and heat loss effectors. The rapid reversal of thermoregulatory effects upon PGE_1 infusion contrasts with the slow decline of the thermoregulatory effects of a single injection of ACH. PGE_1 may not exert similar influences at the same points in the neuronal complex upon which the central control of body temperature depends.

After the work of Feldberg et al. in 1970, Myers and Veale (42) showed that body temperature of unanesthetized cats could be raised or lowered by varying the ratio of sodium to calcium in the tissue of the posterior hypothalamus, and suggested that alteration of this ratio may be produced by pyrogens. It has been shown in cats that the rise in temperature occurring during profusion of the ventricular system with a calcium-free fluid is unlikely to be attributed to the increased synthesis and release of PGs in the hypothalamus [Dey et al. (43)]. Since sheep have been shown to respond to ionic changes in the CSF with changes in body temperature, the possibility exists that the effect of pyrogens given intravenously in the newborn lamb may be through this postulated ionic mechanism and not involving PGE_1. One possible explanation for these changes in body temperature is that the drug may have an influence on the synapsis lying within the pathways mediating thermoregulatory responses. PGs could modulate synaptic function through influences on the release of neurotransmitter substances. Therefore, the flooding of the ventricular system with relatively large quantities of PGE_1 may have no specific effects on the normal thermal regulatory patterns of the animal. The PGE_1 injected may have entered the tissue of the brain and exerted an effect. The results would suggest that the newborn lamb may be able to develop a fever independently of the central involvement of PGE_1 since lambs that are capable of responding to bacterial pyrogen often fail to develop fever after ventricular PGE_1. Alternatively, the intraventricular approach may not be a useful method for the study of central involvement of PGs in pyrogens in the control of body temperature of the newborn lamb.

Baird et al. (44) studied the thermoregulatory responses to monoamines, acetylcholine, and PGs in the lateral cerebral ventricle of the echidna. Briefly, placental animals tested to date invariably exhibit a hyperthermic response to PG, and the hypothermic responses of this monotreme that is the echidna is therefore unique. The present study included the confirmation of a hyperthermic response of PGE_1 and PGE_2 in cats and rats. Therefore, the concept of thermoregulation by amines and other substances in the hypothalamus of placental animals may also be applicable to monotremes that have evolved separately from the marsupials and placental animals. 5-HT, NE, ACH, and PGE_1 and PGE_2, after being injected into the lateral cerebral ventricle of the conscious echidna, caused deep body temperature to fall by peripheral vasodilation and/or reduced metabolic rate due to a decrease in shivering or to gentle relaxation. The responses of many placental mammals to 5-HT, NE, and ACH vary widely and the echidna appears to exhibit responses most like those of the rat.

Ford (45) suggests that PGE_1 has a selective action on hypothalamic neurons which respond to small changes in brain temperature. The possibility was tested by applying PGE_1 from multibarreled micropipettes directly onto the hypothalamic neurons using the technique of inotophoresis. The results obtained from 46 neurons showed stable mean firing rates at 38°C. The results suggest that PGE_1 selectively excites cold responsive neurons which are presumed to drive heat production and heat conservation mechanisms. This selective action may be the means by which PGE_1, when injected, causes body temperature to rise. It may also be part of the process by which pyrogens act, since PGs of the E series are known to be released into the third ventricle during pyrogen fever.

Stitt et al. (46) have demonstrated preoptic and anterior hypothalamus thermosensitivity in rabbits prior to enduring fevers produced by intrahypothalamic injections of PGE_1 at various ambient temperatures. Stitt et al. concluded that fever is produced by an upward displacement of a central "reference point" rather than by any changes in the central thermosensitivity. Veale and Cooper (47) observed that by using push-pull cannulas and perfusing hypothalamic tissue and the ventricular and the lateral ventricle at the same time, they could measure the passage of PGE_1 into the CSF. PGE_1 was perfused through the tissue of the anterior hypothalamus and produced a sharp increase in body temperature. Their results indicate that after PG is placed into the anterior hypothalamus and a febrile response is produced, the PGE_1 can find its way quickly into the ventricular system. It thus supports the suggestion that the CSF may be important in the passage of PGE_1 from the brain. Further, they support the theory that leukocyte pyrogen may produce fever by releasing PG within the tissue of the hypothalamus. Cooper and Veale (48) produced fever by intravenous bacterial pyrogen after injection of reserpine into the lateral ventricle of the rabbit. Body temperature was also shown to fall following the injection of atropine into the lateral ventricle. It has been suggested that the fever produced by intravenous pyrogens may be mediated by the release of PGEs within the hypothalamus. Briefly, Cooper and Veale compared the effects of reserpine injected into a lateral cerebral ventricle and of intraventricular reserpine on fever due to either intravenous leukocyte pyrogen or to PGE_1 injected into the PO/AH area. Atropine delayed the onset and reduced the extent of fever due to leukocyte pyrogen and brought the body temperature down.

There was a similarity in the effects of reserpine and atropine on the fevers due to leukocyte pyrogen and PGE_1. This is consistent with the hypothesis that PGE_1 is released in the hypothalamus during pyrogen-induced fever. Laburn et al. (49),studied the mechanism of action of PGE_1 on the hyperthermic effect of NE injected in rabbits. They investigated the possible role for NE and cyclic AMP in the febrile PGE_1 response. They used unilateral injections of PGE_1 into the PO/AH area on either side of the midline. The NE nerve terminals of the opposite side of the hypothalamus were destroyed by 6-hydroxydopamine, and the response to PGE_1 on that side was reduced. In addition, phenoxybenzamine reduced the febrile response to PGE_1, whereas propranolol had no effect. When they injected dibutyl cyclic AMP into the anterior hypothalamus, they produced a febrile response. Also, theophylline injected into the anterior hypothalamus produced a greater fever than that induced by the same dose of PGE_1 into the control side. Nicotinic acid, on the other hand, attenuated the febrile response to PGE_1. Laburn et al. (49) therefore suggest that the full febrile response to PGE_1 is dependent on an intact noradrenergic system in the hypothalamus and second, that varying the levels of endogenous cyclic AMP in the hypothalamus affects the response of PGE_1. This suggests that PGE_1 could act via a monoaminergic system to increase the activity of adenyl cyclase in certain hypothalamic neurons, and thus produce fever.

Rudy and Viswanathan (50) suggest a cholinergic involvement in the hypothermic action of PGE_1 injected into the PO/AH region. They injected either atropine or mecamylamine into the cerebral ventricle prior to the injection of PGE_1 and this did not attenuate the hyperthermia. Both atropine and mecamylamine produced a rise in body temperature. It thus seems unlikely that PGE_1 evokes hyperthermia in the rat by releasing endogenous acetylcholine at synapses in the rostral hypothalamus. However, the possibility of acetylcholine release in this region requires additional investigation. Until the selectivity of the cholinergic blockage provoked by these agents can be demonstrated, the possibility that PGE_1 evokes hypothermia through inhibition of cholinergic function within the PO/AH cannot be discounted. It may also be the case that PGE_1 acts directly or through a mechanism involving a neurotransmitter other than acetylcholine.

Pittman et al. (51) suggested that pyrogens may produce their febrile response by the release of PGs into the hypothalamus (a popular theory). They injected PGE_1 into the lateral ventricle of conscious newborn lambs and got a rise in body temperature. Several injections of 300 ng of pyrogen caused fever. The results suggest that newborn lambs need to be able to develop a fever independently of the central involvement of PGE_1. Alternatively, the intraventricular approach may not be useful for the simple control of body temperature in the newborn lamb. It has been suggested that pyrogens could elevate body temperature independently of PGE_1 release. Again, some workers suggest that the hyperthemia is due to an action of sodium together with the absence of calcium on the cells in the hypothalamus and not on the monoaminergic neurons that innervate these cells. It has been postulated that one of the actions of a pyrogen may be to lower the level of calcium or to prevent its action within the hypothalamus.

Cranshaw and Stitt (52) injected PGE_1 into the PO/AH area in the squirrel monkey and recorded increases in body temperature. When the ambient temperature was below the thermoneutral zone, increases in body temperature were produced entirely by increases in metabolic rate. When the ambient temperature was at the upper end of the thermoneutral zone, increases in body temperature were produced by vasoconstriction in addition to lesser increases in metabolic rate. During sessions of behavioral temperature regulation, PGE_1 injections were followed by selection of a higher ambient temperature, an increase in skin temperature, and subsequent increases in body temperature. PGE_1 injections produce dose-dependent increases in body temperature which are similar regardless of ambient temperature or whether behavioral or autonomic means are utilized to raise the heat content of the body. Veale and Wishaw (53) produced fever by pyrogens applied directly to the PO/AH area of unanesthetized rats at various ambient temperatures. They have determined that this is the region of the brain of the rat from which temperature responses can be produced by local injection. They also suggest that the responses to local injections of PGE_1 are relatively unaffected by environmental temperatures, whereas those in response to injections of NE are influenced by ambient temperature.

These are similar findings with respect to the response to pyrogens in that it is relatively unaltered by ambient temperature. Their work lends further support to the hypothesis that pyrogens act in the hypothalamus by releasing PGs. Myers and Waller (54) chronically implanted push-pull cannulas into the diencephalon of a Rhesus monkey which was accustomed to a primate chair. Skin temperatures were measured during the experiment, in which a site in the hypothalamus had been labeled by microinjection of tritiated 5-HT or tritiated NE. Consecutive push-pull profusions with an artificial CSF were carried out for 10 min. PGE_1 was added to the artificial CSF during the third and fifth successive profusions. Nonlabeled PGE_1 failed to exert a precise and consistent effect on the characteristic pattern of efflux of either tritiated 5-HT or NE when profusion sites were distributed widely throughout the hypothalamus. In some experiments, however, an enhanced efflux of 5-HT label did occur after the temperature had begun to rise following a profusion with PGE_1. These findings indicate that PG injected into the brain does not evoke hyperthermia by way of a pathological disturbance to the balance in the presynaptic release of 5-HT and NE within nerve endings in the rostral hypothalamus of the monkey. Conversely, neither 5-HT nor NE influences the PG activity within the hypothalamus, at least insofar as a functional change in the body temperature of the primate concerned.

Antipyretics

The antipyretic activity of paracetamol has been shown by Flower and Vane (55) to be due to the inhibition of PG synthetase in brain. The inhibition of PG biosynthesis by aspirinlike drugs has now been confirmed in several systems. The theory that this antienzyme action is the basis of the clinical effects of aspirinlike drugs has recently been reviewed. One of the few anomalies was that paracetamol was inactive against dog spleen synthetase. A possible explanation for this discrepancy is that synthetase systems from different regions of the body show different sensitivities to drugs. PGs are pyrogenic, as we have stated. Paracetamol produces a prompt reduction in fever produced by intravenous pyrogens and reduces the PG substances in the CSF. It seems clear that paracetamol acts centrally as an antipyretic.

Flower and Vane (55) further studied the effect of paracetamol on the PG synthetase system derived from rabbit brain. They compared the dog spleen synthetase and rabbit brain synthetase and the effects of paracetamol, aspirin, and indomethacin and found that aspirin had similar activities in both systems. However, indomethacin was much less active as an inhibitor of PG production in brain tissue than in spleen and paracetamol was a more potent inhibitor of brain enzyme than of spleen enzyme. All three compounds are antipyretic (a central effect) and all have an inhibitory effect on the brain enzyme in concentrations found in the plasma after therapeutic doses. Both as antipyretics and as inhibitors of brain PG synthetase, the descending order of potency is indomethacin; aspirin; paracetamol. Unlike indomethacin and aspirin, which are anti-inflammatory, paracetamol has no anti-inflammatory activity and is not active against the dog's spleen synthetase in therapeutic concentrations. The results illustrate that the mechanism by which the clinical actions of the aspirinlike drugs are determined is by the differential sensitivity of the PG synthetase systems of the "target tissues." They support the idea that a study of PG synthetase systems from different tissues will lead to aspirinlike drugs with a greater specificity of action.

Milton (56) studied the effects of these same three drugs in PGE_1 and endotoxin-induced fever. They produced the fever in the conscious cat by intracerebral ventricular injection of bacterioendotoxin of PGE_1. The three antipyretic drugs indomethacin, aspirin, and paracetamol all suppressed the fever produced by endotoxin but were ineffective in suppressing a fever produced by PGE_1. The results provide evidence for the idea that PGE is a mediator in endotoxin fever and that antipyretic drugs act by preventing PG synthesis and release. The hypothermic action of antipyretics in afebrile animals is unlikely to be due to inhibition of PGE synthesis, and it is questionable whether a PGE is involved in normal thermal regulation. The evidence that Milton has shown is compatible with the concept that release of a PG of the E series is responsible for hyperthermia of fever. The observation that all three antipyretic drugs studied were without effect on PGE_1 hyperthermia is in accord with the view that antipyretics act by producing PG synthesis or release. Feldberg et al. (57) collected samples of CSF from unanesthetized cats while recording rectal temperature. They produced fever by injecting the bacterial pyrogen Shigella dysenteriae into the third ventricle, cysternia magna, or intravenously. In each experiment, PGE_1 activity increased in samples of CSF collected during the pyrogen fever, irrespective of the route of administration of the pyrogen. However, 1000 times larger doses of the pyrogen were required on intravenous injection than an injection into the cysternal space. The antipyretic drugs indomethacin, aspirin, and paracetamol, injected intraperitoneally during the pyrogen fever, brought down the body temperature and the PGE activity of the cysternal CSF became low. These findings support the theory that pyrogens produce fever by increasing synthesis and release of PGs in the PO/AH area and that antipyretics of the aspirin type bring down this fever since they inhibit the synthesis of PGs. It is concluded that the pyrogen increases PG synthesis not only in the PO/AH area, but when injected into the intracysternal space there is an increased synthesis of PGEs near the surface of the brain stem, and possibly other parts of the CNS. But to produce fever, the PG has to act on the PO/AH area.

Feeding

Davis et al. (58) reported evidence for a humoral factor which is present in rats that reduces food intake when the rats are hungry. This factor is apparently an inhibitor of feeding but is present only in ad lib fed rats or in rats only after several hours following a scheduled meal. Such a factor in the blood may be related to a long-term control of feeding, or energy balance, or to act as a signal for satiety. Davis et al. (58) reported experiments to test a hypothesis relating PGs and the hypothalamus in energy balance regulation. PGs may play a role in reducing the rate of lipolysis of adipose tissue, especially following activation of lipolytic processes over their basal levels. The assumption is that PGs produced in adipose tissue act on hypothalamic centers to modulate long-term control of feeding, and thus play a role in the maintenance of energy balance. This hypothesis requires the PG to be transported via blood, a portion of which escapes degradation in the lung and which can penetrate to hypothalamic areas, affecting feeding.

Baile et al. (59) studied the modulation of food intake possible by signals arising in adipose tissue that are concerned with theories of energy balance regulation. Their experiments tested the effects of some PGs produced in adipose tissue on food and water intake in rats. They postulate that some PGs may be components of a signal, relating fat depots and energy balance regulation. Previous work has reported that there are relationships between the state of energy balance and feeding behavior. However, the components of the proposed regulatory system are not known. It was proposed that the production in the fat depots of a (steroidlike) structure which stimulates feeding by acting on the hypothalamus could act as a feedback for regulating fat deposition. The concentration in plasma of the factor could vary inversely with the size of the fat depot. If the effect on feeding of PGs injected subcutaneously is mediated by the hypothalamus, then PGs injected into the hypothalamus result in decreased feeding. They postulate that the PG level may modulate the level of adiposity and modulate hypothalamic activity in such a way as to function as a component of a regulator signal for energy balance. Genetic obesity may be the result of insensitivity of a receptor to an endogenous PG. The rate of degradation resulted in less PG reaching the receptor and/or decreased production of endogenous PG. High levels of PGE_1 maintained by subcutaneous injections provided information concerning the proficiency of PGE as a long-term regulator of energy balance. Ten micrograms per 24 hr of PGE_1 resulted in a significant reduction of food intake. They have also shown that injections of PGE_1 in some areas of the medial hypothalamus decreased feeding and that a PG antagonist, polyphloretin phosphate, injected into the same site triggers feeding. Also, the PGE_1 injection blocks the feeding stimulated by NE injected into the same locus.

Martin and Baile (60) found that when PGE_1 was injected into the anterior hypothalamus, feeding decreased. PGE_1 and PGE_2 antagonized the NE effect on cerebellar Purkinje cells and reduced NE release from the sympathetic nerves; this is a possible explanation of the mechanism involved in the PG-elicited hypophagia. A series of experiments was designed to test the effects of PGE_1 and of an α and β, agonist and antagonist, on feeding behavior in sheep. Isoproterenol will elicit feeding in sheep injected intrahypothalamically, but if injected into the hypothalamus of rats will cause hypophagia. Injections of PGE_1 into the sheep hypothalamus will cause marked feeding and is blocked by propranolol. Polyphloretin phosphate, injected at α or β loci was similar to that of isoproterenol. The feeding effect produced by PGE_1 at the β loci was similar to that of isoproterenol. It has been suggested that a receptor modulating substance is either a PG or a substance promoting the synthesis of PG. The various effects are known to be associated with activation of adenyl cyclase. Whether the feeding effects in sheep following PGE_1 injection at β loci is related to change in adenyl cyclase level has not been shown.

Baile and Martin (61) have proposed that PGs may play a modulating role on hypothalamic areas controlling feeding and energy balance. In the medial hypothalamus of sheep they looked for an interaction between α- and β-receptors, PGE, and a PG antagonist, PPP. Sheep were prepared with six cannuli guides in the hypothalamus. In each sheep following preliminary injection of NE and isoproterenol, loci were selected that showed preferentially α- or β-receptor bound feeding. In a subsequent experiment, PGE_1 blocked NE-elicited feeding at the α-bound feeding loci but PGE_1 elicited the feeding when injected into the β-bound feeding loci. The PGE_1-elicited feeding was specifically blocked by a β antagonist (LB-46). The PPP elicited feeding in both α- and β-bound feeding loci, but the responses were blocked only by the α antagonist (phentolamine) in the α loci and by the β antagonist in the β loci. These responses lend support to our previous conclusions that injection of an α agonist into some, and a β agonist into other hypothalamic sites will elicit feeding. PGE_1, injected into loci showing differences in sensitivity to adrenoreceptor agonists which elicit feeding, results in increased feeding or decreased feeding, as shown previously. Thus we conclude that although it is unlikely that systemically produced PGs modulate hypothalamic controls on feeding and energy balance because of the dual effect on feeding, there may be an interaction of endogenous hypothalamic PG and adrenoreceptors.

Wishaw and Veale (62) studied the effect of PGE_1 and norepinephrine on the ingestive behavior of the rat. Norepinephrine or PGE_1 were injected directly into the hypothalamus in unrestrained, unanesthetized rats. The animals had free access to food and water. NE injected into the perifornical area of the hypothalamus, the hippocampus, and the amygdola elicited vigorous eating. PGE_1 did not produce eating, which differed from that observed following control injections of a physiological control solution. Drinking was not observed following injections of either saline or PGE_1. These data indicate that PGE_1 does not play a direct role in the hypothalamic and limbic control of eating behavior.

Pituitary

Zor et al. (63) indicate that there is a growing body of evidence suggesting that cyclic AMP may be involved in the regulation of the release and synthesis of some of the anterior pituitary hormones. Thus cyclic AMP enhanced the release of luteinizing hormone (LH), growth hormone (GH), thyroid-stimulating hormone (TSH), and prolactin, as indicated by several authors. There is consistent evidence that cyclic AMP is indeed the mediator of LH as well as of PG action on ovarian steroid oogenesis. However, although PGs mimic many of the actions of LH on the ovary, there is no conclusive evidence that the PGs provide an essential link in the causal chain connecting LH with adenyl cyclase activation. To establish the physiological role of the PGs, more information is required on the changes in ovarian PG production rate in response to LH and on the effects of inhibitors of the action of PG biosynthesis. The ovarian adenyl cyclase in the newborn rat responds very feebly to LH in vitro, although it is fully responsive to PG. It is possible that the regulatory subunits of both the ovarian adenyl cyclase and of the protein kinase are produced later than the catalytic portions of these enzymes in the course of postnatal development.

Varavudhi and Chobsieng (64) have done stereotaxic implantation of $PGF_{2\alpha}$ in the posterior part of the anterior pituitary and in the vicinity of the median eminance during various intervals of the active phase of pseudopregnancy. The anterior pituitary implantation on various sites showed significant shortened normal duration of pseudopregnancy of animals without $PGF_{2\alpha}$ implantation. The median eminance implant of the drug ($PGF_{2\alpha}$) failed to show clear-cut statistically shortened periods of pseudopregnancy. The mean duration of pseudopregnancy of these animals was 12 days. These results favor the possibility of a direct stimulating effect of $PGF_{2\alpha}$ on the release of pituitary LH in rats. Spies and Norman (65) infused PGE_1 into the third ventricle of rats on the afternoon of vaginal proestrus and reversed the pentobarbital blockade of ovulation in the majority of rats. Plasma levels of LH were higher in the PGE_1-infused females than in the pentobarbital-blocked controls, but the peak concentrations were only half as high and lasted only half as long as comparable values in normal proestrus females. PGE_1 was a more potent stimulator of ovulation in pentobarbital-blocked females than either PGE_2 or $PGF_{2\alpha}$. If infused into the pituitary or injected subcutaneously, however, PGE_1 failed to induce ovulation in pentobarbital-blocked animals. The data indicate that PGE_1 stimulates LH release and ovulation in the pentobarbital treated rat by activating a neurally controlled gonadotropin releasing mechanism.

Carlson et al. (66) indicate that studies might suggest that PGs of the E and F series may cause release of the adenohypophysial hormones, LH, GH, and prolactin. Indirect evidence exists that $PGF_{2\alpha}$ may stimulate LH release in the rat as cited in Ref. 64. Systemic infusion of $PGF_{2\alpha}$ in sheep with autotransplanted ovaries resulted in an increase in the progesterone secretion rate. This increase might have resulted from a direct or indirect effect of $PGF_{2\alpha}$ on the pituitary. Further evidence for a pituitary effect was obtained following the subcutaneous injection of $PGF_{2\alpha}$ into normal ewes while studying the estrus-cycle control. In four ewes $PGF_{2\alpha}$ brought about small increases in the concentration of LH in the venous plasma. In each ewe the rise in plasma $PGF_{2\alpha}$ concentration preceded the increase in plasma LH concentration.

In view of these findings, the effects of intracarotid infusions of $PGF_{2\alpha}$ on LH release were examined at midcycle and during anestrus. Between days 5 and 10 of the estrus cycle, a sharp increase in LH concentration in the venous plasma was noted following the intracarotid infusion of $PGF_{2\alpha}$. Similar amounts of $PGF_{2\alpha}$ infused into the carotid artery of two ovariectimized ewes during anestrus failed to elicit a release of LH. Intracarotid infusions given to four ewes during anestrus in small doses failed to increase plasma LH levels. The finding of a second LH peak in the cycling ewe 10.5 hr after $PGF_{2\alpha}$ infusion was unexpected.

In order to determine whether estrogen secretion by the ovary was stimulated by the initial LH release, estradiol concentration from the jugular vein was measured following an intracarotid infusion of $PGF_{2\alpha}$. It is possible that the initial peak of LH released during $PGF_{2\alpha}$ infusion stimulated the ovary to secrete estrogen, which in turn brought about a secondary release of LH by a positive feedback mechanism. Alternatively, the pituitary-hypothalamic response to $PGF_{2\alpha}$ may have released FSH and/or other trophic hormones, in addition to LH, resulting in estrogen synthesis by the ovary. These results indicate that small doses of $PGF_{2\alpha}$ can trigger LH release from the anterior pituitary of the ewe only during the breeding season. It would, therefore, appear that $PGF_{2\alpha}$ may act primarily at the level of the hypothalamus, although at this time it is not possible to rule out a direct action of $PGF_{2\alpha}$ on the pituitary. The evidence for PG-mediated ACTH release, however, indicates an indirect route through the hypothalamus. Since previous studies in the sheep indicate that the peripheral levels of $PGF_{2\alpha}$ do not show any significant elevation at the time of ovulation, it is unlikely that circulating levels of $PGF_{2\alpha}$ are directly responsible for LH release. It is not known whether synthesis of either $PGF_{2\alpha}$ or PGE_1 is required at the pituitary-hypothalamic level for the normal release of LH in ewes, as has been postulated for the rat. It is possible that the observation may represent a pharmacological effect of $PGF_{2\alpha}$ on the pituitary-hypothalamic system; nevertheless, the results suggest that synthesis of PG at the pituitary/hypothalamic level may be involved in the process of LH release.

Labhsetwar and Zolovick (67) suggest that the hypothalamic tissue contains a relatively higher concentration of catecholamines and PGs than do other regions of the brain. Both catecholamines and PGs have been reported to promote gonadotropic secretions in appropriate conditions, but whether or not they interact in any other way in the CNS to modulate gonadatropin secretion for ovulation is not known. Following their initial finding that $PGF_{2\alpha}$ stimulates LH synthesis in the pituitary gland, these authors thought that PG may potentiate the adrenergic transmission in the hypothalamus which is normally required for the secretion of gonadotropins. If this hypothesis is true, a direct application of aspirin to the hypothalamus but not to other brain areas or to the pituitary gland should result in inhibition of ovulation, and this blockade should be reversible not only by excess PGs, but also by a catecholamine such as dopamine. The results indicate that hypothalamic injection of aspirin interferes with progesterone-induced ovulation by blocking PG synthesis in the anterior hypothalamic area. As the stimulatory effects of progesterone on ovulation are transmitted through the α-adrenergic pathway in the hypothalamus, they also indicate that catecholamines and $PGF_{2\alpha}$ interact to potentiate the adrenergic transmission for gonadotropin secretion. The results indicate that there is a functional significance for a high level of PGs in the hypothalamus for the first time.

Harms et al. (68) injected PGs intravenously, intraventricularly, or into the anterior pituitary gland to evaluate the possible participation in the control of gonadotropin release. The effect on plasma LH was determined by radioimmunoassay. Intravenous injection of PGE_2 produced a slight increase in plasma LH in ovariectimized animals. Other PGs were ineffective. The third ventricular injections of PGE_2 produced a marked increase in plasma LH in ovariectimized animals (80). The increase was much greater than that observed following intravenous injection (81). Ovariectimized animals were injected prior to an experiment with estradiol benzoate to sensitize the pituitary to the gonadotropin releasing factors. In these animals injections in the third ventricle of PGE_2 produced a dose-related increase in plasma LH. A significant increase was also obtained with PGE_1. The results indicate that

PGE_2 and to a lesser extent PGE_1 had a specific effect in stimulating the release of LH by the adenohypophysis. The principal site of action appears to be in the central nervous system, with another, less important site on the anterior pituitary itself. The findings suggest that PGE_2 and possibly PGE_1 are involved in neural control of the pituitary gonadotropin release.

Poulain and Carette (69) studied the release of adenohypophyseal hormones in rats. For example, PGE_2 elicits a rise in serum LH. In the sheep, $PGF_{2\alpha}$ increases the level of LH. There is some evidence that the endogenous synthesis of PGs at the hypothalamohypophyseal level may be involved in the process of LH release (82). In order to determine a possible effect of PGE_2 and PGF_2 of the site of recording, these substances were applied by iontophoresis for electrophysiological recording from single cell bodies located in preoptic and septal areas and the arcuate area of the guinea pig. These neurons both contain LH releasing factor, have axons terminating in the median eminance, and may be involved in the control of ovulation. Experiments were performed on 12 female guinea pigs, and of the 77 cells studied, 38 showed antidromic activation. Of the total number of units investigated, 57 responded significantly to brief applications of PGE_2 or $PGF_{2\alpha}$ by a prolonged increase in their firing rate. The discharge of some cells was inhibited; 13 neurons failed to exhibit any marked response.

Most cells tested with PGE_2 or $PGF_{2\alpha}$ responded with an increase in their firing rate, but the time course of this activation was not uniform and the excitation could be divided into three types according to the latency of onset: (1) excitation is slow in onset and long-lasting, which was the most characteristic feature of PG activation; (2) excitation was rapid in onset; and (3) strong excitation, slow in onset. In the three types, desensitization was frequently observed in subsequent applications when PG failed to excite neurons to the same extent as the first application. Although the role of PGs in the brain is not yet clear, certain general observations were reported: iontophoretic activation outlasts the time of application, and tachyphylaxis often occurs. This study was the first documented example of the characteristic features of PG activation at the hypothalamic level. There is no significant difference between the excitatory effects of both PGs in the different areas of the hypothalamus. The data suggest that the discharge of most cells in the preoptic and septal areas and the arcuate area are affected by PGE_2 or $PGF_{2\alpha}$ and the predominant influence is a long-lasting activation with very small amounts of substances. Although no correlation can presently be established between iontophoretic activation of these neurons and their possible function with respect to the adenohypophysis, it could be argued that PGs might have the capacity for firing the hypothalamic neurons implicated in the control of gonadotropic secretions.

Ojeda et al. (70) injected PGE_2 into the third ventricle of intact or castrated conscious male rats and found markedly increased plasma LH titers 30 min after its injection. PGE_1 injected at a similar dose slightly increased plasma LH in intact rats. These results indicate that PGE_2 and to a lesser extent PGE_1 specifically stimulate gonadotropin release in the male rat, possibly by a direct action on the central nervous system. They support the hypothesis that PGE_2 and perhaps PGE_1 play a physiological role in the neural control of pituitary gonadotropin release.

Sato et al. (71) designed a study to ascertain whether or not PGs act directly on the pituitary. In one experiment, the plasma LH levels were decreased 24 hr after the production of hypothalamic lesions in ovariectimized mature rats. Ten minutes after the injection of PGE_1, PGE_2, or $PGF_{2\alpha}$, the plasma LH levels increased significantly. Following direct microinjection of PGE_1 or PGE_2 into the rat pituitary, plasma LH was increased. However, $PGF_{2\alpha}$ failed to increase the plasma LH levels. In the last experiment, the effect of PGE_1, PGE_2, or $PGF_{2\alpha}$ on in vitro pituitary release was studied. The addition of all three PGs to the incubation medium produced a significant increase in LH release. These observations indicate that sufficient dosages of PGs can also stimulate LH secretion by acting directly on the pituitary. A major site of action of PGs appears to be at the hypothalamus, as indicated by their observations of the decreased LH releasing hormone content in the hypothalamus, and the increased plasma LH levels following intravenous injection of PGs and the increased plasma LH levels following microinjection of PGs into the third ventricle or the median eminence in rats. The plasma LH levels in rats with hypothalamic lesions are lower than those of rats with an intact hypothalamus following PG treatment. It is possible that a major site of action of the PG-induced plasma LH secretion may be on the hypothalamic-pituitary access rather than in the pituitary. These authors indicate that PGE may act by mediating or modulating the action of synaptic transmitters such as NE or DA, since PG has been implicated in transmission of adrenergic ganglia in the cerebellum. PGs may also bring about the effect via cyclic AMP as PGs augment the anterior pituitary adenyl cyclase.

Chobsieng et al. (72) studied the stimulatory effect of PGE_2 on LH release in the rat and give evidence for a hypothalamic site of action. Intravenous PGE_2 was administered to immature male and female rats and an increase in the serum level of LH was observed. The effect was presented by prior administration of an antiserum to the hypothalamus LH releasing hormone. LH release from rat pituitary in vitro was not stimulated by PGE_2. It is inferred that the stimulatory effect of PGE_2 on LH is not a direct one on the pituitary gland, but is exerted at the level of the hypothalamus. Chobsieng et al. (72) suggest that further study is required to determine whether PGE_2 is merely exerting a pharmacological effect on the hypothalamic secretions of the gonadotropin releasing hormone.

Anti-LH releasing hormone serum may also prove to be a useful tool in studying the site of action of neurotransmitters in other substances affecting gonadotropin release. Sato et al. (73) have studied the effects of indomethacin on hypothalamic pituitary system in rats. Previous to their study, injections of indomethacin did not block LH release but exerted its antiovulatory action directly on the ovary. It is also accepted that PGs have stimulatory effects at various levels of the hypothalamic pituitary system.

Sato et al. (73), using adult female rats 5 weeks after ovariectomy, determined plasma and pituitary levels of LH using radioimmunoassay. After treatment with 3 mg of indomethacin, for 5 days, the serum LH level was significantly decreased compared to control group. The decreased serum LH induced with indomethacin covered half the administration of $PGF_{2\alpha}$. There was no change in pituitary level content after the injection of indomethacin, whereas implantation of the drug into the median eminance induced a significant increase in pituitary LH content as well as a decrease in serum LH. The response of the pituitary to exogenous LH releasing hormone was significantly lowered in the indomethacin-treated group than in the control group, although plasma LH level in the treated rats was not significantly different from those of the control animals. PGE_2 injected into the third ventricle of spayed rats produced a rise in plasma LH, 15 min after treatment, and this was maintained throughout the period studied. However, this effect was abolished by pretreatment with indomethacin. It appears that the release of LH releasing hormone from the hypothalamus and LH from the anterior pituitary is affected by indomethacin, and it is suggested that PGs may serve as one of local regulatory agents of cell function and are involved in the control of the hypothalamus and pituitary system.

Exogenous $PGF_{2\alpha}$ is luteolytic in many mammalian species and possibly considered to be the physiological luteolytic agent in some species. However, the mechanism(s) of $PGF_{2\alpha}$-induced luteolysis is less clear. Hypotheses which have been proposed thus far to explain the luteolytic action of $PGF_{2\alpha}$ include: (1) reduction of ovarian blood flow as a result of constriction of the utero-ovarian vein; (2) reduction of luteal blood supply due to an increase in shunt flow in the arteriovenous (A-V) anastomoses in the corpus luteum; (3) release of a luteolytic level of LH by the pituitary; (4) antagonism of gonadotropin maintenance of luteal function; and (5) $PGF_{2\alpha}$-dependent inhibition of gonadotropin uptake in vivo is due to restricted access of luteal cells to gonadotropin caused by a decrease in capillary permeability or impaired interstitial diffusion of gonadotropin within the corpus luteum (74).

Warberg et al. (75) reviewed the structure-activity relationships of PG-induced relationships of PG-induced release of anterior pituitary released hormones. PGs of the E, F, A, or B series were infused into a lateral ventricle of the brain of adult male rats and the efficacy of each PG to stimulate the discharge of LH, prolactin, and TSH from the pituitary gland was determined. PGE_2, $PGF_{2\alpha}$, and $PGF_{2\beta}$ were found to be potent stimulators of LH release. The release was considerably less when PGE_1, $F_{1\beta}$, A_2, and B_2 were infused. The basal release of LH was not altered by others. It is suggested that the cis double bond and the 5, 6-position and the 11-hydroxy group are essential for the LH releasing activity of PGs and that these functional groups may be important for activation of a receptor at the level of the brain. Prolactin secretion was stimulated six- to sevenfold by the infusion of PGE_2. $PGF_{2\beta}$ caused a three- to fourfold increase in plasma prolactin concentration. It was the only other PG-stimulating prolactin release. None of the PGs infused intraventricularly affected TSH secretion.

Kuhl et al. (76) studied the effect of PGs on hypothalamic cysteine arylamidase activity (CAA) and on LH secretion in the rat. The effect of intravenous injections of several PGs of CAA in the hypothalamus in the rat was investigated. PGA_1, PGE_1, and $PGF_{2\alpha}$, and PGE_2 stimulated the enzyme activity within 30 min by approximately 60-100%. In contrast to LH, which stimulated hypothalamic arylamidase only in synergism with sex steroids, the enzyme activity with both intact and ovariectomized female rats and of immature rats was increased when the animals were treated with PGE_2. LH and PGE_2 at suboptimal doses were additive in their effect, whereas optimal doses failed to do so. Aspirin did not block the stimulatory action of LH on CAA, indicating that this effect of LH was not mediated by the PGs. CAA had previously been shown to inactivate LH-releasing hormone in all probability to be involved in the short feedback mechanism of LH. PGs seem to act as modulators in this system, since they were found to mimic the effect of LH on this enzyme. An intravenous dose of 15 μg of PGE_2 caused a significant increase in plasma LH within 7.5 min in intact diestrus rats, whereas ovariectomized, estrogen-progesterone treated rats showed the effect between 7.5 and 30 min after the intravenous injection, when the plasma LH values were significantly higher. Thus LH is capable of stimulating CAA in the rat hypothalamus. This enzyme could also be shown to inactivate LH releasing hormone.

Growth Hormone

Szabo and Frohman (77) sought to develop a sensitive in vivo model for GH-releasing activity in porcine median eminence extracts to compare the GH releasing effects of the median eminence of PGE_2 and to study the effect of somatostatin on the foregoing stimuli. The use of the 1-day estrogen-primed male rat is a model sensitive to an injection of extracts from the median eminence of the porcine stock. Neither increasing the duration of estrogen pretreatment nor reserpine resulted in a greater response. The GH-releasing effects of porcine stock-related eminence extracts were related directly to the preinjection of GH level. Two successive injections of somatostatin at 30-min intervals evoked similar responses; in contrast to PGE_2, effects were not potentiated by estrogen pretreatment and were independent of the preinjection level. The GH-releasing effect of somatostatin is not related to its content of TRH. These results provided evidence for the direct inhibitory effect of somatostatin on GH secretion in vivo and suggest that somatostatin is capable of blocking a variety of different stimuli to GH release.

Sundberg et al. (78) studied the effect of various PGs and a PG synthetase on rat anterior cyclic AMP levels and hormone release in vitro. They suggested that PGs might mediate the effect of some hormones via adenyl cyclase activity of their target organs. It has already been shown that several PGs stimulate the pituitary adenyl cyclase and increase cyclic AMP concentrations in the intact gland, while they have also been shown to increase GH release in vitro. Furthermore, it has been shown that a PG antagonist (7-oxy-13-prostanoic-acid) inhibits GH release and TSH release in vitro. The effects of PGEs E_1, E_2, $F_{1\alpha}$, $F_{2\alpha}$, and indomethacin were studied on rat anterior cyclic AMP levels and the concomitant levels of LH, GH, TSH, and prolactin in vitro. In summary: (1) PGs E_1, E_2, $F_{1\alpha}$, or $F_{2\alpha}$ increased the release of GH with a parallel increase in cyclic AMP, intracellularly; and (2) none of the PGs consistently affected either the basal release of LH or prolactin. Indomethacin inhibited GH release and at high doses inhibited prolactin release. It had no significant effect on intracellular cyclic AMP concentration.

TSH

Brown and Hedge (79) reviewed several PGs for effects on basal and TSH secretion in anesthetized female rats. The PGs were given intravenously or were stereotaxically directed into the medial basal hypothalamus or anterior pituitary. Plasma TSH levels were measured by radioimmunoassay. PGs A_1, B_1, E_1, and $F_{1\alpha}$ were tested. These PGs were without effect on TSH secretion; however, all of the PGs potentiated the response of the pituitary to subsequent administration of TRH, the releasing hormone. This effect was observed only when PGs were injected directly into the anterior pituitary. When administered intravenously, all the PGs failed to exhibit this effect. One, PGE_1, inhibited the response to TRH. This appears to be secondary to the cardiovascular effects of the PGE that are evident at the dose used intravenously. It is concluded that the PGs may play a more subtle role in the control of the regulation of TSH secretion, as indicated by the potentiation of the stimulatory effect of TRH.

DISTRIBUTION OF PROSTAGLANDINS AND ITS EFFECT ON THE CENTRAL AND PERIPHERAL NERVOUS SYSTEM

Prostaglandins are extremely ubiquitous substances affecting almost every tissue or cell type and generally accompanied by an increase in intracellular cyclic nucleotide levels of cyclic AMP.

One distinguishing phenomenon of these compounds from the physiologically accepted neurotransmitters is that neither the classical prostaglandins, endoperoxides, thromboxanes, or prostacyclin seem to be stored in any measurable quantities in cells. Instead, the release of these fatty acid molecules from cells or tissues represents neosynthesis and not the release of preformed stored substances (83, 84). However, the synthesis of prostaglandinlike molecules by the fatty acid cyclooxygenase (i.e., prostaglandin synthetase) appears to depend on substrate availability. The addition of prostaglandin precursor fatty acids rapidly stimulates prostaglandin biosynthesis. Interestingly, considerable amounts of precursor acids are found in membrane phospholipids (85), and the rate of synthesis can be stimulated by substances that contain high concentrations of phospholipase A, which can selectively remove the fatty acid from the 2-position of the phospholipid. Agents such as snake venom can increase the rate of synthesis. Triglycerides have been reported to serve also as a precursor for prostaglandin biosynthesis (86). Evidence suggests that prostaglandins are synthesized and released coincident with hormonal or by mechanical stimulation of cells and that they act as either positive or negative regulators of hormone action (87-89); the prostaglandins are then metabolized at or near their original site of biosynthesis (90-92). These properties suggest that the prostaglandins can serve as local hormones or modulators in the central and peripheral nervous systems. That the prostaglandins have a limited effect is also observed by their very short half-life in the circulation. Most of the prostaglandins are almost totally metabolized by a single passage through the lungs (93).

Prostaglandins appear to be naturally occurring constituents of normal mammalian central nervous tissue and are also found in perfusates of cerebral cortex and in cerebrospinal fluid (94,95). Gray matter appears to have the highest overall concentration, and the medulla was subsequently reported to have the lowest concentration of E-type prostaglandins (96). Generally, prostaglandin $F_{2\alpha}$ has been shown to predominate. This is of particular interest since endorphins and the phenomenon of stimulus-produced analgesia (SPA) has been demonstrated in the mesencephalic periacqueductal gray area. The possible role of prostaglandins acting as a modulator or neurotransmitter in affecting analgesia produced by the endorphins or by SPA awaits further scientific clarification. Wolfe et al. (97) have shown, in vitro, that the endogenous biosynthesis of prostaglandins in rat cerebral cortex is stimulated by dopamine, norepinephrine, and adrenochrome. Serotonin has also been shown to increase prostaglandin output in dog cerebral ventricles (8) and by afferent nerve stimulation, release from frog spinal cord, and cerebral cortex in the cat. SPA and morphine analgesia can be altered by pharmacologically manipulating central pools of dopamine, serotonin, and norepinephrine (98). Serotonin has also been shown to alter prostaglandins in dog cerebral ventricles (97).

Stimulation of sympathetic or parasympathetic nerves in adipose tissue (99), rat stomach (100,101), spleen, and other tissues and organs has been shown to release prostaglandins, especially E_2 and $F_{2\alpha}$. Data suggest that the postsynaptic effector cell membrane is the site of synthesis and release by peripheral nerve stimulation. Hedqvist (102) has suggested that prostaglandin E_2 might act as a negative feedback regulator of norepinephrine release from the presynaptic terminals. Prostaglandins of the F type have been shown to have a facilitating action (103,104). In addition, there are studies in which PGE_1 and PGE_2 have antagonistic effects (105,106), lending further support of a problem presented in the context of the Yin-Yang hypothesis (107).

The amount of norepinephrine released from sympathetic nerves is considered to be controlled by the frequency of nerve impulses arriving at the nerve ending, whereas the quantitative release per impulse is subject to neuronal and humoral regulation via presynaptically located receptors (108, 109). Modulators include the transmitter itself acting via presynaptic α- and β-adrenergic receptors, angiotensin, acetylcholine, adenosine triphosphate (ATP), and E-type prostaglandins. Prostaglandins can inhibit norepinephrine release due to nerve stimulation or depolarization by K^+ (110). Additionally, prostaglandins are released from many tissues during sympathetic nerve stimulation or infusion of adrenergic agonists (111, 112). It has thus been postulated that E-type prostaglandins may regulate norepinephrine release and hence modulate sympathetic neurotransmission (113). Evidence to support PGE modulation of norepinephrine release from CNS preparations are contradictory, possibly related to differences in preparations and methods of evoking norepinephrine release. However, it has been demonstrated that there is a reduction in norepinephrine release from rat brain slices by PGE_2 (114), that PGE_2 can also decrease norepinephrine overflow from rat hypothalamic synaptosomes (115) and that PGE_2 may not induce a reduction in norepinephrine overflow in similar preparations (116, 117), and that PGE_2 can reduce, dose dependently, the evoked overflow in rat cerebral cortex slices (118).

Prostaglandins can alter the local nervous tissue milieu by the role played by the ability of various vascular regions to convert arachidonic acid to prostaglandins. The relative distribution of the locally formed prostaglandins differs between the regions, indicating the existence of a certain tissue specificity in the expression of the biosynthesis of prostaglandins. For example, prostacyclin appears to be the quantitatively most important prostaglandin in the human coronary and skeletal muscle vasculatures, whereas in the renal medulla, prostaglandins of the D, E, F, and I series appear to be formed in mainly equal amounts (119). However the prostaglandins affect nervous tissue, it is presently thought that their biological activity is due to their rapid metabolism within the tissues, rather short lasting and accordingly confined to the vicinity of the sites of synthesis. However, the most interesting prostaglandin from a physiological point of view is PGI_2 (6, 9α-epoxy-11α, 15S-dihydroxyprosta-5, 13-dienoic acid) prostacyclin, isolated by Moncada et al. in 1976 (120). PGI_2 is a possible candidate for the role of a naturally occurring systemic vasoregulating agent. By this action PGI_2 can have widespread effects in the central and peripheral nervous systems. It is not inactivated in the lung (121, 122) and is almost as potent as PGE_1 in its vasodilating activity (121). Its synthesis is widespread, being undertaken actively by arterial vascular tissue (123). In addition, PGI_2 is a potent inhibitor of platelet aggregation (120).

Thus it appears that the prostaglandins can affect the peripheral and central nervous system primarily through their local vasoregulating action, possibly directly by altering neurotransmitter release or by receptor interaction and indirectly through some local feedback system. PGE_1 and PGE_2 have been shown to reduce the vasoconstrictor responses of the perfused cat hind limb induced by sympathetic nerve stimulation (124). In contrast to this inhibitory effect of the PGEs, Kadowitz et al. (103) have found that $PGF_{2\alpha}$ enhanced transmitter release from adrenergic nerve terminals in the cutaneous vascular bed. PGE_2 and $PGF_{2\alpha}$ have also been found to be ineffective at altering the release of neurotransmitter in a number of preparations (124). Bergstrom et al. (114) have shown that PGE_2 (1×10^{-6} M) reduced the stimulation-induced outflow of [^{3}H]NE from rat brain slices. However, Roberts and Hillier (125) have reported that similar concentrations of PGE_2 (1×10^{-6} M) induced an increase in [^{3}H]NE release from synaptosomes. Wendel and Strandhoy (115) have shown that the release of [^{3}H]NE from synaptosomes isolated from rat hypothalami is multiphasic, with an initial fast release phase followed by a slower release phase. PGE_2 (1×10^{-6} M) attenuated [^{3}H]NE release during the fast phase and reduced the amount of [^{3}H]NE released due to KCl stimulation. At lower concentrations of PGE_2 there was no change in the release profile. $PGF_{2\alpha}$ was without effect on [^{3}H]NE release at several concentrations tested.

Prostaglandins, especially prostacyclin and thromboxane A_2, interact with the neurotransmitter serotonin through the mechanism of hemostasis. The importance of serotonin in the neurophysiology of pain is well documented and it is now thought that morphine analgesia is partially produced by activation of a descending inhibitory serotonergic tract from the raphe cell bodies located in the pons and upper brain stem. Further, afferent nerve endings are stimulated by bradykinin, which can concomitantly cause a release of E-type prostaglandins (126). Prostaglandins, particularly those of the E type, have been shown to reproduce several signs of acute inflammation, including vasodilatation, increased permeability, local edema, and pain. Prostaglandins at physiological doses have also been shown to produce sensitization to the inflammatory properties of other mediators, such as histamine and serotonin (127). Collier and Schneider (128) found $PGF_{2\alpha}$ to lack a nociceptive effect following intraperitoneal injection in mice. Further studies concluded that $PGF_{2\alpha}$ does not inhibit the effect of the algesic substance E-type prostaglandins, only the pain-enhancing action of the PGE released by bradykinin (129).

Paravascular nociceptors have been described by electron microscopic studies (130, 131) to have thin myelinated or nonmyelinated afferent fibers (132) and are thought to exist in two subdivisions, the mechanical and the thermal nociceptors (133). It has been suggested (134) that some substances, such as serotonin, may be presensitizing the tissue so that bradykinin and other algogens become more effective stimulators of nociceptors.

Thromboxane A_2, prostacyclin, and prostaglandin endoperoxides have been shown to be involved in the inflammatory process. Of particular interest, evidence in the last few years has shown that slow-reacting substance in anaphylaxis (SRS-A) could be a product of arachidonic acid (135). The name leukotriene has been introduced as a generic name for eicosanoids such as SRS, which are noncyclyzed C-20 carboxylic acids with one or two oxygen substituents and three conjugated double bonds (136, 137). Leukotrienes share certain structural features with some oxygenated products of arachidonic acid in human and rabbit PMNs (138). It is not presently known whether these compounds are identical to SRS-A released from the lungs, but these findings highlight the importance of the products of the different lipoxygenases in cell migration, inflammation, and in other conditions, such as increased mediator release and airway reactivity during asthma or anaphylaxis (139). The study of interactions between lipid peroxides, the newly described leukotrienes, and the prostacyclin/thromboxane A_2 system with neurotransmitters will undoubtedly lead to further research to elucidate their function and role in the peripheral and central nervous systems.

ACKNOWLEDGMENT

Stan Greenberg's contribution to this chapter is the result of research conducted as a recipient of Research Career Development Award NHLBI, HL-00231-01, and HL-00428-02.

REFERENCES

1. Coceani, F. Prostaglandins and the central nervous system. Arch. Intern. Med. 133:119-129, 1974.
2. Wolfe, L. S. Possible roles of prostaglandins in the nervous system. In Advances in Neurochemistry, Vol. 1, B. W. Agranoff and M. H. Aprison (Eds.). Plenum Press, New York, pp. 1-49, 1975.
3. Coceani, F., Puglisi, L., and Lavers, B. Prostaglandins and neuronal activity in spinal cord and cuneati nucleus. Ann. N.Y. Acad. Sci. 180: 289-301, 1971.
4. Ramwell, P. W., and Shaw, J. E. Spontaneous and evoked release of prostaglandins from the cerebral cortex of anesthetized cats. Am. J. Physiol. 211:125-134, 1966.
5. Bradley, P. B., and Elkes, J. The effect of some drugs on the electrical activity of the brain. Brain 80:77-117, 1957.
6. Bradley, P. B., Samuels, G. M. R., and Shaw, J. E. Correlation of prostaglandin release from the cerebral cortex of cats with electrocorticogram following stimulation of the reticular formation. Br. J. Pharmacol. 37:151-157, 1969.
7. Raffel, G., Peskar, B. A., Hertting, G., and Clarenba, P. Synthesis and release of prostaglandin by rat brain snaptosomal fractions. J. Neurochem. 26:493-498, 1976.
8. Holmes, S. W. The spontaneous release of prostaglandins into the cerebral ventricles of the dog and the effect of external factors on this release. Br. J. Pharmacol. 38:653-658, 1970.
9. Berti, F., Trabucchi, M., Bernareggi, V., and Fumagalli, R. The effects of prostaglandins on cAMP formation in cerebral cortex of different mammalian species. Pharmacol. Res. Commun. 4(3):253-259, 1972.

10. Berti, F. and Fumagalli, R. The effects of prostaglandins on cAMP formation. Adv. Biosci. 9:475-480, 1973.
11. Collier, H. O. J., and Roy, A. C. Morphine-like drugs inhibit the stimulation of E-prostaglandins of cAMP formation in rat brain homogenate. Nature (Lond.) 248:24-27, 1974.
12. Abdulla, Y. H., and McFarlane, E. Control of adenyl kinase by PGE_2 and PGE_3. Biochem. Pharmacol. 20:1726-1730, 1971.
13. Abdulla, Y. H., and McFarlane, E. Control of PG biosynthesis in rat brain homogenates by adenine nucleotides. Biochem. Pharmacol. 21: 2841-2847, 1972.
14. Wellman, W., and Schwabe, U. Effects of PGs E_1, E_2 and F_{2a} on cAMP levels in brain in vivo. Brain Res. 59:371-378, 1973.
15. Dismukes, K., and Daly, J. W. Accumulation of adenosine 3',5'-monophosphate in rat brain slices: effects of PGs. Life Sci. 17:199-210, 1975.
16. Tell, G. P., Pasternak, G. W., and Cuatrecases, P. Brain and caudate nucleus adenylate cyclase: effects of dopamine, GTP, PGEs and morphine. FEBS Lett. 51(1):242-245, 1975.
17. Goldberg, N. D., O'Dea, R. F., and Haddox, M. K. Cyclic AMP. Adv. Cyclic Nucl. Res. 3:156-223, 1973.
18. Horton, E. W. Actions of PGE_1, E_2 and E_3 on the central nervous system. Br. J. Pharmacol. 22:189-192, 1964.
19. Hedqvist, P. Control by PGE_2 of sympathetic neurotransmission in the spleen. Life Sci. 9:269-278, 1970.
20. Steiner, L., Forester, D. M. C., Bergvall, U., and Carlsson, L. A. Effect of PGE_1 on cerebral circulatory disturbances. Proc. 5th Int. Symp. Part II. Eur. Neurol. 8:23-31, 1972.
21. Yamamoto, Y. L., Feidel, W., Wolfe, L. S., Katoh, H., and Hodge, C. P. Effects of PGs on cerebral blood flow. Proc. 5th Int. Symp. Part I. Eur. Neurol. 6:144-152, 1972.
22. Pickard, J. D. The mechanism of action of $PGF_{2\alpha}$ on cerebral flow in the baboon. J. Physiol. (Lond.) 234(2):46P-47P, 1973.
23. Pickard, J. D., and Mackenzie, E. T. Inhibition of PG synthesis and the response of baboon cerebral circulation to carbon dioxide. Nature (New Biol.) 245(145):187-188, 1973.
24. Emerson, T. E., Jr., Radawski, D., Veenendaal, M., and Daugherty, R. M., Jr. Effects of cerebral ventricular, systemic, and local administration of $PGF_{2\alpha}$ on canine cerebral hemodynamics. Prostaglandins 8(6):521-530, 1974.
25. Staszewska-Barczak, J., and Vane, J. R. Role of prostaglandins in the local control of circulation. Clin. Exp. Pharmacol. Physiol. Suppl. 2: 71-78, 1975.
26. Collier, H. O. J., and Roy, A. C. Inhibition of PGE-sensitive adenyl cyclase as the mechanism of morphine analgesia. Prostaglandins 7(5): 361-376, 1974.

27. Collier, H. O. J., McDonald-Gibson, W., and Saeed, S. A. Morphine and apomorphine stimulate PG production by rabbit brain homogenate. Br. J. Pharmacol. 52(1):116P, 1974.
28. Ferri, S., Santagostino, A., Braga, P. C., and Galatulas, I. Decreased antinociceptive effect of morphine in rats treated intravenously with PGE_1. Psychopharmacologia 39(3):231-235, 1974.
29. Singh, K. P., and Bhandari, D. S. Neuropharmacological study of $PGF_{2\alpha}$. J. Indian Med. Assoc. 61(10):423-427, 1973.
30. Ferreira, S. H., Moncada, S., and Vane, J. R. Prostaglandins and the mechanism of analgesia produced by aspirin-like drugs. Br. J. Pharmacol. 49:86-97, 1973.
31. Kakunaga, T., Kaneto, H., and Hano, K. Pharmacologic studies of analgesia. J. Pharmacol. Exp. Ther. 153:134-144, 1966.
32. Haubrich, D. R., Perez-Cruet, J., and Reid, W. D. PGE_1 causes sedation and increases in 5-HT turnover in rat brain. Br. J. Pharmacol. 48:80-87, 1973.
33. Milton, A. S. PGE_1 and endotoxin fever, and the effects of aspirin, indomethacin and paracetanol. Adv. Biosci. 9:495-500, 1973.
34. Milton, A. S., and Wendlandt, S. A possible role for PGE_1 as a modulation for temperature regulation in the CNS of the cat. J. Physiol. (Lond.) 20:76P-77P, 1970.
35. Veale, W. L., and Cooper, K. E. Species differences in the pharmacology of temperature regulation. In The Pharmacology of Thermoregulation, E. Schonbaum and P. Lomax (Eds.). Karger, Basel, pp. 1-583, 1973.
36. Feldberg, W., and Saxena, P. N. Further studies on PGE_1 fever in cats. J. Physiol. (Lond.) 219(3):739-745, 1971.
37. Hales, J. R., Bennett, J. W., Baird, J. A., and Fawcett, A. A. Thermoregulatory effects of prostaglandins E_1, E_2, F_1, and F_2 in the sheep. Pfluegers Arch. 339(2):125-133, 1973.
38. Bligh, J., Cottle, W. H., and Maskrey, M. Influence of ambient temperature on the thermoregulatory response to 5-HT, NE, and ACh injected into the lateral cerebral ventricles of sheep, goats and rabbits. J. Physiol. (Lond.) 212:377-392, 1971.
39. Avery, D. D. Thermoregulatory effects of intrahypothalamic injections of adrenergic and cholinergic substances at different environmental temperatures. J. Physiol. (Lond.) 222:257-266, 1972.
40. Lipton, J. M., Welch, J. P., and Clark, W. G. Changes in body temperature produced by injecting PGE_1, EGTA and bacterial endotoxins into the PO/AH region and the medulla oblongata of the rat. Experientia 29:806-808, 1973.
41. Bligh, J., and Milton, A. S. The thermoregulatory effects of PGE_1 when infused into the lateral cerebral ventricle of the Welsh Mountain sheep at different ambient temperatures. J. Physiol. (Lond.) 229(1): 30P-31P, 1973.

42. Myers, R. D., and Veale, W. L. The role of sodium and calcium ions in the hypothalamus in the control of body temperature of the unanesthetized cat. J. Physiol. (Lond.) 212:411–430, 1971.
43. Dey, P. K., Feldberg, W., Gupta, K. P., Milton, A. S., and Wendlant, S. Further studies on the role of prostaglandins in fever. J. Physiol. (Lond.) 241:629-646, 1974.
44. Baird, J. A., Hales, J. R. S., and Lang, W. J. Thermoregulatory responses to the injection of monoamines, ACh and prostaglandins into a lateral cerebral ventrical of the echidna. J. Physiol. (Lond.) 236(3): 539-548, 1974.
45. Ford, D. M. A selective action of PGE_1 on hypothalamic neurons in the cat which respond to brain cooling. J. Physiol. (Lond.) 242(2):142P-143P, 1974.
46. Stitt, J. T., Hardy, J. D., and Stolwijk, J. E. PGE_1 fever: its effects on thermoregulation at different low ambient temperatures. Am. J. Physiol. 227(3):622-629, 1974.
47. Veale, W. L., and Cooper, K. E. Prostaglandin in cerebro spinal fluid following perfusion of hypothalamic tissue. J. Appl. Physiol. 37:942-945, 1974.
48. Cooper, K. E., and Veale, W. L. The effects of reserpine and atropine, injected into the lateral cerebral ventricle, on fever due to intravenous leukocyte pyrogen and hypothalamic injection of PGE_1 in the unanesthetized rabbit. J. Physiol. (Lond.) 241(1):25P-26P, 1974.
49. Laburn, H. P., Rosendorff, C., Williams, G., and Woolf, C. A role for NE and cAMO in PGE_1 fever. J. Physiol. (Lond.) 240(2):49P-50P, 1974.
50. Rudy, T. A., and Viswanathan, C. T. Effect of central cholinergic blockade on the hyperthermia evoked by PGE_1 injected into the rostral hypothalamus of the rat. Can. J. Physiol. Pharmacol. 53:321-324, 1975.
51. Pittman, Q. J., Veale, W. L., and Cooper, K. E. Temperature responses of lambs after centrally injected prostaglandins and pyrogens. Am. J. Physiol. 228:1034-1038, 1975.
52. Cranshaw, L. I., and Stitt, J. T. Behavioral and autonomic induction of PGE_1 fever in squirrel monkeys. J. Physiol. (Lond.) 244(1):197-206, 1975.
53. Veale, W. L., and Wishaw, I. Q. Body temperature responses at different ambient temperatures following injections of PGE_1 and NE into the brain. Pharmacol. Biochem. Behav. 4:143-150, 1976.
54. Myers, R. D., and Waller, M. B. Is prostaglandin fever mediated by the presynaptic release of hypothalamic 5-HT or norepinephrine? Brain Res. Bull. 1:47-56, 1976.
55. Flower, R. J., and Vane, J. R. Inhibition of prostaglandin synthetase in brain explains the antipyretic activity of paracetamol (4-acetamidophenol). Nature (Lond.) 240 (381):410-411, 1972.

56. Milton, A. S. PGE_1 and endotoxin fever, and the effects of aspirin, indomethacin and paracetamol. Adv. Biosci. 9:495-499, 1973.
57. Feldberg, W., Gupta, K. P., Milton, A. S., and Wendlandt, S. Effect of pyrogen and antipyretics on prostaglandin activity in cisternal CSF of unanesthetized cats. J. Physiol. 234:279-303, 1973.
58. Davis, J. D., Gallagher, R. J., Ladove, R. F., and Turauski, A. J. Inhibition of food intake by a humoral factor. J. Comp. Physiol. Psychol. 67:407-414, 1969.
59. Baile, C. A., Simpson, C. W., Bean, S. M., McLaughlin, C. L., and Jacobs, H. L. Prostaglandins and food intake of rats: a component of energy balance regulation. Physiol. Behav. 10:1077-1085, 1973.
60. Martin, F. H., and Baile, C. A. Feeding elicited in sheep by intrahypothalamic injections of PGE_1. Experientia 29:306-307, 1973.
61. Baile, C. A., and Martin, F. H. Relationship between PGE_1, polyphloretin phosphate and alpha and beta adrenoceptor-bound feeding loci in the hypothalamus of sheep. Pharmacol. Biochem. Behav. 1(5):539-545, 1973.
62. Wishaw, I. Q., and Veale, W. L. Comparison of the effect of PGE_1 and norepinephrine injected into the brain on ingestive behavior in the rat. Pharmacol. Biochem. Behav. 2:421-425, 1974.
63. Zor, U., Lamprecht, S. A., Kaneko, T., Schneider, H. P., McCann, S. M., Field, J. B., Tsafriri, A., and Lindner, H. R. Functional relations between cyclic AMP, prostaglandins, and luteinizing hormone in rat pituitary and ovary. Adv. Cyclic Nucleotide Res. 1:503-520, 1972.
64. Varavudhi, P., and Chobsieng, P. Biological evidence for the direct stimulating effect of PGF_2 alpha on the release of pituitary luteolytic agent(s) of pseudopregnant rats. Prostaglandins 2(3):199-205, 1972.
65. Spies, H. G., and Norman, R. L. Luteinizing hormone release and ovulation induced by the intraventricular infusion of prostaglandin E_1 into pentobarbital-blocked rats. Prostaglandins 4(1):131-141, 1973.
66. Carlson, J. C., Barcikowski, B., and McCracken, J. A. Prostaglandin F_2 alpha and the release of LH in sheep. J. Reprod. Fertil. 34(2):357-361, 1973.
67. Labhsetwar, A. P., and Zolovick, A. Hypothalamic interaction between prostaglandins and catecholamines in promoting gonadotropin secretion for ovulation. Nature (New Biol.) 246(150):55-56, 1973.
68. Harms, P. G., Ojeda, S. R., and McCann, S. M. Prostaglandin-induced release of pituitary gonadotropins: central nervous system and pituitary sites of action. Endocrinology 94(5):1459-1464, 1974.
69. Poulain, P., and Carette, B. Iontophoresis of prostaglandins on hypothalamic neurons. Brain Res. 79(2):311-314, 1974.
70. Ojeda, S. R., Harms, P. G., and McCann, S. M. Effect of third ventricular injections of prostaglandins (PGs) on gonadotropin release in conscious free moving male rats. Prostaglandins 8(6):545-552, 1974.

71. Sato, T., Hirono, M., Jyujo, T., Iesaka, T., Taya, K., and Igarashi, M. M. Direct action of prostaglandins on the rat pituitary. Endocrinology 96:45-49, 1975.
72. Chobsieng, P., Naor, Z., Koch, Y., Zor, U., and Lindner, H. R. Stimulating effect of PGE_2 on LH release in the rat: evidence for a hypothalamic site of action. Neuroendocrinology 17(1):12-17, 1975.
73. Sato, T., Jyujo, T., Hirono, M., and Iesaka, T. Effects of indomethacin, an inhibitor of prostaglandin synthesis on the hypothalamic-pituitary system in rats. J. Endocrinology 64(2): 395-396, 1975.
74. Pang, C. Y., and Behrman, H. R. Acute effects of prostaglandin $F_{2\alpha}$ on ovarian and luteal blood flow, luteal gonadotropin uptake in vivo, and gonadotropin binding in vitro. Endocrinology 108:2239-2244, 1981.
75. Warberg, J., Eskay, R. L., and Porter, J. Prostaglandin-induced release of anterior pituitary hormones: structure-activity relationship. Endocrinology 98:1135-1141, 1976.
76. Kuhl, H., Frey, W., Rosniatowski, C., Bericks-Tan, J., and Taubert, H-D. The effect of prostaglandins on hypothalamic 1-cystine arylamidase activity and on LH secretion in the rat. Acta Endocrinol. 82:15-28, 1976.
77. Szabo, M., and Frohman, L. A. Effects of porcine stalk median eminence and prostaglandin E_2 on rat GH secretion in vivo and their inhibition by somatostatin. Endocrinol. 96:955-961, 1975.
78. Sundberg, D. K., Fawcett, C. P., Illner, P., and McCann, S. M. The effect of various prostaglandins and a prostaglandin synthetase inhibitor on rat anterior pituitary cyclic AMP levels and hormone release in vitro. J. Proc. Soc. Exp. Biol. Med. 148:54-59, 1975.
79. Brown, M. R., and Hedge, G. A. In vivo effects of prostaglandins on TRH induced TSH secretion. Endocrinology 95(5):1392-1397, 1974.
80. Harms, P. G., Ojeda, S. R., and McCann, S. M. Prostaglandin involvement in hypothalamic control of gonadotropin and prolactin release. Sciene 181(101):760-761, 1973.
81. Ojeda, S. R., Harms, P. G., and McCann, S. M. Central effect of prostaglandin E_1 (PGE_1) on prolactin release. Endocrinology 95(2):613-618, 1974.
82. Coceani, F., and Vita, A. Actions of PGE_1 on spinal neurons in the frog. Adv. Biosci. 9:481-487, 1973.
83. Eliasson, R. Studies on prostaglandin; occurrence, formation and biological actions. Acta Physiol. Scand. 46(Suppl. 158): 1-73, 1959.
84. Pace-Asciak, C., and Wolfe, L. S. Inhibition of prostaglandin synthesis by oleic, linoleic and linolenic acids. Biochim. Biophys. Acta 152: 784-787, 1968.
85. Haye, B., Champion, S., and Jacquemin, C. Control by TSH of a phospholipase A_2 activity; a limiting factor in the biosynthesis of prostaglandins in the thyroid. FEBS Lett. 30:253, 1973.
86. Haye, B., Champion, S., and Jacquemin, C. Stimulation by TSH of prostaglandin synthesis in pig thyroid. Adv. Prostaglandin Thromboxane Res. 1:29-34, 1976.

87. Palmer, M. A., Piper, P. J., and Vane, J. R. Release of rabbit aorta contracting substance (RCS) and prostaglandins induced by chemical or mechanical stimulation of guinea pig lungs. Br. J. Pharmacol. 49:226, 1973.
88. Needleman, P., Minkes, M. S., and Douglas, J. R., Jr. Stimulation of prostaglandin biosynthesis by ademine nucleotides. Profile of prostaglandin release by perfused organs. Circ. Res. 34:445, 1974.
89. Gimbone, M. A., Jr., and Alexander, R. W. Angiotensin II stimulation of prostaglandin production in cultured human vascular endothelium. Science 189:219-220, 1975.
90. Anggard, E., and Jonsson, C. E. Studies on the analysis and metabolism of the prostaglandins. Ann. N.Y. Acad. Sci. 180:200-217, 1971.
91. Hamberg, M., Israelsson, U., and Samuelsson, B. Metabolism of prostaglandin E_2 in guinea pig liver. Ann. N.Y. Acad. Sci. 180:164-180, 1971.
92. Samuelsson, B., Granstrom, E., Green, K., and Hamberg, M. Metabolism of prostaglandins. Ann. N.Y. Acad. Sci. 180:138-163, 1971.
93. Ferreira, S. H., and Vane, J. R. Prostaglandins: their disappearance from and release into the circulation. Nature (Lond.) 216:868, 1967.
94. Coceani, F., and Wolfe, L. S. Prostaglandins in brain and the release of prostaglandin-like compounds from the rat cerebellar cortex. Can. J. Physiol. Pharmacol. 43:445-450, 1965.
95. Horton, E. W., and Maine, I. H. M. The identification of prostaglandin in central nervous tissues of the cat and the fowl. J. Physiol. (Lond.) 185:13-37, 1966.
96. Horton, E. W. Hypotheses on physiological roles of prostaglandins. Physiol. Rev. 49:122-161, 1969.
97. Wolfe, L. S., Pappius, H. M., and Marion, J. The biosynthesis of prostaglandins by brain tissue in vitro. Adv. Prostaglandin Thromboxane Res. 1:345, 1976.
98. Liebskind, J. C. Pain modulation by central nervous system stimulation. Adv. Pain Res. Ther. 1:445-453, 1976.
99. Shaw, J. E., and Ramwell, P. W. Release of prostaglandin from rat epididymal fat pad on nervous and hormonal stimulation. J. Biol. Chem. 243:1498-1503, 1968.
100. Coceani, F., Pace-Asciak, C., Volta, F., and Wolfe, L. S. Effect of nerve stimulation in prostaglandin formation and release from the rat stomach. Am. J. Physiol. 213:1056-1064, 1967.
101. Bennett, A., Friedmann, C. A., and Vane, J. R. Release of prostaglandin E_1 from the rat stomach. Nature (Lond.) 216:873-876, 1967.
102. Hedqvist, P. Studies on the effects of prostaglandins E_1 and E_2 on the sympathetic neuromuscular transmission in some animal tissues. Acta Physiol. Scand. (Suppl.) 345, 1970.
103. Kadowitz, P. J., Sweet, C. S., and Brody, M. J. Influence of

prostaglandin on adrenergic transmission to vascular smooth muscle. Circ. Res. 31:36-50, 1972.
104. Brody, M. J., and Kadowitz, P. J. Prostaglandins as modulators of the autonomic nervous system. Fed. Proc. 33:48-60, 1974.
105. Salzmann, E. W. Prostaglandins and platelet function. Prostaglandin Thromboxane Res. 2:767, 1976.
106. Manku, M. S., Mtabaji, J. P., and Horrobin, D. F. Effects of prostaglandins on baseline pressure and responses to noradrenaline in a perfused rat mesenteric artery preparation. PGE_1 as an antagonist of PGE_2. Prostaglandins 13(4):701-709, April 1977.
107. Goldberg, N. D., Haddox, M. K., Hartle, D. K., and Hadden, J. W. The biological role of cyclic 3',5'-guanosine monophosphate. Proc. Int. Congr. Pharmacol. (5th) 5:146-169. Karger, Basel, 1972.
108. Starke, K. Regulation of noradrenaline release by presynaptic receptor systems. Rev. Physiol. Biochem. Pharmacol. 77:1-124, 1977.
109. Westfall, T. C. Local regulation of adrenergic neurotransmission. Physiol. Rev. 57:659-728, 1977.
110. Hedqvist, P. Basic mechanisms of prostaglandin action on autonomic neurotransmission. Annu. Rev. Pharmacol. Toxicol. 17:259-279, 1977.
111. Ramwell, P. W., and Shaw, J. E. Biological significance of the prostaglandins. Recent Prog. Horm. Res. 26:139-187, 1970.
112. Piper, P., and Vane, J. The release of prostaglandins from lung and other tissues. Ann. N.Y. Acad. Sci. 180:363-385, 1971.
113. Hedqvist, P. Modulating effect of prostaglandin E_2 on noradrenaline release from the isolated cat spleen. Acta Physiol. Scand. 75:511-512, 1969.
114. Bergstrom, S., Farnebo, L., and Fuxe, K. Effect of prostaglandin E_2 on central and peripheral catecholamine neurons. Eur. J. Pharmacol. 21:362-368, 1973.
115. Wendel, O. T., and Strandhoy, J. W. The effects of prostaglandins E_2 and $F_{2\alpha}$ on synaptosomal accumulation and release of ^{3}H-norepinephrine. Prostaglandins 16:441-449, 1978.
116. Roberts, P. J., and Hillier, K. Facilitation of noradrenaline release from rat brain synaptosomes by prostaglandin E_2. Brain Res. 112:425-428, 1976.
117. Gilbert, J. C., Davison, D. V., and Wyllie, M. G. Studies on the physiological roles of prostaglandins in the central nervous system. Neuropharmacology 17:417-419, 1978.
118. Hillier, K., and Templeton, W. Regulation of noradrenaline overflow in rat cerebral cortex by prostaglandin E_2. Br. J. Pharmacol. 70:469-473, 1980.
119. Nowak, J. Prostaglandins in the cardiovascular system in man. Acta Physiol. Scand. (Suppl. 467), 1979.
120. Moncada, S., Gryglewski, R. J., Bunting, S., and Vane, J. R. An enzyme isolated from arteries transforms prostaglandin endoperoxides to unstable substance that inhibits platelet aggregation. Nature (Lond.) 263:663-665, 1976.

121. Armstrong, J. M., Chapple, D., Dusting, G. J., Hughes, R., Moncada, S., and Vane, J. R. Cardiovascular actions of prostacyclin (PGI_2) in chloralose anaesthetized dogs. Br. J. Pharmacol. 61:136, 1977.
122. Dusting, G. J., Moncada, S., and Vane, J. R. Disappearance of prostacyclin (PGI_2) in the circulation of the dog. Br. J. Pharmacol. 62:414-415, 1978.
123. Moncada, S., Higgs, E. A., and Vane, J. R. Human arterial and venous tissues generate prostacyclin (prostaglandin X), a potent inhibitor of platelet aggregation. Lancet 1:18-20, 1977.
124. Horton, E. W. Prostaglandin at the adrenergic nerve ending. Br. Med. Bul. 29:148-151, 1973.
125. Roberts, P. J., and Hillier, K. Facilitation of noradrenaline release from rat brain synaptosomes by prostaglandin E_2. Brain Res. 112: 425-428, 1976.
126. Lembeck, F., Popper, H., and Juan, H. Release of prostaglandins by bradykinin as an intrinsic mechanism of its algesic effect. Naunyn-Schmiedeberg's Arch. Pharm. 294:69-73, 1976.
127. Flower, R. J. Prostaglandins and related compounds, in Inflammation—Mechanisms and Their Impact on Therapy, I. L. Bonta, J. Thompson, and K. Brune (Eds.). Ag. Act. Suppl. 3, p. 99, 1977.
128. Collier, H. O. J., and Schneider, C. Nociceptive response to prostaglandins and analgesic actions of aspirin and morphine. Nature (New Biol.) 236:141-143, 1972.
129. Juan, H., and Lembeck, F. Prostaglandin $F_{2\alpha}$ reduces the algesic effect of bradykinin by antagonizing the pain-enhancing action of endogenously released prostaglandin E. Br. J. Pharmacol. 59:385-391, 1977.
130. Pritz, W., and Stockinger, L. Über den Zahnschmerz. Ost. Z. Stomat. 5:170-178, 1971.
131. Stockinger, L., and Pritz, W. Morphologische Aspekte der Schmerzempfindung im Zahn. Dtsch. Zahnarztl Z. 25:557-565, 1970.
132. Zotterman, Y. The peripheral nervous mechanism of pain: a brief view. In Ciba Foundation Study Group No. 1. Pain and Itch. Nervous Mechanisms, G. E. W. Wolstenholme and M. O'Connor (Eds.). Churchill, London, pp. 13-34, 1959.
133. Iggo, A. Peripheral and spinal "pain" mechanisms and their modulation. Adv. Pain Res. Ther. 1:381-394, 1976.
134. Sicuteri, F. Sensitization of nociceptors by 5-hydroxytryptamine in man. In Pharmacology of Pain, Vol. 9, Proc. 3rd Int. Congr. Pharmacol., R. K. Lim, D. Armstrong, and E. G. Pardo (Eds.). Pergamon, Oxford, pp. 57-68, 1968.
135. Bach, M. K., Brashler, J. R., and Gorman, R. R. On the structure of slow reacting substance of anaphylaxis: evidence of biosynthesis from arachidonic acid. Prostaglandins 14:21-38, 1977.
136. Murphy, R. C., Hammarström, S., and Samuelsson, B. Leukotriene C: a slow-reacting substance from murine mastocytoma cells. Proc. Natl. Acad. Sci. USA 76:4275-4279, 1979.

137. Samuelsson, B., Borgeat, P., Hammarström, S., and Murphy, R. C. Introduction of a nomenclature: leukotrienes. Prostaglandins 17(6): 785-787, 1979.
138. Borgeat, P., and Samuelsson, B. Metabolism of arachidonic acid in polymorphonuclear leukocytes. Structural analysis of novel hydroxylated compounds. J. Biol. Chem. 254:7865-7869, 1979.
139. Moncada, S., and Vane, J. R. Pharmacology and endogenous roles of prostaglandin endoperoxides, thromboxane H_2 and prostacyclin. Pharmacol. Rev. 30:293-331, 1979.

Author Index

Numbers in parentheses are reference numbers and indicate that an author's work is referred to although his name is not cited in the text. Underscored numbers give the page on which the complete reference is listed.

A

B

C

E

F

G

I

J

L

M

N

S

U

V

W

Subject Index